Contested Cures

Edinburgh Studies in Religion in Antiquity

Series editors: Matthew V. Novenson, James B. Rives, Paula Fredriksen

Edinburgh Studies in Religion in Antiquity publishes cutting-edge research in religion in the ancient world. It provides a platform for creative studies spanning time periods (classical antiquity and late antiquity), geographical regions (the Mediterranean and West Asia), religious traditions (Greek, Roman, Jewish, Christian, and more), disciplines (comparative literature, archaeology, anthropology, and more) and theoretical questions (historical, philological, comparative, redescriptive, and more). Deconstructing literary canons and confessional boundaries, the series considers and questions what we moderns call "religion" as a prominent feature of the human past and a worthy object of historical enquiry.

Advisory Board

Helen Bond, University of Edinburgh
Kimberley Czajkowski, University of Edinburgh
Benedikt Eckhardt, University of Edinburgh
Martin Goodman, University of Oxford
Oded Irshai, Hebrew University of Jerusalem
Timothy Lim, University of Edinburgh
Yii-Jan Lin, Yale University
Candida Moss, University of Birmingham
Paul Parvis, University of Edinburgh
Matthew Thiessen, McMaster University
Philippa Townsend, University of Edinburgh
Greg Woolf, University of California-Los Angeles

Books published in the series

Megan S. Nutzman, *Contested Cures: Identity and Ritual Healing in Roman and Late Antique Palestine*
Matthew T. Sharp, *Divination and Philosophy in the Letters of Paul*

Visit the series webpage: https://edinburghuniversitypress.com/series-edinburgh-studies-in-religion-in-antiquity

Contested Cures

Identity and Ritual Healing in Roman and Late Antique Palestine

Megan S. Nutzman

EDINBURGH
University Press

Edinburgh University Press is one of the leading university presses in the UK. We publish academic books and journals in our selected subject areas across the humanities and social sciences, combining cutting-edge scholarship with high editorial and production values to produce academic works of lasting importance. For more information visit our website: edinburghuniversitypress.com

© Megan Nutzman, 2022, 2024

Edinburgh University Press Ltd
The Tun – Holyrood Road
12(2f) Jackson's Entry
Edinburgh EH8 8PJ

First published in hardback by Edinburgh University Press 2022

Typeset in 11/13 Bembo Std by
IDSUK (DataConnection) Ltd, and
printed and bound by CPI Group (UK) Ltd
Croydon, CR0 4YY

A CIP record for this book is available from the British Library

ISBN 978 1 3995 0273 3 (hardback)
ISBN 978 1 3995 0274 0 (paperback)
ISBN 978 1 3995 0275 7 (webready PDF)
ISBN 978 1 3995 0276 4 (epub)

The right of Megan Nutzman to be identified as the author of this work has been asserted in accordance with the Copyright, Designs and Patents Act 1988, and the Copyright and Related Rights Regulations 2003 (SI No. 2498).

Contents

List of Illustrations		vi
Preface and Acknowledgements		viii
List of Abbreviations		xii
Introduction: Roman and Late Antique Palestine		1

Part I Miraculous Objects

1	One God Who Conquers Evil: Gemstone and Jewelry Amulets	15
2	For I Am Yahweh Who Heals You: *Lamellae* and Amulets with Biblical Quotations	38

Part II Miraculous Places

3	In This Holy Place: Hot Springs as Sites of Ritual Healing	71
4	In Which Many Miracles Are Worked: Ritual Continuity at Healing Sites	92

Part III Miraculous People

5	In the Name of Jesus of Nazareth the Crucified: Ritual Practitioners Who Offered Cures	117
6	Working Such Wonders and Signs: Charismatic Wonderworkers Who Offered Cures	149

Part IV Elite Rhetoric

7	It Is Better to Die: Elite Rhetoric and Communal Identity	181
	Epilogue: It Is Better to Live	209

Bibliography	214
Index of Ancient Sources	241
Subject Index	247

Illustrations

Frontispiece

Map of Palestine (Drawing by D. Weiss)   xviii

Figures

1.1	A reaper gemstone from Caesarea (Hamburger 1968)	21
1.2	A brass ring from Hammat Gader (Drawing by D. Weiss)	25
1.3	A bronze pendant from Gush Halav (Photo by Clara Amit, Courtesy of the Israel Antiquities Authority)	29
2.1	An octagonal ring from Khirbet Kusieh (Drawing by D. Weiss)	39
2.2	A silver *lamella* from Tiberias (Drawing by Ada Yardeni in Naveh and Shaked 1993; with permission of Magnes Press)	47
2.3	A copper *lamella* from 'Evron (Kotansky 1991, with permission of Roy Kotanksy)	58
2.4	A bronze bracelet from Caesarea (Hamburger 1959; Israeli and Mevorah 2000)	62
3.1	Partial reconstruction of Hammat Gader (Hirschfeld 1997, fig. 51; with permission of the Israel Exploration Society)	76
4.1	Plan of the Pool of Bethesda (Drawing by D. Weiss, after Gibson 2011)	96
4.2	Plan of the Shuni and 'Ein Tzur (Drawing by D. Weiss, after Hirschfeld 1995 and Shenhav 1997)	104

Tables

1.1	Circumstances of finds	17
1.2	Types of amulets	18

1.3	Language of amulets	19
1.4	Language according to amulet type	20
2.1	Samaritan biblical quotations on amulets	43
2.2	Biblical quotations on amulets by language	53
2.3	Biblical quotations on amulets by amulet type	54

Preface and Acknowledgements

There were two starting points for this project. The first was the Archaeology and the World of the New Testament seminar at Harvard Divinity School. I was assigned the site of Epidauros and I spent the semester researching the cult of the healing god Asklepios in preparation to lead the group's tour at Epidauros, sight unseen. This was my first trip to Greece, and while there I quickly found myself drawn to the similarities between votive offerings dedicated by grateful visitors at ancient Asklepieia and the *tamata* that continue to be strung up in front of icons in Orthodox churches across Greece. *Tamata* are small metal plaques embossed with a stylized representation of a body part or a person. Comparisons between these votive offerings in contexts separated by more than two thousand years sparked my interest in how the search for divine cures can transcend time and place.

A second origin story for this book was my introduction to the study of ancient "magic" at the University of Chicago. Through coursework with Chris Faraone and David Martinez, who would become my advisor and a member of my dissertation committee respectively, I learned about the range of practices that scholars label "magic," including the Greek Magical Papyri and ancient gemstones. Given my prior interest in the cult of Asklepios, it was perhaps no surprise that I was particularly drawn to forms of "magic" associated with healing and protection. When it came time to prepare my dissertation proposal, I wanted to find a way to bring evidence from the cult of Asklepios into dialogue with that from healing "magic," but I became increasingly disappointed by scholarly conventions that resulted in these two interests rarely being examined alongside each other. I knew that, in part, this reflected the chronological and geographic limitations of our evidence. My thinking shifted when I ran across an article by S. Vernon McCasland (1939a), who in just a few short pages laid out the evidence for a range of ritual healing options in Roman Palestine, including amulets, exorcisms, the hot springs, and the Pool of Bethesda. With this, the pieces fell into place. My focus narrowed to

Palestine, the region that first sparked my interest in the ancient world and where I had my first exposure to archaeology, digging at Tel Kedesh with Andrea Berlin.

In the intervening years, my research has been funded by the American Council of Learned Societies, the National Endowment for the Humanities, the Albright Institute of Archaeological Research in Jerusalem, and the Frankel Institute for Advanced Judaic Studies at the University of Michigan. Without the assistance of these programs, this book would not have been possible. Many people have spent countless hours discussing the project with me and reading drafts. Their insightful comments and questions have repeatedly made me see my work from new angles and have pushed me to make more convincing arguments. My reading group colleagues at Old Dominion University have enthusiastically waded through material centuries, and even millennia, removed from their own research, and have helped me see the big picture when I was lost in the weeds. My thanks go out to Nick Abbott, Brett Bebber, Marvin Chiles, Elizabeth Fretwell, Erin Jordan, Tim Orr, Jelmer Vos, John Weber, and Elizabeth Zanoni. The year that I spent in Ann Arbor at the Frankel Institute transformed this project from a dissertation into a monograph, thanks in no small part to the fantastic cohort of fellows assembled there under the direction of Rafe Neis: Todd Berzon, Rick Bonnie, Ra'anan Boustan, Sean Burrus, Mike Chin, Deborah Forger, Chaya Halberstam, Daniel Picus, Michael Swartz, Juan Tebes, and Rebecca Wollenberg. I am particularly indebted to the rabbinics scholars in the group who patiently answered questions and directed this classicist toward resources that were critical for my project. I also owe a sincere debt of gratitude to my advisor at the University of Chicago, Chris Faraone, without whose direction the original dissertation would never have been possible. The unwavering support and productive feedback of Chris and my other committee members, David Martinez and Jonathan Hall, shaped me into the scholar that I am today. Others from the University of Chicago saw me through the early stages of this project with their steadfast moral support, including my dissertation writing partners, Jessica Seidman, Kristine Hess Larison, and Monica Crews, and our departmental administrator, Kathy Fox. And finally, my students at ODU, who were always excited to hear about my book, provided the encouragement that I needed as I completed it.

My dad used to say that I cut my proverbial candle in half and burned all four ends. If this was true in my younger years, then it has been all the more true in the years that it has taken to bring this project from conception to its final form. That candle would not have kept burning without all the support from my family – my mom and my sister, and most especially my husband, Chris. Without his tireless patience and encouragement, love and laughter, I never would have finished this book. Thank you.

I produced my final manuscript with the help of a number of people. First and foremost, I want to thank everyone at Edinburgh University Press: the Edinburgh Studies in Religion in Antiquity series editors, James Rives, Matthew Novenson, and Paula Fredriksen, for believing in this project, and the fabulous editorial staff including Carol MacDonald, Rachel Bridgewater, Louise Hutton and Fiona Conn. I am in awe of Jane Burkowski's work as a copyeditor and her corrections of my many inconsistencies, omissions, and mistakes. Any remaining errors are, of course, my own. I also want to thank everyone who has helped with the illustrations and image permissions for the book: Dan Weiss for his beautiful drawings and site plans, Marfa Heimbach and Werner Eck with *Corpus inscriptionum Iudaeae/Palaestinae*, Atalya Fadida at the Israel Antiquities Authority, Yael Klein at Magnes Press, His Grace, Bishop Joachim (Cotsonis) of Amissos, and the V. Rev. Archimandrite Maximos Constas. Finally, I appreciate the detailed work that David Zwick has done as my research assistant as I prepared the manuscript for publication. An earlier version of Chapter 3 was presented at a Society for Ancient Mediterranean Religions conference and subsequently became a chapter in *Gods, Objects, and Ritual Practices*, published by Lockwood Press. I am grateful to Sandra Blakely, the volume's editor, and the anonymous reviewers for their constructive feedback, and to other dialogue partners whom I have gotten to know through SAMR conferences.

This book is situated at the intersection of several distinct fields of study: classics and religion, history and archaeology, early Christianity and ancient Judaism. The divisions between modern academic disciplines mean that specialists in these fields often work in different languages, teach in different departments, and write for different audiences. To make this book accessible across the disciplinary boundaries that subdivide the study of religion in antiquity, I have chosen to provide transliterations wherever a reference to the original language is necessary. Hebrew and Aramaic transliterations use the Society of Biblical Literature's academic style for transliteration, except for words that are more commonly known in English using the general-purpose style (e.g. *genizah, miqveh, Shema, tefillin*). My preference is to transliterate Greek directly (e.g. Asklepios instead of Asclepius), but in the case of well-known authors and figures, I have kept the more familiar Latinized forms of Greek names.

I completed this manuscript in the world of Covid-19. Writing during the pandemic, with library closures and the scramble to find new ways to teach, presented a unique set of challenges. However, writing *this* book during a global health crisis, a book about the measures that people in antiquity took to be cured, also invited reflection on the universality of health and healing. Social media offered windows into various communities' ritual responses to the pandemic. My own community added special prayers at every service, specifying "the peril of the coronavirus against us" in a petition for "deliverance from all affliction, wrath, danger and distress," and including the extra petition, "For our brethren, those who lead the fight against the coronavirus, the doctors, the medical workers and the scientists, let us pray to the Lord." The service of unction, or anointing with oil, whose origins can be traced to some of the material discussed in Chapter 5, was offered more frequently, and, at least for me, took on special meaning. While I found comfort in these rituals, I also had confidence in the work being done by the medical community to improve treatments and to develop an effective vaccine. Others, however, rejected science, and many did so in the name of religion. They drew boundaries between "us" and "them," with mask-wearing, social distancing, and acceptance of vaccines as litmus tests advanced by religious leaders who used their platforms to decry such measures. Where Chrysostom in the fourth century denounced people who wore amulets to protect against disease, his modern counterparts directed their ire against those who wore masks to protect against the coronavirus. This intertwining of history and our lived experience of Covid-19, from ritual responses to the virus to the religious rhetoric that defined the boundaries of communal responses, repeatedly demonstrated the timelessness of the material that I explore in *Contested Cures*.

M.N., Norfolk, VA
September 2021

Abbreviations

Journals and Series

AJA	*American Journal of Archaeology*
AncW	*Ancient World*
ANF	*The Ante-Nicene Fathers: Translations of the Writings of the Fathers Down to A.D.* 325. Edited by Alexander Roberts and James Donaldson. 10 vols. 1885–1887. Repr., Grand Rapids: Eerdmans.
ANRW	*Aufstieg und Niedergang der römischen Welt*
AnSoc	*L'Année sociologique*
ARG	*Archiv für Religionsgeschichte*
BAIAS	*Bulletin of the Anglo-Israel Archeological Society*
BAR	*Biblical Archaeology Review*
BASOR	*Bulletin of the American Schools of Oriental Research*
BASP	*Bulletin of the American Society of Papyrologists*
BJPES	*Bulletin of the Jewish Palestine Exploration Society*
BN	*Biblische Notizen*
CBQ	*Catholic Biblical Quarterly*
CCSL	Corpus Christianorum: Series latina. 1953–. Turnhout: Brepols.
CH	*Church History*
CIIP 2	Cotton, Hannah, Eran Lupu, and Walter Ameling. 2010. *Corpus inscriptionum Iudaeae/Palaestinae: A Multi-Lingual Corpus of the Iscriptions from Alexander to Muhammad.* Vol. 2: Caesarea and the Middle Coast. Berlin: De Gruyter.
ClAnt	*Classical Antiquity*
DOP	*Dumbarton Oaks Papers*

LIST OF ABBREVIATIONS xiii

DSD	*Dead Sea Discoveries*
ErIsr	*Eretz-Israel*
ESI	*Excavations and Surveys in Israel*
GR	*Greece and Rome*
GRBS	*Greek, Roman and Byzantine Studies*
HR	*History of Religions*
HS	*Hebrew Studies*
HTR	*Harvard Theological Review*
HUCA	*Hebrew Union College Annual*
IEJ	*Israel Exploration Journal*
IG	*Inscriptiones graecae. Editio minor.* 1924–. Berlin: De Gruyter.
JA	*Journal asiatique*
JAC	*Jahrbuch für Antike und Christentum*
JAJ	*Journal of Ancient Judaism*
JAOS	*Journal of the American Oriental Society*
JBL	*Journal of Biblical Literature*
JECS	*Journal of Early Christian Studies*
JEH	*Journal of Ecclesiastical History*
JJS	*Journal of Jewish Studies*
JPOS	*Journal of the Palestine Oriental Society*
JQR	*Jewish Quarterly Review*
JRS	*Journal of Roman Studies*
JSJ	*Journal for the Study of Judaism in the Persian, Hellenistic and Roman Period*
JSNT	*Journal for the Study of the New Testament*
JSS	*Journal of Semitic Studies*
LASBF	*Liber annuus Studii biblici franciscani*
MdB	*Le Monde de la Bible*
MUSJ	*Mélanges de l'Université Saint-Joseph*
NEASB	*Near Eastern Archaeological Society Bulletin*
NovT	*Novum Testamentum*
NPNF	*A Select Library of Nicene and Post-Nicene Fathers of the Christian Church.* Edited by Philip Schaff and Henry Wace. 28 vols. in 2 series. 1886–1889. Repr., Grand Rapids: Eerdmans.
NTS	*New Testament Studies*
OrChr	*Oriens christianus*

PEFQS	*Palestine Exploration Fund Quarterly Statement*
PEQ	*Palestine Exploration Quarterly*
PG	*Patrologia graeca.* Edited by J.-P. Migne. 161 vols. Paris: Migne, 1857–66.
PGM	*Papyri magicae graecae*
PL	*Patrologia latina.* Edited by J.-P. Migne. 217 vols. Paris: Migne, 1844–65.
PrOrChr	*Proche-Orient Chrétien*
Qad	*Qadmoniot*
QDAP	*Quarterly of the Department of Antiquities in Palestine*
RB	*Revue biblique*
REG	*Revue des études grecques*
REJ	*Revue des études juives*
RTL	*Revue théologique de Louvain*
SCI	*Scripta Classica Israelica*
SEG	*Supplementum epigraphicum graecum*
SM	*Supplementum magicum*
SR	*Studies in Religion*
TA	*Tel Aviv*
TAPhS	*Transactions of the American Philosophical Society*
TynBul	*Tyndale Bulletin*
VT	*Vetus Testamentum*
ZDPV	*Zeitschrift des deutschen Palästina-Vereins*
ZPE	*Zeitschrift für Papyrologie und Epigraphik*

Ancient Texts and Authors

1 *Apol.*	*Apologia I* by Justin Martyr
Adv. haer.	*Adversus haereses* by Irenaeus
Adv. Iud.	*Adversus Iudaeos* by John Chrysostom
Ant.	*Antiquitates judaicae* by Josephus
b.	Babylonian Talmud
Ber.	*Berakot*
C. Cels.	*Contra Celsum* by Origen
C. Hier.	*Contra Hieroclem* by Eusebius

Catech. 1–23	*Catechetical Lectures* by Cyril of Jerusalem
Catech. illum.	*Catecheses ad illuminandos* by John Chrysostom
CD	*Damascus Document*
Cod. Theod.	*Codex Theodosianus*
Comm. Isa.	*Commentariorum in Isaiam* by Jerome
Const. ap.	*Apostolic Constitutions*
Cyril Hier.	Cyril of Jerusalem
Cyril Scyth.	Cyril of Scythopolis
Dem. ev.	*Demonstratio evangelica* by Eusebius
Dial.	*Dialogue with Trypho* by Justin Martyr
Ep.	*Letter*
Ep. Arist.	*Letter of Aristeas*
ʿ*Erub.*	ʿ*Erubin*
Fr. de amul.	*De amuletis* (frag) by Athanasius
HA	*Historia Augusta*
Hist. Eccl.	*Ecclesiastical History*
Hom. Col.	*Homiliae in epistulam ad Colossenses* by John Chrysostom
Ḥul.	*Ḥullin*
Itin. Burd.	*Itinerary* by the Bordeaux Pilgrim
Itin. Eger.	*Itinerary* by Egeria
Itin. Plac.	*Itinerary* by the Piacenza Pilgrim
John Chrys.	John Chrysostom
Jub.	*Jubilees*
Ketub.	*Ketubbot*
Lev. R.	*Leviticus Rabbah*
LXX	Septuagint
m.	Mishnah
Menaḥ.	*Menaḥot*
NRSV	New Revised Standard Version
Onom.	*Onomasticon* by Eusebius
Orig. Hom. Lev.	*Origenis Homiliae in Leviticum* by Rufinus
Pan.	*Panarion* (*Against Heresies*) by Epiphanius
Prat.	*Pratum spirituale* (*Spiritual Meadow*) by John Moschos
Ps.-Clement	Pseudo-Clement
Šabb.	*Šabbat*

Sanh.	*Sanhedrin*
Spec.	*De specialibus legibus* by Philo
t.	Tosefta
T. Sol.	*Testament of Solomon*
Ta'an.	*Ta'anit*
Trad. ap.	*Apostolic Tradition*
V. Abr.	*Life of Abraamius* by Cyril of Scythopolis
V. Apoll.	*Life of Apollonius* by Philostratus
V. Cyriac.	*Life of Cyriacus* by Cyril of Scythopolis
V. Euthym.	*Life of Euthymius* by Cyril of Scythopolis
V. Georg. Choz.	*Life of George of Choziba* by Antony of Choziba
V. Hil.	*Life of Hilarion* by Jerome
V. Jo. Hes.	*Life of John the Hesychast* by Cyril of Scythopolis
V. Petr. Ib.	*Life of Peter the Iberian* by John Rufus
V. Procli	*Life of Proclus* by Marinus of Neapolis
V. Pyth.	*Life of Pythagoras*
V. Sab.	*Life of Sabas* by Cyril of Scythopolis
V. Soph.	*Lives of the Sophists* by Eunapius of Sardis
y.	Jerusalem Talmud

Σῶσον, Κύριε, τὸν λαόν σου

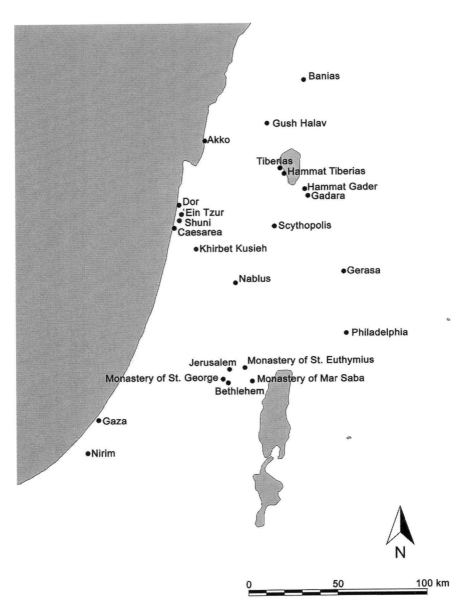

Map of Palestine (Drawing by D. Weiss)

INTRODUCTION

Roman and Late Antique Palestine

Imagine, if you will, a woman living in Caesarea in the early fourth century CE. Caesarea is a bustling metropolis, the provincial capital. It is home to a cross section of Palestine's inhabitants: Roman officials, Greek-speaking polytheists, Jews, Samaritans, and Christians. This woman has a young son who regularly gets sick. One day he will be shivering uncontrollably, and the next his body will be consumed with fever. Bad headaches and vomiting complicate the child's situation. The woman's husband is a skilled artisan, and so they have a little money to spend on physicians, but none of the prescribed remedies have had any lasting effect. He seems to get better, only to have the symptoms return with a vengeance sometime later. Our mother is desperate. She fears that her son does not have the strength to survive another episode. Only divine intervention will save him.

This woman's son has malaria, a disease that was endemic throughout the region. Illnesses and injuries of all sorts were ubiquitous in the ancient Mediterranean world. Manual labor resulted in traumatic injuries. Poor hygiene and sanitation led to outbreaks, and contagious diseases spread rapidly. Put simply, physical infirmities of one sort or another were inescapable. People lived under continuous threat of severe bodily harm and were well acquainted with death from a young age. The same impulse that drives people to the Internet today to research symptoms and find possible treatments would have also motivated those in the ancient world to look for answers. Casual conversations at wells, along roads, and in markets would have inevitably turned to the health and well-being of one's family. One woman might be tired because she had been up all night caring for an elderly relative, while another might question a friend as to why they had not seen a particular neighbor recently. And we can imagine that our woman from Caesarea would talk about little but her fears for her ailing son. In each of these situations, responses would have contained a mixture of sympathy and advice: Have you tried this herb? My cousin visited a holy man who cured him. Did you hear about my brother's son who was healed after wearing an amulet? I know a poultice that will work. You should bathe in the hot springs. In a world where disease and death were omnipresent, these conversations would have been common.

To which of Caesarea's diverse communities does our woman belong? I would suggest that it does not matter. In Roman and late antique Palestine, these exchanges crossed the notional lines that divided Greeks from Romans, Jews from Christians, and Samaritans from the followers of local deities. The inevitability of sickness and injury would have made people willing to experiment with seemingly beneficial forms of healing, even if they originated in a foreign cultural or religious tradition. Within circumstances of close cultural contacts such as prevailed in cities like Caesarea, the setting was ripe for neighbors to borrow rituals perceived to be efficacious and to alter them to fit their own cultic framework. As a result, they all employed related means of seeking miraculous cures. The similarities of these rituals, despite changes in the identity of the divine healers whom they invoked, made them the subject of polemical discourse among elite authors trying to police collective borders. The resulting intersection of ritual healing and communal self-understanding is the space that *Contested Cures* explores. The purpose of the book is twofold: first, to delineate categories of ritual healing that transcended the boundaries of ethnic and religious groups, and second, to use these rituals as a lens to examine the rhetoric by which Jewish and Christian authors differentiated themselves from each other and from their Samaritan, gentile, and "pagan" neighbors.

Diverse communities

Alexander the Great's conquests brought the land of Israel within the Greek world roughly two centuries after the Israelite exiles began their return from captivity in Babylon. The Seleucid Empire, a successor state set up by one of Alexander's generals, would come to control Palestine, but its treatment of the Jews led to an uprising against foreign rule. The victorious Jews set up an independent state and embarked on a campaign of Judaizing parts of Palestine with little or no Jewish presence. Dynastic disputes among later Hasmonaean rulers eventually resulted in Roman intervention in the person of Pompey Magnus in 63 BCE, at which point the Hasmonaean king, now ruling a much smaller territory, became a client of Rome. The most famous of these client kings was Herod the Great, an Idumaean who married into the Hasmonaean royal family, and who successfully switched his allegiance from Antony to Octavian after the battle of Actium and solidified his position as a client of Rome. With Herod's death, his territory was divided among his sons, whose kingdoms would all come under direct Roman rule by the conquest of Jerusalem by Vespasian in 70 CE during the Jewish revolt.[1] A second revolt, named for its leader Bar Kokhba, again brought Jews into conflict with the Roman Empire, with the result that Hadrian forbade Jews from the city of Jerusalem, which he refounded as the Roman colony Aelia Capitolina. The conversion of Constantine to Christianity two centuries later led to imperial patronage of the region, as the emperor's mother, Helena, implemented a building program that transformed Palestine into a Christian Holy Land. Samaritan unrest in the late fifth and sixth centuries reflected religious tensions between Samaritans and Christians on both the local and imperial scale. In 614 CE, the Persians laid siege to Jerusalem and, with the help of local Jews, took control of Byzantine Palestine. It would return briefly to Byzantine control in 628, before the Muslim conquest a decade later. The boundaries, and even the name, of the province changed over time. Known as Judaea until Hadrian, it was renamed Palestine in the second century CE before being divided into smaller provinces in the late fourth century.[2]

A complex network of ethnic, cultural, and religious groups inhabited Palestine throughout this period. The Jews and the Samaritans are best understood as ethnic groups, with identities rooted in their ancestral homeland, language, customs, and worship. At the same time, a shared culture could unite people across multiple ethnicities, as happened with the introduction of Greek language, political functions, architectural styles, and cults in the centuries following the conquest of Alexander the Great. It was only with the rise of Christianity that a concept of "religion" as something separate from ethnicity or culture emerged.[3] Each of these ethnic, cultural, and religious groups was shaped by its interaction with the others and by the governments that ruled them. The Jewish encounter with Hellenism, for example, and the later Jewish response to the Roman destruction of the Temple were transformative.[4] Likewise, the birth of Christianity and its subsequent growth cannot be understood outside the contexts of Jewish Palestine, Greek culture, and the Roman

---

[1] For the history of Palestine as part of Rome's empire in the Near East, see Millar 1993.

[2] For the sake of consistency, I will use "Palestine" to refer to the region throughout the book, regardless of the precise time period under discussion. As Nicole Belayche articulated in the introduction to her 2001 book, provincial boundaries are just one way of conceptualizing ancient Palestine, alongside the rabbinic concept of *Eretz Israel* and Christian understandings of the Holy Land. For her detailed survey, see Belayche 2001, 13–25. Another invaluable resource for studying the region in this period is Tsafrir et al. 1994.

[3] For two influential studies on the concept of "religion," see Smith 1982; Nongbri 2013.

[4] The body of scholarship on these topics is immense, including Levine 1989; Sanders 1992; Levine 1998, 3–32; Gruen 1998; Schwartz 2001; Rajak 2001; Friedheim 2006; Lapin 2012.

4 CONTESTED CURES

Empire. This is particularly true, for the purposes of this book, when it comes to understanding the miracle stories that pervade early Christian texts.[5]

Abundant literary evidence written by Jews and Christians in the Roman and late antique periods and the centrality of these centuries for the subsequent histories of Jews and Christians have resulted in a particularly rich body of scholarship. However, neither the Samaritans nor the Greek, Roman, and Semitic cults of Palestine have received the same level of scrutiny. In part, this is due to a dearth of sources. Few Samaritan literary works survive from late antiquity, and evidence for Samaritans in the Roman and late antique periods is often pieced together from archaeological remains, much later Samaritan works, and accounts of Samaritans written by non-Samaritan authors. The last are particularly problematic since Samaritans were a perennial "other" to both Jews and Christians. There remains considerable disagreement about the context, and even the date, for the formation of a unique Samaritan identity, but as with Jews and Christians it was solidified and maintained in opposition to other groups.[6] A similar lack of sources also characterizes the non-Jewish, non-Samaritan, and non-Christian cults of the region, such that most of our evidence comes from archaeological remains, including architecture, sculpture, inscriptions, and coins. Devotees of these cults, as polytheists, did not construct identities for themselves in opposition to their neighbors in the same way that Jews, Christians, and Samaritans did. However, their presence in Palestine has also received considerably less attention in the scholarship.[7] All too often the non-Christian and non-Jewish inhabitants of Palestine got lumped together as the conglomerate "other" that existed for polemical flourish in the writings of Christian and Jewish authors, and modern scholars have at times followed suit, investigating them as part of the historical background of texts written by Jews and Christians, but less frequently as objects of study in and of themselves.[8] The result is that many regional studies of Palestine in

---

[5] Among the many books that could be mentioned here, see Smith 1978; Kee 1983; Davies 1995; Reed 2000; Eve 2009; Horsley 2014; Fredriksen 2018.

[6] For example, see discussions in Purvis 1968; Di Segni 1998; Kirkpatrick 2008; Kartveit 2009; Knoppers 2013; Pummer 2016. The word "identity" can signify a number of different concepts. As Rogers Brubaker and Frederick Cooper (2000) have argued, these senses are, at times, conflicting and need to be differentiated wherever possible. In general, my use of "identity" and "identity formation" in this book aligns with Brubaker and Cooper's first set of alternative terms: "identification and categorization," which emphasize that someone is doing the identification. In this book, the identifiers are typically the elites who want to define the communal boundaries of their group. Brubaker and Cooper's second set of alternative terms, "self-understanding and social localization," are also relevant. The inflexibility of elite identifications is, I would argue, at odds with the more fluid self-understandings of the people who made use of various healing rituals.

[7] For an overview of local cults in the Hellenistic and Roman Near East, and relationships between local, Semitic cults and Greek and Roman ones, see Kaizer 2008.

[8] Two notable, but by no means the only, exceptions are Belayche 2001; Graf 2015, 66–86.

the Roman and late antique periods prioritize the history of just one of the region's constituent groups. In contrast, *Contested Cures* seeks to understand the populations that made up the mosaic of Palestine as a whole and the ideological borders that these groups created surrounding ritual healing.

Several related avenues of inquiry pertain to the presence of these diverse groups in the same territory. One key set of questions relates to the demographics of Palestine. Archaeological surveys and excavations have enabled scholars to trace settlement patterns and identify where members of different communities had their strongest concentrations, such as Jews in the Galilee and devotees of various Greek cults in the Decapolis cities. As a number of scholars have demonstrated, devotion to Greek and Roman gods did not disappear with Constantine's conversion to Christianity but rather persisted throughout late antiquity.[9] Demographics were of course not static, and so this research has also traced the Christianization of Palestine, and how the settlement patterns changed over time. The transformation of Palestine into a Christian Holy Land made visible changes to the physical contours of the region, with the construction of new churches, monasteries, and amenities to accommodate the influx of pilgrims. We should not underestimate the importance of these pilgrims from across the late Roman Empire and beyond as key components of the social fabric of the region.[10] With this transformation, Christians shaped an image of the Jews and their presence in the land that would fit into the new, Christianized ritual landscape.[11]

This book also raises questions related to scholarship on the "parting of the ways," where the articulation of communal boundaries is a central theme. Scholars have offered various explanations for when and why a definitive break took place between Jews and Christians.[12] As has become clear in recent scholarship, the self-definition that emerged in these centuries was neither uniform nor fixed, but rather the product of an ever-evolving series of contacts. *Contested Cures* makes no attempt to articulate precisely how and why the divisions between Jews and Christians became insurmountable, but rather offers ritual cures as one component of a complex matrix that eventually resulted in the delineation of clear boundaries. In his introduction to *Religious and Ethnic*

---

[9] Meyers 1985; Van Dam 1985; Horsley 1995; Gregg and Urman 1996; Dauphin 1998; Holum 1998; Geiger 1998; Tsafrir 1998; Gregg 2000; Bar 2003; Aviam 2004; Friedheim 2006; Friedheim and Dar 2010.

[10] For the identity of these pilgrims, many of whom took up residence in the region around Jerusalem, see Di Segni and Tsafrir 2012.

[11] Jacobs 2004.

[12] One of the most prominent voices in this scholarship is Daniel Boyarin, including his 1999 and 2004 books. For other work being done on the "parting of the ways," see for example Robinson 2009; Schremer 2010 and the studies in Becker and Reed 2003; Shanks 2013.

6   CONTESTED CURES

Communities in Later Roman Palestine, Hayim Lapin proposed that "we will have to take seriously both the ways in which the religious and ethnic communities remain in contact with and influenced by each other and the ways that they maintain boundaries between themselves and other groups."[13] This is precisely the approach that I take in the present book. By examining the ways in which forms of ritual healing were shared by the diverse populations of Roman and late antique Palestine, we see the ongoing contact between communities mentioned by Lapin. At the same time, as will be explored in Chapter 7, such points of contact are critical for making sense of the rhetoric used to create and perpetuate space between communities, at least as those communities were defined by elite authors. This does not mean that every individual making use of one of these cures had personal interaction with someone outside his or her community. As Lapin again argued in his introduction, "the cultural world that the individuals and the communities of later Roman Palestine inhabited on a daily basis was wider than the horizons of their everyday life."[14] In other words, a Jewish woman living in rural Galilee in a small village of fellow Jews need not have personal experience with purveyors of foreign cures to learn and make use of a prayer for healing that, to our modern eyes, invoked divine names from other traditions. These ideas and types of rituals would have spread, even to individuals whose routine contacts were limited to those within a given community.

The foregoing has referred to "Christians," "Jews," and "Samaritans" as groups that can be easily identified, but they should not be imagined as either monolithic or even necessarily as mutually exclusive. Any given individual might have identified with one or more of these labels, and to varying degrees that could change over time or that could depend on the people with whom they were interacting at a particular moment. Considerable space has been devoted in the recent scholarship to the diversity of both Judaism and Christianity in antiquity. I will argue in Chapter 2 that even among the Samaritans we should not exclude the possibility for either multiple identities or diversity within the community, despite the attempts I expect Samaritan leaders made to circumscribe acceptable practice. In his 1999 article "Identifying Jews and Christians in Roman Syria-Palestine," Reuven Kimelman addressed both the problem of determining who should be labeled a "Jew" and who a "Christian" and the way that the identities claimed by individuals may or may not have reflected those that elite authors tried to maintain:

---

[13] Lapin 1998, 8.
[14] Lapin 1998, 14.

INTRODUCTION   7

It is easy to see such people as crossovers from Judaism to Christianity or from Christianity to Judaism, but this would be adopting the perspective of the victors in this issue, who of course opposed the blurring of boundaries. From the perspective of the participants, it was clear that the alternative to either/or was both/and, especially if the best of both worlds was attainable.[15]

Health and healing, as I argue in this book, is precisely one of those concerns where the "both/and" approach would have been particularly attractive. My use of the labels "Jewish" and "Christian" therefore is not meant to be prescriptive or absolute. When I apply such labels to healing rituals, calling one, for example, a Christian ritual, it is not to say that everyone who used it would have identified as a Christian. Even if they did identify as a Christian, this does not mean that they identified thus to the exclusion of all other possible identities, or that Christian authorities would have necessarily recognized them as such. Rather, labeling a ritual as Christian simply indicates that the content of the ritual reflects Christian ideas, perhaps exclusively or perhaps not. As Raʿanan Boustan and Joseph Sanzo have argued, "The scholarly predilection to label isolated elements and to formulate abstract rules governing the limits of what a practitioner from a given religious community might do . . . builds unwarranted definitions into the very phenomena that a scholar has set out to study."[16] This book, therefore, repeatedly questions assumptions about the identity of the individuals participating in these rituals.

The label "pagan" is particularly problematic, originating in *paganus*, a pejorative term used by Christian authors in Latin to create "others" out of non-Christians.[17] Additional terms that similarly designate outsiders include *goyim* (gentiles) and *minim* (heretics) among Jewish authors and Hellenes or *ethnikoi* among Christian authors writing in Greek. "Pagan" may therefore be the appropriate term to use when discussing ancient Christians' attempts to circumscribe religious boundaries by assigning certain healing practices to "pagan" others. Ideally, I would not use it beyond its original function as a way to label outsiders, and to the degree that it is possible I avoid it in favor of greater specificity regarding particular cults. Nevertheless, with some hesitation I do follow other scholars who choose to use it as a neutral term, without the late antique Christian connotations, to refer collectively to non-Christians, non-Jews, and non-Samaritans if for no other reason than unwieldiness of specifying each of these negative identities at every turn.[18]

---

[15] Kimelman 1999, 327.
[16] Boustan and Sanzo 2017, 218.
[17] See discussion in Remus 2004.
[18] For example, Belayche 2001; Friedheim and Dar 2010.

8   CONTESTED CURES

Religion and magic

Evidence for healing rituals in antiquity is diverse both chronologically and geographically. Amulets and sympathetic remedies are already known in Homer, while incubation at healing shrines survived into the Middle Ages. A wealth of evidence for the cult of Asklepios comes from Greece, while Egypt has yielded an abundance of inscribed amulets and formularies. Considerable efforts have been made to collect and systematize this evidence and to excavate and publish the remains from local healing cults.[19] Without such projects, a book such as this would not be possible. Of necessity, many of these works have focused on discrete corpora, defined by traits such as language, medium, and site. At the same time, such publications have reinforced the categories in which healing practices are studied, even if not intentionally. At issue are the labels "religion" and "magic." A putative divide between the two was popularized by James Frazer in the late nineteenth and early twentieth centuries. Since then, generations of scholars have proposed various models of the relationship between magic and religion, from the evolutionary approach, to the argument that magic is socially deviant, to the equation of magic with coercion versus supplication in religion.[20] Much space has been devoted to the validity of the very term "magic" itself to describe ancient practices.[21] One of the questions revealed by this ongoing debate is whether the rituals collected by modern scholars in the category of "magic," including activities as diverse as healing, aggressive curses, erotic spells, agnostic pursuits, necromancy, and divination, formed a unique, integrated system in the minds of those who used them, or whether they were part of a magic–religion continuum into which all such rituals fit. As insightful as these studies are for reconstructing the relationship between various types of rituals, they foreground questions that I would argue were, for the most part, of little interest to the sick and injured in the ancient world whose primary concern was a cure in whatever form it presented itself.

This book therefore takes an approach to healing rituals that prioritizes local ritual practices. The goal has been to gather from Roman and late antique

---

[19] To mention just a few, Bonner 1950; Delatte and Derchain 1964; Preisendanz and Henrichs 1973; Naveh and Shaked 1985; Philipp and Büsing 1986; Daniel and Maltomini 1990; Naveh and Shaked 1993; Kotansky 1994; Barrett-Lennard 1994; Brashear 1995; LiDonnici 1995; Edelstein and Edelstein 1998; Meyer and Smith 1999; Renberg 2016. For specific site reports, see Chapters 3 and 4.

[20] Important contributions to this debate include Mauss and Hubert 1902; Frazer 1911–15; Durkheim 1912; Evans-Pritchard 1937; Lévi-Strauss 1962.

[21] For example, see Aune 1980; Versnel 1991; Smith 1995; Graf 1997; Braarvig 1999; Thomassen 1999; Dickie 2001; Bremmer 2002; Smith 2002; Frankfurter 2019a; Sanzo 2020. For work on the concept of ancient Jewish "magic" and its relationship to other Jewish practices, see Bohak 2008; Harari 2017.

INTRODUCTION   9

Palestine a wide variety of approaches to preserving health, healing injury, and curing illness that presuppose some form of divine intervention to bring about the desired result, without exclusions based on the categories of "religion" and "magic" or based on the cultural or religious tradition in which the ritual emerged.[22] To the degree that they can be differentiated, surgical, pharmacological, and other forms of medical cures have been omitted, along with those that draw on what was understood to be the inherent characteristics of natural elements.[23] This leaves us with an assortment of practices that are frequently not studied together. That is not to say, of course, that none of them are ever studied together. Ways that the miracles of Jesus and early Christians were seen to challenge the popularity of Asklepios, for example, have been a frequent topic of scholarly interest.[24] In contrast, similarities between the goals of people using amulets and those visiting a sanctuary of Asklepios – a desire to be healed – have not. To avoid the labels of "magic" and "religion," and the presuppositions that come with them, I refer collectively to the remedies explored in this book as "ritual healing."[25] Beyond a simple desire to circumvent the bifurcation of scholarship that has resulted from the labels "magic" and "religion," a further reason for eschewing them is that they run the risk of reifying the category of "magic" as defined by elite authors in antiquity who used it in their constructions of communal identity. Ancient conceptions of "magic," chiefly as a ritual performed by someone outside or on the fringes of one's group, do of course play a key role in shaping our understanding of certain healing rituals. As will be explored in depth in Chapter 7, ancient authors used labels such as "magic" to circumscribe their community's own practices and to restrict their members from participating in others.

* * *

This book is divided into four parts; each of the first three focuses on a different medium used in ritual healing: objects, places, and people. In the first part, Chapters 1 and 2, I argue that amulets from Roman and late antique Palestine

[22] My focus on "local religion" and on reading evidence for "popular religion" alongside more institutionalized rituals and in light of the "discourse of ritual censure" promulgated by elites reflects the groundwork laid by Frankfurter 2005.

[23] For medicine see Nutton 2004; for natural elements see Faraone 2018, 79–101. Medicine and ritual healing cannot be entirely separated in the ancient world, as can be seen, for example, in the presence of physicians at Asklepieia and Galen's acknowledgement of the power of amulets. Stories of Asklepios as a deified physician further blur these categories.

[24] For example, Yeung 2002, 83–97; Weissenrieder and Etzelmüller 2015; Flannery 2017.

[25] For a similar justification for using the phrase "ritual healing," see Ildikó Csepregi's preface to Csepregi and Burnett 2012. However, Csepregi uses the term somewhat more broadly than I do, since she also includes medical cures within this rubric.

were considerably more diverse than the impression given by studies that compartmentalize them according to language or medium, and that it is only by looking at the corpus as a whole that we can understand the similarities and differences of amulet use across the region's communities. Chapter 1 focuses on gemstone and jewelry amulets, which are by far the most common types to survive from Roman and late antique Palestine. The chapter considers three amulets in depth and uses them to investigate others with similar components: a reaper gemstone from Caesarea, a brass *boēth(e)i* ("help") ring from Hammat Gader, and a bronze pendant from Gush Halav with the acclamation *heis theos* ("one god") and the Holy Rider image. Chapter 2 investigates the use of biblical quotations on amulets from Roman and late antique Palestine. Two case studies, a Samaritan octagonal ring from Khirbet Kusieh and an Aramaic silver *lamella* from Tiberias, permit an investigation of the different choices that Samaritans and Jews made with regard to the use of biblical material on amulets. They also invite a comparison with Jewish *tefillin*, as both allowed people to wear biblical texts on their body.

The book's second part, Chapters 3 and 4, examines sacred sites that drew visitors in search of divine cures. Chapter 3 looks at the thermal-mineral springs of Palestine and their reputation for healing. Votive offerings at the hot springs demonstrate that some visitors understood the healing that took place there to be ritual, rather than medical, in nature. I argue that the process of seeking a divine cure at the hot springs involved some form of incubation, and that devotees of various healers, including Asklepios, Elijah, and Jesus, could have awaited healing theophanies in the springs at the same time. Chapter 4 examines two additional sites of ritual healing in Palestine: the Pool of Bethesda in Jerusalem and Shuni/'Ein Tzur a short distance northeast of Caesarea. While neither one is a hot spring, water still figured prominently at both. These sites changed hands with the transformation of the political and religious landscape, but their association with healing persisted. The Pool of Bethesda was a large *miqveh* (ritual bath) that was the setting for Jesus' miraculous raising of the man suffering from paralysis in John 5. The site became a sanctuary of Serapis-Asklepios, likely dating to the foundation of Aelia Capitolina, and later people visited a church built on this site in search of their own miraculous cures. The literary evidence for Shuni/'Ein Tzur is extremely limited, and the investigation must be based primarily on archaeological remains. It may have been particularly associated with women who wanted to become pregnant. I propose that earlier, non-Christian fertility rituals at Shuni were supplanted by Christianized rituals at 'Ein Tzur, the spring that supplied water to Shuni.

The book's third part, Chapters 5 and 6, considers ritual practitioners and charismatic wonderworkers who performed exorcisms and miraculous cures. Unlike the first two parts of the book, which rely heavily on archaeological remains, this section is mostly limited to textual evidence. The rhetoric that elite authors used to circumscribe their communal identity complicates our readings of these texts, as it portrays the authors' coreligionists as the purveyors of miracles and accuses outsiders of magic. I argue that despite these exclusionary tactics, it is possible to distinguish between two broad categories of cures ascribed to people, addressed in Chapters 5 and 6 respectively. Chapter 5 examines healings that were understood to take place through a wonderworker's performance of prescribed words and actions. Some of the people who performed these rituals were acting in an official capacity on behalf of their community, while other practitioners could be called freelancers. Chapter 6 looks at wonderworkers who were understood by their coreligionists to have a personal ability to perform miracles; no specific prayers or rituals were required. Ancient authors describe the wonderworkers' power in a variety of ways. In some cases, they seem to have an intrinsic healing power that can be conveyed by touch or speech. Other stories point to their extraordinary knowledge, their ability to persuade God to act, or their particularly close relationship with the divine.

The book's final part argues that the rejection of various methods of ritual healing by patristic and rabbinic authors represent attempts to demarcate acceptable practices within their communities and, in many cases, to consolidate power within their own social networks. In Chapter 7, I show that all three categories of ritual healing explored in this book – miraculous objects, miraculous places, and miraculous people – drew the criticism of elite authors. In some cases, such as John Chrysostom's condemnation of incubation in Daphne or the Yerushalmi's rejection of Jacob of Kefar Sama, specific sites or individuals were the focus of these critiques. In both of these examples, the rejection deliberately engaged the boundary being constructed between Jews and Christians, since incubation in Daphne took place at a synagogue and Jacob of Kefar Sama's method of healing involved an invocation of Jesus. Even in cases where the prohibitions by Jewish or Christian authors described categories of rejected practices, rather than specific sites or individuals, I argue that they demonstrate knowledge of healing practices outside their community and reflect a deliberate desire to deny these practices to their coreligionists.

While Chapter 7 demonstrates that these cures were indeed contested, the rhetoric of elite authors should not overshadow the picture of intertwined and shared forms of healing explored in the first six chapters. The countless nameless and faceless people of Roman and late antique Palestine, like our hypothetical woman from Caesarea, were simply looking for relief. Although rabbinic and patristic condemnations may have deterred some people from pursuing certain practices, there is no reason to expect that this was any concern, let alone the most important factor, to everyone who identified as a Jew or a Christian.

PART I

Miraculous Objects

CHAPTER I

One God Who Conquers Evil: Gemstone and Jewelry Amulets

In 1957, nineteen rolled metal amulets were found in the apse of a late antique synagogue near Kibbutz Nirim in southern Israel, near the border with Gaza. Of these nineteen amulets, three have been unrolled and the texts on them read. The best preserved is a bronze amulet that can be read nearly in its entirety:

> An amulet proper for Esther, daughter of Ṭ'tys, to save her from evil tormentors, from evil eye, from spirit, from demon, from shadow-spirit, from [all] evil tormentors, from evil eye, from . . . from imp[ure] spirit, . . . "If you will diligently hearken to the voice of Yahweh your God, and will do that which is right in his sight, and will give ear to his commandments, and keep all his statutes, I will put none of these diseases upon you, which I have brought upon the Egyptians. For I am Yahweh that heals you." . . .[1]

Written in a combination of Aramaic and Hebrew, the amulet identifies Esther as the person for whom it was made. It also includes the name of her mother and the conditions from which Esther sought protection. The extant portion of the amulet concludes with a quotation from Exod 15 that promises God's protection against disease.[2] Each of these components are common on amulets from Palestine, and especially among the amulets that will be considered in Chapter 2. One of the things that makes this Nirim amulet

---

[1] For the publication and translation of this amulet, see Naveh and Shaked 1985, 98–101, no. 13. This translation has been modified slightly to update archaic pronouns and verb tenses and to include the vocalization "Yahweh" instead of "the Lord."

[2] This amulet lists the ailments from which Esther requires healing twice – the first time in Aramaic, and the second time in Hebrew.

particularly noteworthy, however, was its discovery in a secure archaeological context. Its deposition in a synagogue, together with its use of Aramaic, means that we can be reasonably certain that the user considered herself a Jew. The vast majority of amulets from Roman and late antique Palestine lack archaeological context, which means that, unlike the Nirim amulets, it is difficult to interrogate the religious or ethnic self-understanding of the practitioner who crafted the object and the person who originally used it. This is particularly true for the amulets with the inscription *heis theos* ("one god") or its extended form *heis theos ho nikōn ta kaka* ("one god who conquers evil"). As I will argue below, the *heis theos* acclamation could have appealed to members of disparate communities.

The purpose of this chapter is twofold. The first is to outline varieties of amulets known from Roman and late antique Palestine, the languages in which they were written, and the relative frequency of each. Inscribed amulets from the ancient Mediterranean world came in a variety of forms including thin metal sheets called *lamellae*, jewelry, gemstones, and perishable materials, most notably papyri. The first three categories are well attested in Roman and late antique Palestine; only the last is lacking.[3] This absence is regrettable, as the ready availability of perishable materials such as papyri and leaves would have made these amulets cheaper to acquire and likely quite common. The second objective of this chapter is to look at three examples of gemstone and jewelry amulets in detail. Such amulets are often relegated to specialized studies and are overlooked in broader treatments of amulets, which tend to focus on media that permit lengthier texts, namely papyri and *lamellae*. Nevertheless, as I demonstrate in Chapter 7, the amulets of this chapter were likely among those targeted by elite rhetoric. In order to understand how elite authors used amulets to construct collective identity, it is necessary to explore the varieties known from Palestine and to identify wherever possible the religious and cultural milieux in which they were fashioned.

A few words are necessary at the outset about the amulets on which this chapter and the next will focus. First, they are all previously published amulets, and they all have either a confirmed or a reported provenience of ancient Palestine, including the immediate Transjordan region. Reported

---

[3] Papyri amulets survive in abundance in Egypt, where they give tantalizing hints about what might have been lost in the wetter climate of Israel (e.g. Daniel and Maltomini 1990; De Bruyn and Dijkstra 2011). We know that perishable amulets were used in Palestine since they are mentioned in rabbinic literature (*m. Šabb.* 8.3; *y. Šabb.* 8:3 [10d]), and we can infer their presence from the discovery of empty metal amulet cases that originally held perishable amulets that have long since been lost (e.g. Macalister 1912, 1:365; Baramki 1932, pl.V, no. 15; Gudovitch 1996, 68–9, 67: fig. 3, no. 9; Kogan-Zehavi 2006, 66* and 72* (fig. 7, no. 28); Eshel and Leiman 2010, 194; Jakoel 2013, 37–8, 220, fig. 28.5; Ashkenazi 2015, 120–1; Jackson-Tal 2015b, 190). For introductions to the papyri from Egypt, see, for example, Brashear 1995; Dieleman 2019.

Table 1.1 Circumstances of finds

	Excavated	Surface	Reported provenience	Unprovenienced
Lamellae	11	1	8	0
Gems	8	21	17	12
Jewelry	19	12	20	2
Total	**38 (29%)**	**34 (26%)**	**45 (34%)**	14 **(11%)**

provenience is far more common. The discovery of amulets in controlled archaeological excavations, such as at Nirim, is rare. For many of these amulets, details of provenience are extremely problematic (see Table 1.1).[4] Without secure provenience, scholars are left in the dark regarding an object's precise date and the circumstances in which it fell out of use, or even whether it was deliberately deposited, such as in a grave or a rubbish pit, or whether it was lost in the abandonment of a settlement.[5] A second caveat about the types of amulets included in this study must be made. Of necessity, Chapters 1 and 2 focus on inscribed amulets, since uninscribed ones cannot dependably be distinguished in the archaeological record.[6] Examples of the latter could include bells, nails, mirrors, shells, beads, coins, and stones or vegetal matter thought to work on the basis of their natural properties or through some inherent similarity between the material of the amulet and the condition that it was meant to cure.[7] Similarly, objects that include images but

[4] Data for the tables in Chapters 1 and 2 was compiled in the spring of 2018. Many older publications of these amulets provide few details about find location and circumstances, and so my decision on which amulets to include had to be somewhat arbitrary. For example, amulets said to come from either Syria or Palestine have been excluded. In many cases, this provenience information was reported by the antiquities dealers who sold the amulet, making it deeply problematic. Some dealers may have been motivated to say that items came from Palestine in the hopes of a higher sale price. The sixteen Nirim amulets that have not yet been unrolled and deciphered were excluded from these tables, as were the following amulets for which insufficient details have been published: Makhouly 1939, 47, bronze amulet listed in kokh no. 1 without description or image; Patrich and Rafael 2008, 424 and 431, no. 52; Jackson-Tal 2015a, 170, 172. Objects that belong in the category of curses or aggressive "magic" have also been excluded, even if they were intended to be worn on the body (e.g. Naveh and Shaked 1985, 84–9, no. 10; Naveh and Shaked 1993, 43–50, no. 16; Hamilton 1996; Glazier-McDonald and McCollough 2009; Eshel and Leiman 2010, 191–2 and 194–5, nos. 2 and 9).

[5] Jeffrey Spier (2007, 1–9) outlines the history of collecting gemstones from the Renaissance to the twentieth century, a phenomenon that obscured archaeological provenience. As Rangar Cline (2019, 360) observed, the same problem also applies to jewelry amulets.

[6] Uninscribed amulets were particularly common in the pre-Roman Greek world. See discussion in Faraone 2018, 78.

[7] For example, *t. Šabb.* 4:9, *y. Šabb.* 6:2 (8a–b), and *y. 'Erub.* 10:11 (26c) mention roots used as amulets. See discussion of these other types of amulets in Rahmani 1985, 171–2; Nagy 2012, 82–91; Bohak 2017, 172–3; Faraone 2018, 79–101.

lack text or *charaktares* (magical symbols) have also been excluded.[8] There is no doubt that some objects with images – whether inscribed, painted, molded, or carved – functioned as amulets even in the absence of texts. However, it can be difficult to determine when these items were indeed amulets and when they were merely decorative, and so, for the sake of clarity and consistency, they have been excluded.

Published amulets from Roman and late antique Palestine

Of the amulets that survive from Palestine, gemstones comprise the largest category at roughly 45 percent of the corpus, while *lamellae* are by far the smallest category at only about 15 percent (see Table 1.2). Jewelry amulets, a category that includes rings, bracelets, and pendants, comprise roughly 40 percent of the region's amulets. Previous studies of ancient amulets, from Palestine and beyond, have typically been segregated into these categories. To a certain degree, this is logical, as differences in size, shape, and technical expertise mean that the best comparanda for any given object will be found among those within the same category. For example, *lamellae*, like the papyri amulets of Egypt, can contain lengthy texts, while the relatively small surface area of gemstones and jewelry amulets limited the practitioner to inscribing a couple of words or images. However, the tendency to compartmentalize the study of amulets means that even gemstones and jewelry amulets are rarely considered side by side, despite similarities in the size of their writing surfaces. At the same time, this compartmentalization obscures the key characteristic that all shared, namely that any number of objects were thought to offer healing and protection when worn on the body.

Table 1.2 Types of amulets

	N
Lamellae	20 (15%)
Gems	58 (44%)
Jewelry	53 (40%)
Total	**131**

---

[8] As Andrea Berlin helpfully observed, this limits the present study to "talking" amulets. *Charaktares* are signs that look vaguely like letters, sometimes with strokes terminating in a small circle. For more on *charaktares* see Frankfurter 1994, 205–11; Mastrocinque 2004, 90–8; Gordon 2011; Gordon 2014; De Bruyn 2017, 57–8.

Among studies of amulets with longer texts – *lamellae* and the papyri amulets from Egypt – there is a tendency to subdivide the corpus further according to the language of the inscription, a scholarly convention that is sometimes applied to jewelry as well. This use of language as a way to group amulets together reflects the training and disciplinary boundaries that underpin modern academia. Yet these divisions can also guide assumptions about the ethnic and religious identities of the amulets' users. To offset this traditional framework, Chapters 1 and 2 take into account all of the extant varieties of amulets, prioritizing origin – Palestine – rather than language or medium as a diagnostic trait. Nevertheless, it is still useful to understand the relative frequency of different languages. Two-thirds of the amulets from Roman and late antique Palestine are written in Greek, with smaller numbers in Aramaic and Samaritan scripts (see Table 1.3). Some interesting trends emerge when language is mapped onto the different categories of amulets seen in Table 1.2. The vast majority of Greek amulets take the form of gemstones or jewelry; only two Greek *lamellae* have been published from Palestine (see Table 1.4). The opposite is the case among Aramaic amulets, where most are *lamellae*. The Samaritan examples provide a different pattern yet, exclusively taking the form of jewelry. The lack of Greek *lamellae* from Palestine is perhaps most difficult to explain, and it is unclear whether this is simply an accident of preservation or whether it tells us something significant about regional approaches. In contrast, I will argue in Chapter 2 that the high numbers of Aramaic *lamellae* and Samaritan jewelry are suggestive, revealing patterns that can be brought into focus when differences in their use of biblical quotations are considered.

Table 1.3 Language of amulets[a]

	N
Greek	88 (67%)
Aramaic	21 (16%)
Samaritan	18 (14%)
Greek and Samaritan	2 (<2%)
Greek and Hebrew	1 (<1%)
Charaktares without text	1 (<1%)
Total	**131**

[a] For the purposes of this chapter and the next, amulets with Aramaic and Hebrew inscriptions will be considered in a single category. In general, these amulets contain scriptural quotations in Hebrew and any additional text in Aramaic. See discussion in Eshel and Leiman 2010, 194. The Greek total in Table 1.3 includes six pseudo-Greek inscriptions that contain no translatable text, and three reaper gems from Shiqmona whose language is unspecified but presumably Greek like the other examples of this type.

20   CONTESTED CURES

Table 1.4 Language according to amulet type

	Greek	Aramaic	Samaritan	Greek + Samaritan	Greek + Hebrew	Charaktares w/o text
Lamellae	2	17	0	0	1	0
Gems	52	4	0	1	0	1
Jewelry	34	0	18	1	0	0
Total	**88**	**21**	**18**	**2**	**1**	**1**

With this broad outline of the extant corpus of amulets in mind, I turn now to three examples: a reaper gemstone from Caesarea, a brass *boēth(e)i* ("help") ring from Hammat Gader, and a bronze *heis theos* ("one god") pendant from Gush Halav. These exemplars demonstrate not only the range of ritual techniques found in the region, but also points of contact and divergence among amulets made in different media and written in different languages.

A reaper gemstone from Caesarea

The black jasper gemstone shown in Figure 1.1 is roughly 2.5 cm in diameter and was reported as a surface find in Caesarea. It shows on the obverse a man bent over to reap grain; he has already cut off the top of three stalks, and there are three more that remain to be harvested. He reaches out with a sickle in his right hand to cut the next two stalks of grain, with his left hand poised to catch them. On the gem's reverse is an inscription in Greek, *(i)schiōn*, a genitive plural that can be translated "of the hips."[9] The appeal of an amulet such as this one to people engaged in physical labor, such as the agricultural work depicted on the gem, is self-explanatory. The inscription calls to mind sciatica, which takes its name from the Greek word for hips inscribed on the gemstone and which is just one of the conditions that would have troubled laborers. Gems of this type are common in the eastern Mediterranean, including eleven from Palestine, among which there are only minor differences in the composition of the reaper scene on

---

[9] For an extended discussion of the reaper gems, see Bonner 1950, 71–5. For the custom of attaching an amulet as close as possible to the part of the body it was intended to treat, see discussion in Faraone 2018, 247–51. For a recent introduction to gems used as amulets, see Dasan and Nagy 2019. For ease of reading, I use parentheses rather than angle brackets to indicate Attic spellings of words whose later forms were used on amulets. Square brackets indicate letters that are no longer extant but that were supplied in the original or subsequent publications of the amulet.

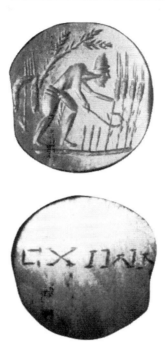

Figure 1.1 A reaper gemstone from Caesarea (Hamburger 1968)

the obverse.[10] A couple of notable inscription variations on the reverse confirm that these gemstones were intended to heal hip pain. The reverse inscription on an oblong steatite gemstone excavated in Beth She'an has been reconstructed to read *(i)schiou therapias*, or "cure of the hip."[11] Two additional gemstones, while not with a known provenience from Israel, include an alternate inscription, *ergazomai ke (kai) ou ponō*, "I work, and I do not suffer."[12]

At first glance, it may seem that these gemstones are intended to represent a reaper who suffered from hip pain himself. However, the alternate inscription known from these last two gems, "I work, and I do not suffer" suggests the opposite is the case. Rather than showing a laborer in pain, the image represents the desired state of the amulet's user – the ability to continue his physical labor unimpeded. Adding weight to this interpretation is the fact that similar

---

[10] Simone Michel lists forty gemstones with the reaper motif. The majority (twenty-eight) have the the *(i)schiōn* inscriptions on the reverse. Michel 2004, 329, no. 47, s.v. Schnitter.

[11] Khamis 2006. Another reaper amulet, originally published by Henri Seyrig (1935, 50) also reads *(i)schiōn therap(e)ia* on the reverse, using the plural for "hips" rather than the singular form found on the Beth She'an gem. See discussion in Vitto 2008, 22*; Bonner 1950, 272–3 and pl. VI, no. 125.

[12] Delatte and Derchain 1964, nos. 261–2. See also Vitto 2008, 22*; Faraone 2009, 248.

22 CONTESTED CURES

reaper images can be traced to Pharaonic tomb paintings, where the reaper represented felicity in the afterlife.[13] The Egyptian concept of the afterlife imagined the deceased in a field of reeds, where there was plentiful grain for reaping. In this reading, the amulet would represent an attempt to secure the same good fortune for physical laborers as the reaper in the afterlife who painlessly harvests grain. The gemstone's felicitous reaper image was likely understood to be augmented by the stone's natural properties, as many reaper amulets are made out of hematite, a stone that was thought to heal a variety of conditions.[14]

The lack of archaeological context for most of the Palestinian reaper gems makes it difficult to say much about the people who used these amulets. For example, one turned up in the debris from the excavation of a late first- or early second-century CE Jewish tomb north of the old city of Tiberias, but its exact relationship to the burials is unknown.[15] Three excavated reaper gemstones from Palestine supply somewhat more information, as they were found in contexts where a Christian user would seem likely.[16] While the archaeological context of

[13] Bonner 1950, 74–5 and pl. XXII, fig. 2; Faraone 2018, 94–5, 149. This Pharaonic motif made its way onto the reverses of some coins minted in Alexandria under Antoninus Pius, where the harvested grain likely alluded to the abundance of agricultural produce that Egypt exported throughout the empire. See Bonner 1950, 74–5 and pl. XXII, fig. 1; Delatte and Derchain 1964.

[14] The reaper gem from Caesarea was made out of jasper, which was sometimes substituted for hematite. Faraone (2018, 95) argues that the image and inscription may have been used to distinguish hematite gemstones intended to cure hip pain from those used to treat other conditions.

[15] Vitto 2008, 7*, 21*–23*.

[16] One was discovered in excavations south of the gate tower on Mount Berenice in the region of Tiberias (Amitai-Preiss 2004, 188). The amulet was found in locus 200; for list of loci, see Hirschfeld and Amir 2004, 230–3. The construction of the city wall on Mount Bernice dates to the sixth century CE, which corresponds to Procopius' testimony that it was built during Justinian's reign to facilitate the construction of a Christian pilgrimage site on the high ground (Hirschfeld 2004a, 77; Hirschfeld 2004b, 220). The date of its deposition, no earlier than the sixth century, and its connection to a pilgrimage site suggest a Christian context. A second reaper amulet was found in a residential area on the north slope of Tel Beth She'an, also in a Byzantine context (Khamis 2006, 675–6; Mazar 2006, 40–2; Applbaum and Mazar 2006, 295). A third gem was discovered in Caesarea in a warehouse complex dating to the fifth to sixth centuries CE (Patrich et al. 1999; Patrich 2002a, 77–8; Patrich 2008; Patrich and Rafael 2008). The warehouse owner's identification as a Christian can be inferred from several frescoes depicting saints and crosses with the Greek letters alpha and omega and the *nomina sacra* for Jesus Christ, and from a partially preserved good luck (*eutychōs*) inscription in a mosaic floor that has been reconstructed with the same type of cross, including *nomina sacra* and the alpha and omega, at the top of the inscription. For the frescoes, see Patrich et al. 1999, 75; Patrich 1996, 169–70; for the crosses, see Patrich 1996, 170–1; Patrich et al. 1999, 78, 80; Patrich 2002a, 77. In addition, small finds from the warehouse complex include a Christian bread stamp, ampullae with images of saints, and a fragment of a marble screen decorated with a cross (Patrich 1996, 170–3; Johnson 2008, no. 618 [pages 58 and 156] and no. 764 [pages 66 and 164]; Patrich 2002b). Patrich (1996, 171–2; 2002a, 77–8) suggests that some of these items might be explained by the presence of a church on an upper floor of the warehouse complex.

these three cannot confirm that the amulets belonged to someone who identified as a Christian, it is certainly suggestive of the milieu in which they were being used. The three additional reaper gems were excavated in Shiqmona, a coastal city near Haifa with a mixed Jewish and Christian population in late antiquity, but insufficient details about their find spot were published to enable any precision about the context in which they were deposited.[17] The remaining four unexcavated amulets were all reportedly found in the diverse city of Caesarea, but without secure archaeological provenience it is impossible to speculate as to the self-understanding of the users.[18]

The appeal of these reaper amulets to those performing hard, physical labor could have crossed the notional lines that separated members of various ethnic, cultural, and religious groups, offering hope to anyone who suffered from chronic pain. While all of the known examples include an inscription in Greek, the vivid imagery on the obverse likely rendered Greek literacy unimportant. The potential for reaper gemstones to be popular in multiple communities may have been facilitated by one of their peculiar features: the examples from Palestine do not name the divine healer from whom help is sought.[19] This opens the possibility that reaper gems could have been shared among members of neighboring communities, despite the attempts of certain Jewish and Christian elites to create space between their ritual practices. Absent any divine names on the gemstones, elites' censure might have been insufficient to prevent their coreligionists from buying such amulets from people outside their community. In towns with heterogeneous populations where several reaper stones were found, such as Caesarea and Shiqmona, the transfer of healing rituals, including these reaper amulets, could have been rather easily accomplished.

Another feature of reaper amulets is the lack of a named user. This is in fact characteristic of gemstone amulets more generally, not simply reaper gemstones. Among Palestinian amulets, gemstones are least likely to be personalized with the name of the user, with only 2 of 58 including a name. In contrast, *lamellae*

---

[17] Elgavish 1994, 140–3.

[18] For the diverse groups that inhabited Caesarea Maritima, see Holum 1998; Donaldson 2000.

[19] Simone Michel identified three exceptions to this, none of which has a reported provenience of Palestine (2004, 329, no. 47.1.c). The first two exceptions have *Sabaō(th)* on the reverse. Because this divine name originated in the Hebrew Bible as an epithet for God ("[God] of hosts"), Erwin Goodenough suggested that the reaper gemstones were Jewish in origin (1953, vol. 2, 289 and vol. 3, no. 1206). However, we now know that the name *Sabaōth* is ubiquitous in Roman and late antique amulets throughout the eastern Mediterranean, often used as a proper name rather than an epithet, and the presence of this name does not necessarily indicate that either the practitioner who created the amulet or the amulet's user was Jewish. A third exception is a reaper gemstone with the *heis theos* ("one god") on the reverse (Michel 2004, 329, no. 47.1.c).

24   CONTESTED CURES

are the category with the largest number of named users (15 of 20), and even jewelry amulets are personalized with greater frequency than gems (13 of 50).[20] It would follow that gemstones were less likely to originate as individual commissions than either *lamellae* or jewelry. Instead, practitioners may have had a premade stock of gemstones from which people could purchase one to meet their needs. A related observation is that only 3 percent of gemstone amulets from Palestine were discovered in funerary contexts, while 15 percent of *lamellae* and 16 percent of jewelry amulets were found in tombs.[21] The relative absence of gemstones in funerary contexts is striking and perhaps related to their lack of personalization. Rather than being buried with the deceased as part of his or her personal effects, these gemstones may have been transferred to new owners where they could continue to be efficacious. This process would have been simplified by the absence of named users. The lack of personalization, coupled with the absence of a named deity, meant that the amulet may have not only been passed to a loved one in need of it, but could have also been sold to someone from a neighboring community.

A brass ring from Hammat Gader

The brass ring pictured in Figure 1.2 was excavated in the synagogue adjacent to the bath complex at Hammat Gader, a thermal-mineral spring in the southern Golan near the Sea of Galilee.[22] As I will argue in Chapter 3, Hammat Gader was itself a site of ritual healing, and it is not difficult to imagine that a visitor who came to the spring in search of a cure might have also sought cures through other means, including amulets. Eleazar Sukenik concluded that the ring post-dated the destruction of the Hammat Gader synagogue, a destruction that is evident from fire damage on the floor and the deliberate demolition of the chancel screen.[23] The ring's oval bezel has a diameter of 1.1 cm, making

---

[20] The reconstruction of the user's name on three amulets is somewhat difficult, but they have still been included in these counts. These include a silver *lamella* from Emmaus (Vincent 1908; Frey 1952, no. 1185; Testa 1962, 64–6; Naveh and Shaked 1985, 60–3, no. 5; Eshel and Leiman 2010, 192, no. 11), a silver *lamella* from Samaria (Eshel and Leiman 2010, no. 10; Müller-Kessler et al. 2007), and a lead ring from Caesarea (Lifshitz 1964, 81, no. 5; Di Segni 1994, 99, no. 9; Belayche 2001, 159; *CIIP* 2, 569, no. 1682). Evidence from Egypt suggests that papyri amulets were likely personalized at a rate closer to that of *lamellae* than that of either gemstones or jewelry.

[21] An additional three *lamellae* were reportedly found in tombs in the vicinity of Irbid in the early 1900s, but no formal excavations were undertaken (Montgomery 1911, 272–3).

[22] Sukenik 1935, 70–1.

[23] Sukenik (1935, 80–1) did not determine a date for this destruction, but Levi Rahmani suggested a destruction in the sixth or early seventh century (1985, 178, no. 15).

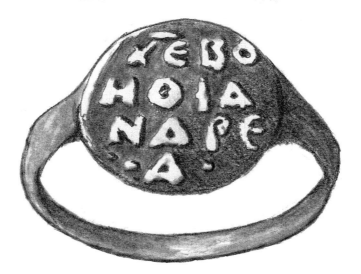

Figure 1.2 A brass ring from Hammat Gader (Drawing by D. Weiss)

it less than half the diameter of the reaper gemstone discussed above (2.5 cm). The Greek text on the ring reads *Ch(rist)e, boēth(e)i Andrea* or "Christ, help Andreas."[24] The use of a *nomen sacrum*, a form of abbreviating divine names, rather than spelling out *Christe*, reflects Christian scribal traditions that were widespread by the fourth century.[25] Whereas reaper gemstones specified the condition being treated but gave no indication of a divine healer or the name of the user, the opposite is true for this brass ring. The Hammat Gader ring specifies both the divine healer and the amulet's user, while the reason this help was needed is left unstated. In fact, it is unclear whether Andreas suffered from a particular condition at the time when he acquired the ring or whether the amulet was meant to protect him from any and all possible afflictions.[26] Whatever his specific circumstances, Andreas' simple plea for help on this ring likely echoes a sentiment that he would have expressed either silently or aloud many times before and after the ring was crafted.

This ring from Hammat Gader is one of six from Roman and late antique Palestine with similarly short, amuletic texts. Each of the rings uses the Greek

---

[24] Sukenik 1935, 70–1; Rahmani 1985, 178 and pl. XLIII, no. 15.
[25] De Bruyn 2017, 60–2.
[26] While some scholars distinguish between amulets that are properly curative and those that are protective, I find this distinction difficult to maintain. Some amulets, such as the reaper gemstones already discussed, cannot be definitively assigned to either category, as someone could conceivably begin carrying one before the onset of symptoms.

imperative *boēth(e)i* or "help," identifies the divine healer, specifies the name of the user, and lacks additional images or texts.[27] Four of the six address the healer in the vocative as *Kyrie* or "Lord," one from Caesarea uses the acclamation *heis theos* or "one god," and the example from Hammat Gader addresses Christ.[28] On all but one of these rings, the inscription is found on the rings' bezel, as on the example from Hammat Gader; on the last one, the text is inscribed around the ring's band.[29] Closely related to these six rings are an additional five that simply say *hygi(ei)a* (health) and the name of the user. The *hygi(ei)a* rings do not identify the divine healer from whom health is requested, nor do they use an imperative verb as the other six do. Despite these differences, the simple texts and lack of other decoration mean that *hygi(ei)a* rings have much in common with those of the Hammat Gader type.[30]

All but one of the *boēth(e)i* rings seem to reflect Christian conventions, since they address *Kyrie* or *Christe*. The religious milieu of amulets with the acclamation *heis theos*, in contrast, is more complicated, and I will return to this issue below. The *hygi(ei)a* rings, lacking a named divine healer, raise the possibility of a wider variety of contexts. The user's name on one of the *hygi(ei)a* rings, Samuel, recalls the prophet from the Hebrew Bible, but since this name was used by both Jews and Christians, the name alone cannot be used to clarify how the user would have identified himself.[31] Unfortunately, only one of the *hygi(ei)a* rings was discovered in the course of archaeological excavations. It was uncovered in a late fifth- or early sixth-century monastic complex on Masada, suggesting that it was used by a Christian, as the *boēth(e)i* rings probably were.[32] Hannah Cotton and Joseph Geiger, who initially published the Masada ring, suggested that it was produced in the same workshop as a similar *hygi(ei)a* ring reportedly found in Apollonia (Arsuf), a coastal site north of Tel

---

[27] A copper ring with a rectangular bezel, reportedly from Caesarea, may have contained a similar inscription, but it also includes an image. The center of the bezel depicts a nimbate bust, facing forward, with an inscription around the edge. Although the reading is not certain, it seems to begin *Kyrie boēth(e)i*. See Amorai-Stark 2016, 394–6, no. 415.

[28] Two of those addressed to *Kyrie* use *nomina sacra*, as does the ring addressed to Christ, while the others write out the name. The *boēth(e)i* ring from Caesarea has *heis theos* in the nominative, rather than the vocative found on the *Kyrie* and *Christe* rings. It is best to read the *heis theos* in this ring not as a grammatical error, using the nominative instead of the vocative, but rather as a declarative statement, followed by a request for healing in the imperative: "[There is] one god. Help Cheromenēs." For the idea that *cheromenēs* should be read as the participle, the woman who has been widowed, see Lifshitz 1964, 81, no. 5; Di Segni 1994, 99, no. 9; *CIIP* 2, 569, no 1682.

[29] *CIIP* 2, 572–3, no. 1686; Lifshitz 1964, 386, no. 5.

[30] A ring in the British Museum collection combines both the *boēth(e)i* formula and *hygi(ei)a*: "Lord, help. Healing of Iakobos" (*K(yri)e, bo(ēthei): Iak(ob)ou hygi(ei)a*). See Perdrizet 1914, 271.

[31] Schwab 1936, 347.

[32] Cotton and Geiger 1995.

Aviv, but this can tell us nothing about the ring's user, since items produced in one workshop could have been marketed to people from different religious communities, a situation that seems to have obtained in Israel for both lamps and the chancel screens for churches and synagogues.[33] Since only one of these *hygi(ei)a* rings has a clear archaeological context, nothing definitive can be said about whether they did, in fact, appeal to a broader range of users than the *boēth(e)i* rings.

The circumstances of the Hammat Gader ring's deposition cannot be determined with confidence, but at least three possibilities exist. Votive offerings are frequent in healing sanctuaries, including, as we will see in Chapter 3, inscriptions and lamps at Hammat Gader. The ring might have been dedicated as a votive once it was no longer needed for protection or healing.[34] If it was left as a votive offering, one might wonder whether the synagogue, which was had already been at least partially destroyed, was the place where the ring was initially deposited or whether it was found in a secondary context. Alternatively, Levi Rahmani hypothesized that some amuletic rings were acquired from shrines as *eulogia*, pilgrimage tokens intended to convey the blessings of the shrine, or its saint, when the visitor returned home.[35] The discovery of one of these rings at Hammat Gader, a site that I argue functioned as a healing shrine, raises the tantalizing possibility that these amulets might have been sold near the hot spring as a way to hold onto the healing benefits of the sacred site when one departed. Absent any evidence for the production or sale of such rings in the area around Hammat Gader, a third possibility must also be considered. It could have simply been lost or discarded by a visitor to the hot spring. There is no reason to suspect that people who came to Hammat Gader exclusively used the hot springs as their method of seeking divine healing. It would make sense that those chronically sick, those with unresolved medical issues, or even just those concerned about the potential for disease would have also employed other forms of ritual cures within their means, such as this *boēth(e)i* ring. Faced with serious concerns about their health, they would have diversified their options.

Unlike the reaper gemstones, whose ritual efficacy seems to be associated with the image and the natural properties of the gemstone, the inscription

---

[33] Cotton and Geiger (1995, 53–4) actually push their conclusion a bit further and suggest that both rings were made for the same client, Babosa, but that an illiterate artisan jumbled the letters to produce Abusob on the ring from Masada.

[34] Gideon Bohak (2008, 315) entertained this possibility when considering the cache of *lamellae* found at the Nirim synagogue. The situation in Hammat Gader does not mirror the Nirim situation precisely, as the dedication post-dates the destruction of the synagogue, but the ring could have originally been dedicated somewhere else in the sanctuary, including at the bath complex itself.

[35] Rahmani 1985, 179–80.

28 CONTESTED CURES

is the key component on the *boēth(e)i* rings. "Lord, help me!" This simple prayer must not have been far from the lips of the people who purchased these amulets. The ring, in fact, can be seen as a way of perpetuating this prayer: the prayer continues to be offered simply by its presence on the ring, even when it is not being spoken aloud. As Chris Faraone has argued persuasively, by inscribing a text that originated as an oral prayer, the promise of healing or protection could be transformed into a tangible object to wear on the body.[36] The short text on *boēth(e)i* rings suggests that users who acquired them may have known what was written, even if they could not read it for themselves. For amulets with longer or more complicated texts, whose contents an illiterate user might not necessarily know, the understanding that the inscribed text created a permanent, tangible prayer for healing would have made them attractive none the less. Low literacy rates combined with the understanding of textual amulets as a form of ongoing, physical prayer may offer some explanation for the existence of amulets with pseudo-inscriptions that look vaguely like a real script, such as Greek or Samaritan, but that cannot be deciphered.[37] In these examples, as in the case of Andreas' *boēth(e)i* ring, wearing an amulet would have been a way to continue praying even when going about one's daily tasks.

A bronze pendant from Gush Halav

In 1937, the bronze pendant shown in Figure 1.3 was excavated in a tomb in Gush Halav (El-Jish), located in the Upper Galilee. The tomb was dated by the excavators to the fourth or fifth century, likely making it somewhat earlier than the *boēth(e)i* ring from Hammat Gader.[38] The two-sided pendant has a suspension loop at the top and is roughly 6.5 cm tall, more than twice the diameter of the reaper gemstone from Caesarea (2.5 cm).[39] The pendant combines detailed images and texts on both sides, distinguishing it from both the reaper gemstones and the *boēth(e)i* rings. On the reverse are inscribed the names *Iaō Sabaōth Michaēl*, followed by the Greek imperative *boēth(e)i* ("help"). The use of *boēth(e)i* echoes the brass ring from Hammat Gader and its analogues, but otherwise this amulet is quite different.[40] While the Hammat Gader ring

[36] Faraone 2018, 177–8.
[37] For examples, see Chapter 2 and Spier 2007, 109–14.
[38] For publication of this amulet, see Makhouly 1939, 49; Di Segni 1994, 96, no. 1b; Israeli and Mevorah 2000, 161, 224.
[39] Israeli and Mevorah 2000, 224.
[40] The same phrase, *Iaō Sabaōth Michaēl boēth(e)i*, is found on a pendant excavated from a grave at Shiqmona. See Elgavish 1994, 152–3.

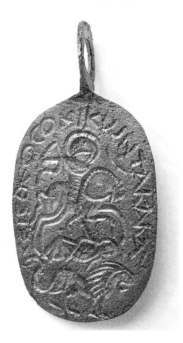 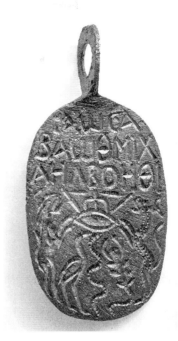

Figure 1.3 A bronze pendant from Gush Halav (Photo by Clara Amit, Courtesy of the Israel Antiquities Authority)

contains a simple request to help a named individual, this pendant includes several divine names and apotropaic images but never specifies the user. The divine names originate in the Hebrew Bible: *Iaō Sabaōth* is a Greek transliteration of the Hebrew *Yahweh Ṣĕbā'ôt* (Yahweh of the Heavenly Hosts),[41] and *Michaēl* appears in the Book of Daniel as the archangel *Mîkā'ēl*.[42]

Below *Iaō Sabaōth Michaēl boēth(e)i* on the reverse is the first of two images that contributed to the amulet's potency: a stylized, lidless eye attacked on all sides by weapons and animals. Directly above the center of the eye is a trident, flanked by two swords, all with points piercing the eye. The lower register of attackers consists of animals, with a leopard to the right of the weapons and a lion to the left. Between the two large cats, from left to right, are a crane, a snake, and a scorpion. Since the 1950s, scholars have associated images such as

---

[41] Among Greek amulets from Palestine, *Sabaōth* always follows *Iaō*. This is in contrast to how *Sabaōth* appears on Greek amulets outside Palestine, where it does not appear exclusively in conjunction with *Iaō*. Rather, it frequently shows up alone or in lists of divine names and seems to function as a proper name rather than as part of an epithet or title (Bonner 1950, 170).

[42] Dan 10:13, 10:21, 12:1. The archangel Michael also appears in the New Testament at Jude 9 and Rev 12:7.

30   CONTESTED CURES

this one, found both on personal and building amulets, with a passage from the *Testament of Solomon*.[43] This first- or second-century CE text attributed to the biblical King Solomon special knowledge that enabled him to restrain affliction-causing demons. The text contains a list of thirty-six demons together with the illnesses they cause and the means of preventing their attacks. The second to the last demon tells Solomon, "I am called Rhyx Phtheneoth. I cast the evil eye (*baskainō*) on every man. But the much-suffering eye (*polypathēs ophthalmos*), when inscribed, thwarts me."[44] The amuletic image of the eye being attacked on all sides can be understood as the much-suffering eye mentioned here. Its presence on amulets would have served to ward off the evil eye.

The obverse of the Gush Halav amulet devotes most of its surface space to the Holy Rider image: a nimbate figure is mounted on a galloping horse, facing right and holding a spear in his right hand. The rider uses the spear to stab a fallen enemy lying on the ground.[45] The Holy Rider is very common on late antique and Byzantine amulets from Palestine and elsewhere, and may have iconographic roots in late classical images of Alexander and Hellenistic kings as armed riders.[46] The identity of the rider is not uniform across examples of this motif and often is not named at all, as in the present case of the Gush Halav pendant. One of the earliest identifications of the rider is Solomon, whom we just saw was noted for his knowledge of how to combat demonic attacks, including the use of the much-suffering eye found on the other side of the Gush Halav amulet.[47] From Palestine, two Holy Rider gems appear to name the rider. The first, a hematite gem reported as a surface find in Caesarea, includes the name Solomon inscribed around the head of the rider; a second surface find from Caesarea is a serpentine gem that depicts the Holy Rider on the obverse with the name *Mich(a)ēl* on the reverse.[48] Regardless of who the Holy Rider was

---

[43] Bonner 1950, 97–100, 211–12; Goodenough 1953, 2.238; Giannobile 2002, 179–80; Faraone 2018, 106–12. Among examples of this image used to protect buildings, one of the most famous is a ceiling tile of the Dura Europos synagogue. For more on the *Testament of Solomon*, see Chapter 5.

[44] *T. Sol.* 18.39. Translations of the *Testament of Solomon* are from Duling 1983. For the evil eye, see Vakaloudi 2000; Wazana 2007.

[45] The fallen enemy whom the rider spears is partially blocked by a striding lion in the foreground. Although this Gush Halav pendant is the only example with a published provenience from Palestine, Bonner (1950, 174, 211–12) pointed out that the combination of the long-suffering eye, the holy rider, and the inscriptions *heis theos ho nikōn ta kaka* and *Iaō Sabaōth Michaēl boēth(e)i* was frequent on amulets.

[46] For published examples and discussion, see Faraone 2018, 113–14, 343–4, n. 40; Cline 2019, 356–8. Faraone recognizes a similarity between the much-suffering eye and the Holy Rider, found on the two sides of the Gush Halav amulet, in that they both represent "action scenes."

[47] Bonner 1950, 208–11; Faraone 2018, 113–14.

[48] For the hematite gem, see Lifshitz 1964, 80, no. 2; Hamburger 1968, 34, no. 119; *CIIP* 2, 576, no. 1692. For the serpentine gem, see Westenholz 2000, 99, no. 67; *CIIP* 2, 577–8, no. 1694.

identified as, and in fact whether he was named at all, there seems little question that this image was used because it was understood as efficacious in some way. The Holy Rider may have been seen, as David Frankfurter argues, as a type of *historiola*, harnessing the power of the figure's mythic or historical past to effect change in the present world.[49]

On the Gush Halav pendant, the text that accompanies the Holy Rider image curves around the edge of the upper two-thirds of the oval and reads *heis theos ho nikōn ta kaka* ("one god who conquers evil"). *Heis theos* ("one god") acclamations have elicited significant scholarly debate, and have been variously attributed to Jews, Samaritans, Christians, "gnostics," and others.[50] The phrase is found on a total of six amulets with a reported provenience from Palestine, including the *boēth(e)i* ring from Caesarea, mentioned above, with *heis theos* rather than *Christe* or *Kyrie*. Other *heis theos* amulets from Palestine include a gemstone from Caesarea published without a drawing or photograph, which is said to depict a standing figure and a large bird with an inscription above the figure: *heis theos LAEPATOO*; the final word is untranslatable.[51] A tin pendant also from Caesarea shows a male figure holding two *kērykeia* (*caducei*), the staff carried by Hermes. The only text on the pendant, *heis theos*, is to the left of the standing figure.[52] The third appearance of *heis theos* is a lead pendant reportedly from Ashkelon, which will be discussed below. Two additional *heis theos* amulets are bilingual Greek–Samaritan examples; they will be considered in Chapter 2. In addition to these amulets, the *heis theos* acclamation appears on a variety of media throughout Israel, mostly in building inscriptions, but also a couple of times in tombs and other contexts. Given the phrase's popularity, previous scholars have tried to identify its origins and dissemination.

The proliferation of *heis theos* evokes the similarly abbreviated phrase *Yahweh 'eḥād* ("Yahweh is one") found on Samaritan amulets, as will be seen in Chapter 2. The Samaritan phrase clearly functioned as an abbreviation for Deut 6:4, and indeed some previous scholars have understood the Greek acclamation *heis*

---

[49] Frankfurter 1995, 464. For more on *historiolae*, see Chapter 2.

[50] Leah Di Segni compiled a very useful catalogue of all the known examples of *heis theos* in Palestine. However, I find her use of labels to categorize these examples somewhat imprecise, as she identifies any amulet that mentions *Iaō* or *Michaēl* or that depicts a mounted rider or the evil eye as "gnostic." While this label was common in early studies of amulets, it has largely fallen out of favor in more recent years. See discussion in Faraone 2018, 295, n. 73. Nicole Belayche expresses a similar concern about Di Segni's catalogue in 2001, 159, n. 399.

[51] Lifshitz 1964, 81, no. 7; Di Segni 1994, 99, no. 10. For problems with the published description of the gemstone, see *CIIP* 2, 569–70, no. 1683.

[52] Lifshitz 1964, 81, no. 4; Di Segni 1994, 98, no. 8; *CIIP* 2, 570, no. 1684.

32 CONTESTED CURES

theos to function in the same way.[53] A related interpretation saw the acclamation as a reflection of the Greek-speaking Jewish community's version of the *Shema* (*Šǝma'*), a central component of daily Jewish prayers that in turn incorporated Deut 6:4–9.[54] The Mishnah permitted people to recite the *Shema* in their vernacular languages (*m. Soṭah* 7.1; cf. *y. Soṭah* 7:1 [20d]).[55] Nevertheless, the relationship between the Greek acclamation *heis theos* and the text of Deut 6:4 is not that simple. The Septuagint version of the last part of Deut 6:4 reads *akoue Israēl, kyrios ho theos hēmōn, kyrios heis esti* ("Hear, Israel: the Lord our God is one Lord"). While *theos* does appear in the verse, it is not modified directly by *heis*. The Septuagint instead uses *kyrios* ("lord") in place of the Tetragrammaton found in the Hebrew text, in keeping with the Jewish practice of not vocalizing the divine name.[56] In other words, *kyrios heis* (or perhaps even *heis kyrios*) would be the more natural abbreviation for the Septuagint text of Deut 6:4. This difference between the acclamation on amulets and the Septuagint passage is the primary reason that Leah Di Segni argues that the *heis theos* formula does not originate in the Jewish community's use of Deut 6:4.[57] Ultimately, however, I am concerned less with the origins of the phrase than with the individuals who would have worn the acclamation as part of an amulet. Even if users knew that it was not a direct quotation of Deut 6:4, this does not preclude the possibility that they understood Deuteronomy's henotheism to lie behind it.

The origin of the second half of the phrase on the Gush Halav pendant, *ho nikōn ta kaka* ("who conquers evil"), is also difficult to determine. It is sufficiently generic that it could be attributed to any number of divinities, although some scholars have suggested that it was particularly popular among Christians.[58] An interesting proposal by Jean Margain understood the second half of the acclamation to be inspired by the Samaritan use of Exod 15:3, "Yahweh is a warrior; Yahweh is his name."[59] As we will see in Chapter 2, this is the most popular

---

[53] For example, Ganneau 1882, 26; Prentice 1908, 18–19; Bonner 1950, 174; Hamburger 1959, 43. In general, quotations from the Hebrew Bible and the New Testament are given in the NRSV. For the sake of clarity in my discussion of divine names and biblical quotations in Chapters 1 and 2, any quotations where the NRSV uses the traditional periphrasis, "Lord," have been replaced with the vocalization "Yahweh."

[54] Dauphin et al. 1996, 312–14; cf. Faraone 2018, 183–4. For a Greek transliteration of the *Shema* on a gold *lamella* found in Halbturn, Austria, see Eshel et al. 2010.

[55] For discussion of the rabbinic texts and the recitation of the *Shema* in languages other than Hebrew, see Eshel et al. 2010, 58–9.

[56] There are, however, examples of *Iaō* being used to transliterate the Tetragrammaton instead of *kyrios*. The most notable example is a Greek manuscript found among the Dead Sea Scrolls, 4QpapLXXLev[b] (4Q120). See Shaw 2014.

[57] Di Segni 1994, 114–15.

[58] Bonner 1950, 46; Pummer 1987, 255.

[59] Margain 1984, 46–7.

verse on polygonal rings and double-sided amulets written in the Samaritan script, but it is completely absent in both Greek and Aramaic amulets. While *ho nikōn ta kaka* is clearly not a quotation of Exod 15:3, Margain's theory about Samaritan influence cannot be ruled out, especially in light of the appearance of *heis theos* in bilingual Greek–Samaritan inscriptions.

With this in mind, let us return to the question of *heis theos* on amulets. As the discussion of the reaper gemstones and *hygi(ei)a* rings demonstrated, in the absence of archaeological provenience (and often even with provenience), it is often difficult to determine with certainty the ethnic, cultural, or religious self-understanding of individuals who used extant amulets.[60] This is particularly true for the *heis theos* amulets. One example, however, invites some speculation. A lead pendant with a *heis theos* inscription, reportedly discovered in Ashkelon, shows on the obverse Helios riding in his horse-drawn chariot; the reverse contains an inscription that reads *heis theos ho boēthō(n). eulogia pasein (pasin)* ("[There is] one god who helps. Blessings for all"). The image of Helios in his chariot is a common motif in the mosaic floors of Palestinian synagogues, and a Jew who frequented such a synagogue might have found an amulet with this depiction particularly appealing.[61] In addition, the phrase *ho boēthō(n)* ("[the one] who helps") evokes Ps 90:1 (MT 91:1), "He who lives by the help of the Most High" (*en boētheia tou hypsistou*), a verse that is found with some frequency on Greek amulets.[62] While neither the depiction of Helios nor the use of *ho boēthō(n)* confirms that the user was Jewish, taken together the two components are suggestive.

Leaving aside the question of whether Jews employed *heis theos* on amulets, Christian use of the phrase is less ambiguous. A passage from 1 Corinthians builds on the henotheism of Deut 6 and, unlike the Septuagint, includes the precise phrase *heis theos*:

---

[60] In his discussion of criteria that can be used to identify an amulet as Jewish, Gideon Bohak (2008, 212–14) considers motifs used by both Jews and Christians, including excerpts from Ps 91:1 (LXX 90:1) and depictions of the Holy Rider or the binding of Isaac. He argues that one should not assume that amulets using one or more of these shared characteristics were Jewish even if identifiably Christian elements are absent.

[61] Di Segni (1994, 104–5, no. 32) suggested that this amulet could have been Jewish or "gnostic". She also identified parallels to the last part of the inscription, *eulogia pasein (pasin)* ("blessing to all"), from Jewish contexts, adding support, although not conclusive proof, to the possibility that the amulet originated in a Jewish context. Among the many treatments of the Helios motif in synagogue mosaic floors, see Magness 2005.

[62] For an amulet from Palestine with a direct quotation of this verse, see Chapter 2. For apotropaic uses of Ps 90:1 from Egypt, see Kraus 2005; Kraus 2007; De Bruyn 2010, 166–74, tables I–II. Many of the amulets from Egypt containing this verse are considered Christian due to their use of the New Testament or Christian symbols, but this does not mean the verse was used exclusively by Christians.

34 CONTESTED CURES

> Hence, as to the eating of food offered to idols, we know that "no idol in the world really exists," and that "there is no God but one" (*kai hoti oudeis theos ei mē heis*). Indeed, even though there may be so-called gods in heaven or on earth – as in fact there are many gods and many lords – yet for us there is one God (*heis theos*), the Father, from whom are all things and for whom we exist, and one Lord, Jesus Christ, through whom are all things and through whom we exist. (1 Cor 8:4–6)[63]

When this passage is read alongside a substantial catalogue of *heis theos* inscriptions that also incorporate identifiably Christian components, the Christian use of the phrase is relatively unproblematic.[64] Indeed, the tomb where the Gush Halav pendant was discovered likely belonged to someone who identified as a Christian, as a second Holy Rider amulet discovered within includes unmistakably Christian iconography on the reverse.[65] It is worth remembering, however, that these amulets do not contain the names of the people who used them. Therefore, we might be able to speculate about the person interred with these amulets as a Christian, but that does not necessarily indicate the context in which the much-suffering eye amulet was originally produced, purchased, or used.

Reinforcing this need for caution are the ever-increasing number of *heis theos* acclamations from Samaritan milieux. Leah Di Segni's 1994 catalogue already revealed a number of inscriptions that could fairly securely be attributed to Samaritans. She even suggested that Samaritans may have been influential in popularizing the use of the phrase in Palestine, in light of its presence on Mount Gerizim and in other Samaritan locales.[66] More recently, excavations in Apollonia have added two additional *heis theos* inscriptions to the Samaritan corpus. In both cases, *heis theos* is modified by *monos* ("alone") and followed by either a participle (*ho boēthōn*) or a finite form (*boēthei*) of the verb "to help" and the names of the people who dedicated the inscriptions.[67]

---

[63] Previous scholars have also connected the 1 Cor passage to this acclamation, including Gregg 2000, 542–3; Trombley 2001, 313–14.

[64] Di Segni's 1994 catalogue of *heis theos* inscriptions notes which inscriptions contain Christian elements.

[65] Makhouly 1939, 49; Di Segni 1994, 95–6. Di Segni, while recognizing that there was a significant Jewish population in the region of Gush Halav, considered these amulets to be straightforward Christian amulets. A few years later, Safrai (1998a, 141–2) suggested that they should be considered "Jewish-Christian," a position which Di Segni had explicitly rejected, but did not explain his hybrid identification.

[66] Di Segni 1994, 113–15.

[67] For the 2006 discovery of an inscription in Area O at the northern end of the site, see Roll and Tal 2008; Tal 2009. For the 2014 discovery of an inscription in Area P1 at the southern end of the site, see Tal 2015.

GEMSTONE AND JEWELRY AMULETS   35

Oren Tal and Israel Roll have argued that these newly discovered inscriptions, together with previously known examples, confirm that the *heis theos monos* version of this acclamation should be considered an exclusively Samaritan variant, while not negating the possibility that simple *heis theos* acclamations were also used by Samaritans.[68]

A final point should be made about the popularity of the *heis theos* acclamation. Two milestones along the Gerasa–Philadelphia road, at eight and nine miles south of Gerasa respectively, include *heis theos* alongside acclamations of the emperor Julian:

> *heis theos n(ika). heis Ioulianos ho augoustos* ("One god conquers. One Julian the emperor")
>> *heis theos: Ioulianos basileus ni[ka]* ("One god. Julian [the] king conquers")[69]

Julian, who reigned from 361 to 363 CE, famously tried to return the Roman Empire to its traditional gods, whose official support had waned following his uncle Constantine's conversion to Christianity. Having been raised within a Christian family, Julian's version of traditional religiosity was influenced by Christian ideas. To that end, Julian and his followers adopted the *heis theos* phrase to assert superiority.[70] Moreover, other inscriptions reveal that the label *heis* ("one") could be applied to the name of a particular god, even – somewhat counterintuitively – to one from a polytheistic pantheon. For example, two aniconic bronze pendants from Israel apply *heis* to Zeus Serapis. The first, from Caesarea, contains the simple acclamation *heis Zeus Sarapis* ("One Zeus Sarapis"), while a second one reportedly found in the Jerusalem area contains a longer inscription: *heis Zeus Sarapis. megas ho epēkoos Sarapis* ("One Zeus Sarapis. Great Sarapis who listens [to prayers]").[71] This indicates that the possible users of *heis theos* amulets need not be limited to monotheistic traditions. Even devotees of Greek and Roman gods may have found them acceptable.

---

[68] Roll and Tal 2008, 145–6; Tal 2009, 323, 327; Tal 2015, 173–4.

[69] Germer-Durand 1895, 393; Germer-Durand 1899, 36–7, nos. 48–9; Welles 1938, 489, no. 345–6; Di Segni 1994, 107, nos. 40–1. A third use of the *heis theos* acclamation in connection to Julian is found in an inscription on a marble column from Ashkelon. See Avi-Yonah 1942, 160–1 and pl. XXXV.1; Negev 1977, 63; Di Segni 1994, 104, no. 31.

[70] See discussion in Avi-Yonah 1942, 160; Negev 1977, 63–4; Di Segni 1994, 95.

[71] For the Caesarea pendant, see Lifshitz 1964, 81–2, no. 8; Di Segni 1994, 99, no. 11; McLean 1999, 25, no. 180; Belayche 2001, 294; *CIIP* 2, 568–9, no. 1681. For the Jerusalem pendant, see Le Blant 1898, 84–6, no. 220; Manns 1977, 234–6; Di Segni 1994, 103, no. 28; Belayche 2001, 158–9; *SEG* 27-1018. For the henotheistic use of *heis theos*, such as in the cults of Isis and Serapis, see Versnel 1990; Versnel 2011, 280–304.

36 CONTESTED CURES

In the end, it is likely that the popularity of *heis theos* on amulets and in other contexts reflects a milieu of religious competition. Its use among Christians, Samaritans, and worshippers of Greek and Roman gods is certain, and its use by Jews is also possible. People employed this phrase to stake a claim to the superiority of their god in comparison to others. Yet at the same time, the appearance of *heis theos* on amulets may have had less to do with competition and more to do with attempts by the sick and injured to call on a divine healer using whatever method they imagined would be powerful. In some cases, the identity of this healer – *heis theos* – might have been deliberately ambiguous, while in others the adjective *heis* might have been added to the deity's name in order to emphasize his unique place in the world or to highlight the relationship between the amulet-wearer and his or her god.

* * *

Returning to the Gush Halav pendant with the much-suffering eye, the Holy Rider, and the *heis theos* inscription, we can conclude that it was deposited in a Christian context. But unlike the Hammat Gader ring, which was straightforwardly Christian, the Gush Halav pendant included components that could have appealed to a variety of ethnic, cultural, and religious communities. As we will see in Chapter 7, rabbinic and patristic authors tried to create space between the practices of their coreligionists and the practices of outsiders. The popularity of the motifs from the Gush Halav pendant on other amulets from ancient Palestine give some indication of the difficult task that these elite authors had to demarcate and maintain this space. The other two amulets considered in Chapter 1, the reaper gemstone from Caesarea and the *boēth(e)i* ring from Hammat Gader, typify two additional types of amulets present in Roman and late antique Palestine. In the first instance, the vivid image of the reaper, the lack of personalization and name of a divinity again open the possibility that these gemstones appealed to a broad cross section of the region's inhabitants, much like *heis theos* inscriptions. The aniconic brass rings, with their simple inscriptions, present the opposite case, naming both the user and the divine healer from whom help was sought, and seem to come predominantly from Christian contexts. The closely related *hygi(ei)a* rings do not identify the god from whom health was sought, and it would be tempting to see this as an attempt to de-Christianize the formula on the *boēth(e)i* rings, but this conclusion cannot be supported by the evidence, as the only one with a clear archaeological context suggests a Christian user.

From the relatively short texts on gemstone and jewelry amulets considered in Chapter 1, Chapter 2 will turn to amulets that have longer texts, frequently involving biblical quotations. Differences between the forms these amulets take – jewelry or *lamellae* – and the types of biblical verses found on them demonstrate some apparent preferences among the people who used Samaritan and Aramaic amulets. Nevertheless, a closer examination will reveal that some of these amulets, particularly the bilingual ones, present just as many ambiguities with regard to their origins and users as those considered in Chapter 1.

CHAPTER 2

For I Am Yahweh Who Heals You: *Lamellae* and Amulets with Biblical Quotations

The bronze *lamella* discovered in the apse of the Nirim synagogue, which was quoted at the beginning of the previous chapter, can again offer a point of departure. In Chapter 1, it drew attention to the issue of an amulet's provenience and how archaeological context offers insight into the amulet's user. While provenience continues to be an underlying concern, we turn now to amulets with longer texts whose contents have the potential to convey more information about the user than the short texts discussed in the previous chapter. Two additional case studies, an octagonal ring from Khirbet Kusieh and a silver *lamella* from Tiberias form the backbone of this chapter. There are a couple of similarities between these two amulets and the one from Nirim. First, they all contain biblical quotations, and in two cases (Nirim and Khirbet Kusieh) these quotations make up a significant portion or even all of the extant text. Second, the community to which the user belonged in all three cases is less ambiguous than some of the examples in Chapter 1. The Nirim amulet was written in a combination of Aramaic and Hebrew and deposited in a synagogue, which has been taken as proof that Esther, the amulet's owner, was a Jew. The silver *lamella* from Tiberias was also written in Aramaic, with a quotation from the Hebrew Bible. While it was found in a tomb rather than a synagogue, it is generally accepted that its user, Ina, was another Jewish woman. The octagonal ring from Khirbet Kusieh, on the other hand, was written in Samaritan script using quotations from the Samaritan Pentateuch. While no user is named on the amulet, it is usually understood as having belonged to a Samaritan.

The use of biblical quotations, such as on these three amulets, is not unique to Palestine, nor is it an aspect of Roman and late antique amulets that has been overlooked in recent scholarship. However, a systematic inquiry into how different communities employed biblical material has not been undertaken. Quantifying the use of biblical quotations within the corpus of published amulets from Palestine reveals distinct trends according to the language in which amulets were composed and by extension the communities in which such amulets were used. A handful of bilingual amulets, in contrast, complicates our understanding, as they do not clearly belong to one group or another. At the same time, the bilingual amulets further illustrate the sorts of practices that religious elites sought to circumscribe. While this chapter argues that these elites were successful in some ways at directing the practices of their coreligionists, using healing rituals to reify the community's borders, they were unable to exert complete control, as amulets that crossed the lines dividing these communities continued to be produced.

An octagonal ring from Khirbet Kusieh

The inscribed bronze ring shown in Figure 2.1 was reportedly found at Khirbet Kusieh ('Ein Kushi), near Caesarea. It is a solid, octagonal band, without a bezel like the ring from Hammat Gader. The inside of the ring is round, while its exterior surface is divided into eight facets, each approximately 5 × 9 mm. Unlike the amulets discussed in Chapter 1, which were all in Greek, the inscription on this amulet uses the Samaritan script. This ring names neither the person who wore it nor the reason the amulet was needed, and while the inscription does identify the divine healer whose help was sought, it does so in a very different way than the direct address seen on the *boēth(e)i* rings or even the invocation of *Iaō Sabaōth Michaēl* and *heis theos* on the Gush Halav pendant. The inscription on the Khirbet Kusieh ring consists entirely of excerpts from

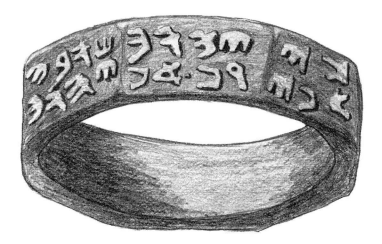

Figure 2.1 An octagonal ring from Khirbet Kusieh (Drawing by D. Weiss)

the Samaritan Pentateuch; no extra-biblical material is present.[1] Quotations from a total of five verses are inscribed across the eight facets, but none are quoted in full. A couple of words were selected from each in order to call to mind a longer passage. Two of the five verses are represented by just two words each; thus, each of these verses was written on a single facet of the ring:

facet 1	Return, Yahweh	*šûbâ Yahweh*[2]	Num 10:36
facet 2	Yahweh is (our) God	*Yahweh 'ēl*	Deut 6:4

The remaining three verses are each spread over two facets, and all but one facet contain two words. The facet with only one word, *Yəšurûn*, has a line break between the *rêš* and the *wāw*:

facets 3–4	For I am Yahweh who heals you	*kî ănî Yahweh rōpə'ekā*	Exod 15:26
facets 5–6	There is none like God, O *Yəšurûn*[3]	*'ên kā'ēl Yəšurûn*	Deut 33:26
facets 7–8	Yahweh conquers, Yahweh is his name	*Yahweh naṣaḥ*[4] *Yahweh šĕmô*	Exod 15:3

The repetition of the Tetragrammaton – the four-letter name for the god of Israel – in four of these five verses is striking. Of the fifteen words on the ring, a full third are the divine name. It is easy to surmise that these particular verses were selected, at least in part, because of the Tetragrammaton. Yet the story told by these verses extends beyond the simple power of Yahweh; they also affirm his uniqueness and his special relationship with Israel. A narrative arc in the verses on the Khirbet Kusieh ring can be articulated, beginning with

---

[1] For the publication of this ring, see Zertal 1977; Zertal 1979, 112–15; Pummer 1987, no. 9; Magen 2008, 253.

[2] The phrase typically used in Samaritan inscriptions to represent this passage is "Arise, Yahweh" from Num 10:35, rather than this phrase from Num 10:36.

[3] *Yəšurûn* is a poetic name for Israel. Some editors construe *'ēl Yəšurûn* as a construct chain, rather than making *Yəšurûn* a vocative. If it is a construct chain, the relationship between God and his people is even more clear, "There is none like the God of *Yəšurûn*."

[4] The quotation found here uses the verbal phrase from the Samaritan Talmud, "Yahweh conquers" (*Yahweh naṣah*) rather than the typical nominal clause, "Yahweh is a warrior" (*Yahweh gibbôr*) from the Samaritan Pentateuch. Another bronze octagonal ring, this one from Nablus, contains the same version of Exod 15:3 as found on the ring from Khirbet Kusieh (Margain 1984; Pummer 1987, no. 15). A bronze pendant from Damascus uses both the version from the Samaritan Talmud and the one from the Samaritan Pentateuch, one after the other (Hamburger 1959, 44–5; Pummer 1987, no. 1).

the story of the exodus from Egypt. Exod 15:3 is part of the Song of the Sea, which Moses and the Israelites sang in thanksgiving after crossing the Red Sea as they escaped Pharaoh's army. The amulet's quotation of this verse deliberately calls attention to the divine name, even repeating it and reinforcing the name's inherent power. The Khirbet Kusieh amulet also quotes a second verse from the same chapter, in which God turned the bitter waters of Marah into fresh water and made the Israelites a promise:

> If you will listen carefully to the voice of Yahweh your God, and do what is right in his sight, and give heed to his commandments and keep all his statutes, I will not bring upon you any of the diseases that I brought upon the Egyptians; for I am Yahweh who heals you. (Exod 15:26)

This passage is particularly appropriate for an amulet, since it affirms God's promise to safeguard his people's physical health, provided they obey his commandments. His provision for the Israelites is seen in the miraculous transformation of the water at Marah, which is contrasted to the plagues that God had sent on Egypt, through Moses, to convince the pharaoh to let the Israelites leave. A conditional promise of benefits for the Israelites, similar to that found in Exod 15, is also present in Deut 6, situated in the period when Israelites were wandering in the desert after their exodus from Egypt. Following the announcement of the Ten Commandments, Deut 6 promises long life for those who keep God's laws. Several verses are worth quoting in full:

> Now this is the commandment – the statutes and the ordinances – that Yahweh your God charged me to teach you to observe in the land that you are about to cross into and occupy, so that you and your children and your children's children may fear Yahweh your God all the days of your life, and keep all his decrees and his commandments that I am commanding you, so that your days may be long. Hear therefore, O Israel, and observe them diligently, so that it may go well with you, and so that you may multiply greatly in a land flowing with milk and honey, as Yahweh, the God of your ancestors, has promised you.
>
> Hear, O Israel: Yahweh is our God, Yahweh alone. You shall love Yahweh your God with all your heart, and with all your soul, and with all your might. Keep these words that I am commanding you today in your heart. Recite them to your children and talk about them when you are at home and when you are away, when you lie down and when you rise. Bind them as a sign on your hand, fix them as an emblem on your forehead, and write them on the doorposts of your house and on your gates. (Deut 6:1–9)

42   CONTESTED CURES

Whereas in Exod 15:26, the Israelites were promised protection from the plagues if they kept God's commandments, in Deut 6 obedience leads to prosperity in the Promised Land. This passage from Deut 6 includes the *Shema*, a key element of Jewish daily prayer that was discussed in Chapter 1. Verse 8 instructs the reader to "bind" God's words onto one's hands, which seems particularly appropriate in the context of this ring.

The Khirbet Kusieh ring continues the story of the Israelites after they received the law with Num 10:35–6. The quotation from Num 10:36 recalled God's constant presence with his people through the Ark of the Covenant and his promise to protect the Israelites from their enemies. The amulet can perhaps be seen as serving an analogous function for the wearer: It was a symbol of God's presence and promise to care for his people. The final verse on the Khirbet Kusieh ring comes from Moses' farewell blessings on the eve of the Israelites' entry into the Promised Land. Once again, the passage affirms the special relationship between God and his people and reinforces his role as their defender: "There is none like God, O Jeshurun, who rides through the heavens to your help . . . Happy are you, O Israel! Who is like you, a people saved by Yahweh, the shield of your help, and the sword of your triumph!"[5] The wearer of this amulet could take comfort in the fact that if God could defeat the Israelites' enemies when they entered Canaan, then he could defeat any and all enemies in the present, including the potentially deadly perils of illness and injury. Taken together, the five passages on the Khirbet Kusieh ring summarize the Israelites' formative years, beginning with the exodus from Egypt, continuing to the institution of the law at Sinai, and culminating in the arrival in Canaan. The repetition of the divine name underscores the fact that it was Yahweh who did these things for his people. Unstated, but implied, is the idea that if God could work these wonders for his people in the past, then he can do the same thing for the wearer of the amulet.

A total of ten polygonal rings with Samaritan inscriptions, including the one from Khirbet Kusieh, are known from Palestine. Closely related to these rings in inscriptional content are six double-sided pendants that are oval or leaf-shaped. Most of the rings are octagonal, like the Khirbet Kusieh example, with two lines of text on each facet, but a couple have either seven or nine facets. Most of the pendants have six lines of text per side, for twelve lines in total, which means they accommodate one or two fewer verses than the sixteen-line octagonal rings. All of the pendants are made up entirely of quotations from the Samaritan Pentateuch, and on all but one these verses are limited to those found on the Khirbet Kusieh ring (see Table 2.1).[6] While

---

[5] Deut 33:26, 29.

[6] The pendant containing Exod 38:8 and Num 14:14 is the one anomaly. For discussion of this amulet, reportedly found in Gaza, see Kaplan 1967, 161–2; Kaplan 1975, 159; Pummer 1987, 257–8.

Table 2.1 Samaritan biblical quotations on amulets

	Polygonal rings[a]	Double-sided pendants[b]	Total
Exod 15:3	5	6	11
Deut 33:26	5	4	9
Num 10:35–6	3	5	8
Exod 15:26	5	3	8
Deut 6:4	3	3	6
Exod 38:8	0	1	1
Num 14:14	0	1	1

[a] Three of the polygonal rings are poorly preserved, leaving multiple facets on each unreadable. Were they in a better state of preservation, we might be able to recognize additional verses to include in Table 2.1. For the ring from Samaria: Westenholz 2007, no. 27. For the two rings from Khirbet al-Hadra: Tal and Taxel 2014, 168–9; Jackson-Tal 2015a.
[b] The readings on a couple of these amulets are not certain. Possible quotations of Deut 33:26 and Deut 6:4 on a pendant from Tel Aviv have been included in these tallies. For other possible readings of this amulet, see Kaplan 1967, 159–60. Similarly, a possible quotation of Exod 15:3 on a pendant from the Tel Barukh cemetery, also in the Tel Aviv area, has been included. For more on the reading of this amulet, see Kaplan 1971; Kaplan 1975, 158; Pummer 1987, 260–1, no. 6; Reich 2002, 295–6, no. 7; Magen 2008, 251–2.

there are a couple of rings that are untranslatable, as we will see below, for the most part the polygonal rings follow the same pattern as the pendants. Two Samaritan amulets, one ring and one pendant, take a different form. The ring has a round bezel, similar to the *boēth(e)i* rings discussed in Chapter 1, and was reported as a surface find from Caesarea.[7] The only text it contains is the Deut 33:26 quotation seen on the Khirbet Kusieh ring, which was written on the bezel. The second anomalous amulet, a pendant, was reportedly found in the region of Bethlehem.[8] Unlike the other Samaritan pendants, it is round, has writing on just one side, and was meant to be strung through a hole pieced on the left side rather than through a suspension loop at the top of the pendant. The placement of this hole, partially atop one of the inscription's letters, indicates that it was pierced after the inscription was written. It quotes Deut 33:26 as well as an excerpt from Num 10:35, both of which are found frequently on Samaritan amulets. These two amulets may reflect experimentation in the otherwise generally fixed format of Samaritan rings and pendants. Yet even while their form is unusual for Samaritan amulets, the content of their inscriptions is not. In fact, the overall consistency of Samaritan amulets suggests some sort of consensus about both the appropriate texts to inscribe and the format that the amulets were to take, perhaps as the result of pressure from elites who were

[7] Ilan 1982, 1, 4; Pummer 1987, 262–3, no. 12; Reich 2002, 299, no. 12; Magen 2008, 253; *CIIP* 2, 597–8, no. 1716.
[8] Farhi 2010.

in a position to create and maintain boundaries between their community and outsiders.

When the Samaritan amulets first came to light, many saw the script as proof of the user's identity, since Samaritan – unlike Greek – was a language whose use was thought to be coterminous with the Samaritan community. This assumption proved to be problematic. Four amulets (two double-sided pendants and two polygonal rings) were excavated in tombs from the northern part of Tel Aviv, which were dated to the second half of the fourth or to the fifth century.[9] Originally the tombs were thought to belong to Samaritans on the basis of these amulets, but the publication two decades later of a Samaritan pendant from Nahariya, a coastal city near the Lebanese border, called this assumption into question. Associated finds in the Nahariya tomb were confidently identified as Christian and dated to the sixth century.[10] Reinhard Pummer explored the implications of this discovery in a 1987 article that examined all the Samaritan amulets discovered to date. Drawing on an earlier article by Anit Hamburger, who had considered two bilingual Samaritan–Greek amulets and argued that they were not used by Samaritans, Pummer pointed to the Samaritans' history of crafting amulets for people outside their community in medieval and modern periods and posited that Roman and Byzantine amulets with Samaritan inscriptions were "'Samaritan' only in the sense that they were produced or partially inscribed by Samaritans; otherwise they are Christian because Christians wore them."[11] Pummer's proposal that all Samaritan amulets were used by Christians was just as problematic as the original assumption that the discovery of a Samaritan amulet automatically confirms the Samaritan identity of a tomb or settlement. Instead, the context of each amulet needs to be examined whenever archaeological provenience is known. More recently, Oren Tal and Itamar Taxel revisited the finds from the Tel Aviv-area tombs, and while they recognized the need for caution in distinguishing Samaritan settlements and burials,

---

[9] The two sites in question are Khirbet al-Hadra and Tel Barukh, which are approximately 3 km from each other. For publication of the amulets, see Kaplan 1967, 158; Kaplan 1971, 255; Kaplan 1975, 158; Ashkenazi 2015, 119–20; Jackson-Tal 2015a; Tal and Taxel 2014.

[10] Reich 1985. Nearby, but beyond the scope of this study, a Samaritan amulet was also found in a Christian cemetery in Tyre (Pummer 1987, 255).

[11] Hamburger 1959, 44–5; Pummer 1989, 257. Pummer (1987, 255) had earlier accepted the identification of the two tombs as Jewish, on the basis of Kaplan 1949–50; Kaplan 1968, 70–1. However, Kaplan's identification of the tombs as Jewish seems to have been due to their presumed connection to a nearby Jewish settlement rather than on the basis of excavated finds. In a recent article, Pummer (2020, 100) revisited his conclusion about who wore the Samaritan amulets: "Who wore these Byzantine amulets with Samaritan writing? In the first place, the Samaritans themselves. There certainly is no literary evidence, either Samaritan or Jewish or Christian, that would preclude such a conclusion."

they made a convincing case that the tombs that had yielded Samaritan amulets were, in fact, used by Samaritans.[12]

Since the probable users of the Samaritan rings and pendants that follow regular patterns can only be ascertained on a case-by-case basis, this is all the more true for Samaritan amulets that do not follow the standard pattern. Several of the polygonal rings, including both with nine facets, are partially or fully untranslatable due to the presence of pseudo-inscriptions that vaguely look like Samaritan text.[13] In his evaluation of one of these rings, Ronny Reich suggested that it was crafted by an artisan who copied letters without understanding what they meant.[14] Transcription errors seem to be the most likely scenario for rings that do contain at least one or two translatable facets. In cases where the entire ring is untranslatable, other options present themselves. While the artisan could have been an insufficiently skilled – or even illiterate – Samaritan who was producing amulets for similarly illiterate Samaritan clients, it is equally possible that the people who created the untranslatable amulets were non-Samaritans trying to capitalize on the perceived power of the distinctive script by creating pseudo-Samaritan inscriptions for Jews or Christians. The resemblance of Samaritan or pseudo-Samaritan inscriptions to archaic Hebrew letters might have suggested to ritual specialists and to users that this script would make the written text, and by extension the amulet as a whole, more efficacious. This is perhaps a phenomenon similar to the proliferation of *charaktares* (magical symbols) on amulets, which were perceived as enhancing an amulet's potency. However, I would cautiously suggest a difference between pseudo-inscriptions and *charaktares*. In the case of pseudo-inscriptions, when a user acquired the amulet, he or she may have been told what was written on it. If users were unable to read the amulet, either because they did not read at all or because they did not read the language in which it was allegedly written, they would have had no reason to doubt that the contents of the inscription were as they were told. Given the amulets seen in Chapters 1 and 2, it is likely that this user would have been told that the pseudo-inscription included a short prayer, an invocation of divine names, or a biblical quotation. The individual might have regularly repeated as a prayer the text that he or she believed was written on the amulet, much as the user of the Hammat Gader amulet in Chapter 1 may have regularly prayed, "Christ,

[12] Tal and Taxel 2014; Tal and Taxel 2015, 193–4.
[13] Ring from Apollonia: Reich 1989; Reich 1994; Reich 2002, 301–2, no. 17; Magen 2008, 254. Ring from Ein ha-Shofet: Reich 2002, 299, no. 13; Magen 2008, 253, fig. 14. Rings from Gelilot: Levy 1991; Reich 1994; Tal 1995, 107–8; Reich 2002, 304–5, no. 20–1; Magen 2008, 254–5. Other pseudo-inscriptions, apparently meant to look like Greek or some other, non-Samaritan script, are also known from the region (e.g. Spier 2007, 109–14).
[14] Reich 2002, 302.

46 CONTESTED CURES

help me." While this scenario may have also been possible for amulets with *charaktares*, with the user being told what the *charaktares* said, it is worth noting that *charaktares* were visually distinct, often marked by small circles decorating the ends of lines. As we will see shortly with the *lamella* from Tiberias, users would have been able to distinguish these *charaktares* from the rest of the inscription due to their visual characteristics, even if they could not read the text. This invites speculation as to whether *charaktares* were understood as powerful images, like the reaper, the much-suffering eye, or the Holy Rider, rather than as an inscribed text.

As suggested in Chapter 1, it is possible that amulets were passed from one user to another after the original owners died or no longer needed them. This was likely more common for amulets whose inscription did not include the name of the user, such as the reaper gemstones, the Gush Halav much-suffering eye amulet, and these Samaritan pendants and rings. Furthermore, just as reaper gemstones could have crossed the notional lines that separated religious and ethnic communities in Roman and late antique Palestine, so too could these Samaritan amulets. We have convincing evidence that this took place with the Samaritan pendant that was deposited in a Christian tomb in Nahariya. While it might be suggested that the Nahariya tomb's occupant had acquired the pendant as a purely decorative object rather than one intended to heal or protect, the presence of a second amulet in the tomb makes this interpretation less likely.[15] What remains uncertain in the case of the Nahariya pendant is whether the amulet itself changed from Samaritan hands to Christian hands, or whether it was only the ritual technology that moved. To put it differently, we cannot determine whether the deceased with whom it was interred was the amulet's original owner, having commissioned it either from a Samaritan or from a Christian practitioner who had begun copying Samaritan amulets, or whether it had been acquired from an original, Samaritan owner. In either case, the Nahariya amulet demonstrates that the boundaries commonly understood by modern scholars to divide ethnic and religious communities from each other could be porous, allowing the transfer of ritual processes and objects.

A silver *lamella* from Tiberias

The silver *lamella* shown in Figure 2.2 measures 4 × 11 cm and was excavated in a tomb in Tiberias. When this amulet was discovered, it was still rolled inside its tubular copper case; such cases would have been attached to the body

---

[15] For this second amulet, see Reich 1985, 386–8; Di Segni 1994, 96, no. 2; *SEG* 37-1524. This amulet is of the *heis theos* and Holy Rider variety, discussed in Chapter 1.

LAMELLAE AND AMULETS WITH BIBLICAL QUOTATIONS

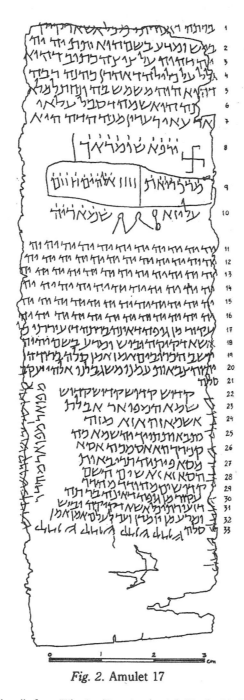

Fig. 2. Amulet 17

Figure 2.2 A silver *lamella* from Tiberias (Drawing by Ada Yardeni in Naveh and Shaked 1993; with permission of Magnes Press)

48   CONTESTED CURES

by a cord. Unlike some gemstones and jewelry amulets, including the reaper gemstones and the Samaritan pendants, which could have writing on two surfaces, *lamellae* are almost exclusively one-sided, as the metal sheets were so thin that incised letters on one side rendered the other side largely unusable. Even one-sided, *lamellae* offered a substantial writing surface; among the varieties of amulets, only those made with papyri, which do not survive from Israel, enabled practitioners to compose similarly lengthy texts. This particular *lamella* is a little less than twice as tall as the Gush Halav much-suffering eye pendant.

The Aramaic text of the *lamella*'s inscription indicates that it was written for a certain "Ina, daughter of Ze'irti," whose name was originally specified three times – once in the first two lines of the text, once in line 17, and finally in lines 30 and 31.[16] As in the Nirim amulet quoted at the beginning of Chapter 1, Ina's mother's name was also included. The consistency of the script around the three occurrences of Ina's name, without changes to the size or spacing of letters, suggests that the amulet was commissioned specifically for this client. In other words, it was not a premade amulet with blanks where the purchaser's name could be filled in. The condition from which Ina sought healing is likewise specified three times: "all hectic fever and illness and sickness" (*mikol 'eša' daqqîqâ ûbûš ûmərā'*). The reference to fever may mean that Ina suffered from malaria.[17] More than a quarter of the *lamellae* from Roman and late antique Palestine mention fevers, making it the most frequently mentioned illness on *lamellae* and perhaps implying widespread concern about malaria. It can be supposed that some of the amulets that do not specify an illness, such as the *boēth(e)i* rings, may have also been used by patients suffering from malaria.

Voces magicae (magical names), nonsensical strings of letters written in a decipherable script such as Greek or Aramaic, are found throughout the Tiberias *lamella*, beginning in line two. *Voces magicae* have long attracted the interests of scholars, and the origins of some have been successfully traced to a particular language or religious context.[18] This scholarly endeavor, however, obscures the fact that by late antiquity many of these *voces magicae* would have been unintelligible to ritual specialists and amulet users alike as anything other than words of power used to secure the desired outcome. The presence of *voces magicae* on the Tiberias *lamella* makes it uncertain whether Ina and the ritual practitioner who created the amulet understood it to address a single

---

[16] For publication and translation of this amulet, see Naveh and Shaked 1993, 50–7, no. 17; Eshel and Leiman 2010, 192, no. 7.

[17] For the prevalence of malaria in the ancient Mediterranean world, see Jones and Withington 1977; Grmek 1989, 245–83; Burke 1995, 75–91; Dauphin 1998, 467–72; Dickie 2001, 130; Scheidel 2001; Sallares 2002; Wandrey 2003; Faraone 2018, 259–60.

[18] For a useful introduction to *voces magicae* and glossary of known *voces*, see Brashear 1995, 3429–38, 3576–603. See also Bohak 2003; Mastrocinque 2004, 98–112; De Bruyn 2017, 55.

LAMELLAE AND AMULETS WITH BIBLICAL QUOTATIONS   49

divine healer, potentially with multiple epithets, or whether multiple distinct powers were being invoked for their healing abilities. The initial appearance of the *voces magicae* immediately follows the first instance of Ina's name and the disease from which she sought healing:

> In the name of HW' YZWT Yah Yah Yah, that was written on his front plate which was unrolled on the wreath of Aaron the High Priest who was serving with it, and he descended in order to fulfill . . . his name, who carries those on high and those below, and all tremble before him. This is it. YRP' ŠWMR'K MRKBY'T ZZZZ the living god 'LYZ' ŠM'RYAH. (lines 2–10)

The last three lines of this section (lines 8–10), beginning with YRP' and continuing to ŠM'RYAH, seem to be particularly important since the scribe used several visual techniques to emphasize them. First, these lines are separated from the rest of the text with wide margins, and a box was drawn around the middle line, "MRKBY'T ZZZZ the living god." Vertical strokes were inserted at the end of the first line and between the first and second words of the second line to further delineate the space, and all but nine of their forty-one letters have short vertical lines or dots placed above them.[19] A final component of these lines is the use of *charaktares*.[20] The first, a swastika, appears at the beginning of line 8. The second two *charaktares* are both ring letters, with small circles on the ends of each stroke, and are positioned in the middle of line 10, centered below the vertical bar in the middle of line 9. The tops of the *charaktares* align with the top of the rest of the text, while the bottoms of the *charaktares* extend below the bottom line of the rest of the text. As a result, the space following lines 8–10 is much greater than the spacing used by the scribe in the rest of the amulet.

Over the next six lines, the first two letters of the Tetragrammaton, YH or *yôd-hê*, which can be vocalized as Yah, are repeated seventy times. Yah had appeared earlier, repeated three times in lines 2–3 among the *voces magicae*. The seventyfold repetition of Yah calls to mind the seventy names of God referenced in some Jewish mystical literature and the seventy names of Metatron, known as Enoch before his transformation into an angel.[21] Yet the significance

---

[19] Similar dots or dashes are found above each letter of the Tetragrammaton in line 18. The use of dots to mark *voces magicae* was common in the ancient Mediterranean world. For an Aramaic example from the Cairo Genizah, see Bohak 1999, 39–41 and pl. 5.

[20] Sixteen amulets from Roman and late antique Palestine contain *charaktares*, including eleven *lamellae* and five gemstones. Since only twenty *lamellae* have been published from Palestine, this means that just over half include *charaktares*, such as on this amulet from Tiberias.

[21] 3 Enoch 48D. See discussion in Dan 1982; Swartz 1990, 173.

50 CONTESTED CURES

of this sevenfold repetition is not strictly textual; it also enhanced the visual impact of the amulet. There is no guarantee that Ina, the amulet's user, was literate and could read the text. However, the layout of the *lamella* would have enabled her to identify key sections of the amulet by their visual characteristics alone. One such section is lines 8–10, with their wide margins and line spacing. The six lines in which Yah is repeated would have also stood out, as the uniformity of these lines distinguishes them from the rest of the amulet.

Following this sevenfold repetition of Yah, Ina's name and her medical condition are repeated. The text requests healing "In the name of Yahweh who is enthroned among the cherubim, Amen Amen Selah. Blessed be he. 'Yahweh of Hosts is with us, the God of Jacob our refuge, Selah.'"[22] The appeal to the cherubic throne recalls the Ark of the Covenant, which was placed in the tabernacle and later inside the Jerusalem temple. The Hebrew Bible contained instructions for crafting the two cherubim with outstretched wings that flanked the Ark of the Covenant's mercy seat, from which God was said to speak.[23] The phrase found on this amulet, "who is enthroned among the cherubim" (*yōšēb hakerûbîm*), is a frequent epithet of God in the Hebrew Bible.[24] The rest of line 19 also recalls biblical texts with the repetition of "amen" (*'āmēn*), "selah" (*selâ*), "blessed be he" (*bārûk hû'*). The amulet's text then shifts to a direct quotation from Psalm 46 that affirms God's constant presence with his people, "Yahweh of Hosts is with us, the God of Jacob our refuge. Selah." The implication is that if God was with his people as far back as Jacob, he would also be with his people today, including the amulet's wearer, who may have identified with the first-person plural speaker in the verse.[25] It is worth noting that God's identity is emphasized in this section, as it contains the only two places in the amulet where the full Tetragrammaton is used, in contrast to the repetition of Yah in the previous lines.

The space that separates the Psalm 46 quotation from the next line is slightly larger than typical on this amulet, which draws attention to another visual component of the *lamella* – a square around the final eleven lines of text. This square is made up not of horizontal and vertical lines but of additional words. The border on the top, right, and bottom sides of the square are all composed of the same word, "holy" (*qādôš*), repeated four times on each side. The writer of the amulet rotated the *lamella* while writing each line, so that

---

[22] Naveh and Shaked replaced the Tetragrammaton in this quotation from Ps 46 with "the Lord," as is common in biblical translations. For the sake of consistency with other amulets discussed in this chapter, I have vocalized the Tetragrammaton as Yahweh.

[23] Exod 25:17–22, 37:1–9. For God speaking from the mercy seat, see Num 7:89.

[24] 1 Sam 4:4; 2 Sam 6:2; 2 Kgs 19:15; 1 Chr 13:6; Ps 80:1, 99:1; Isa 37:16.

[25] In the Masoretic text, verses 8 and 12 of this chapter are identical. The quotation on this amulet comes from these verses. In many English translations, these verses are numbered 7 and 11.

LAMELLAE AND AMULETS WITH BIBLICAL QUOTATIONS   51

the reader must likewise turn the amulet around to read all four sides of the square. Joseph Naveh and Shaul Shaked, who originally published this amulet, posited that the left side of this box was originally two lines deep. The outermost of these two lines is no longer fully extant, as the edges of the silver scroll have deteriorated. However, enough survived for Naveh and Shaked to suggest that this line also repeated *qādôš* four times, which would have brought the total number of repetitions to sixteen. The inner line on the left side of the box is legible, and reads "magnificent, magnificent, splendid" (*məpô'ār məpô'ār mēhădâr*). The repetition of *qādôš* in this word-box should be read alongside the seventyfold repetition of Yah earlier on the amulet; together they recall the engraved metal band or diadem (*ṣîṣ*) that the high priest wore over his turban as part of his official vestments, which was mentioned near the beginning of the amulet in lines 3–4.[26] Exod 28:36 indicates that the phrase "Holy to Yahweh" was engraved on this band, and it is significant that both words appear prominently on the Tiberias amulet with the seventyfold repetition of Yah and the sixteenfold repetition of *qādôš*. The text enclosed within the *qādôš* word-box begins with a reference to "the glorious name" (*šəmā' hāməpô'ār*), followed by four lines of *voces magicae* that conclude with "holy, splendid, splendid" (*qədôšîm mehûdar mēhădâr*) and a final request that Ina be healed from "all hectic fever and illness and sickness from this day to eternity. Amen Amen Selah."

In contrast to some of the other amulets considered in Chapters 1 and 2, the Tiberias *lamella* contains many clues about the user's community. Furthermore, since it specified Ina's name and matronymic three times, it is less likely than some other types of amulets to have been reused once Ina died or no longer needed it. References to the high priestly vestments and the Ark of the Covenant reflect an interest in the temple cult. The quotation of Psalm 46, the use of Aramaic, and the appearance of biblical language such as "amen" and "selah" suggest a Jewish self-understanding of the practitioner who created the amulet or of Ina who wore the amulet – and most likely both. The Jewish use of *lamellae* amulets in late antique Palestine is undeniable. Of the thirty-six *lamellae* known from Palestine, twenty were found in synagogues. Only four of these *lamellae* have been unrolled and read, including three from Nirim and one from Baram. Three additional *lamellae* were found in tombs, including the Tiberias example. These tombs have not been published in sufficient detail for us to be confident about the identity of the tombs' inhabitants. However, unlike the situation with Samaritan amulets, none of the Aramaic *lamellae* from Palestine have been found in contexts that definitively call into question a Jewish identity. In fact, all but two of the *lamellae* from the entire region were

---

[26] Exod 28:36–8. For later rabbinic echoes of these traditions, see Naveh and Shaked 1993, 54–5.

52 CONTESTED CURES

written partially or fully in Aramaic or Hebrew, which underscores a Jewish affinity for this type of amulet.

The use of metal scrolls for amulets, and even their placement in tombs, was not a new phenomenon in Roman and late antique Palestine. In 1979, excavations at a late pre-exilic tomb at Ketef Hinnom in Jerusalem revealed two small silver scrolls inscribed with passages from the priestly blessing of Num 6:24–6:[27]

> Yahweh bless you and keep you;
> Yahweh make his face to shine upon you and be gracious to you;
> Yahweh lift up his countenance upon you and give you peace.[28]

Although neither of the scrolls quotes these verses in their entirety, this passage is clearly the source of amulets' text. Signs of wear indicate that the scrolls were attached to the body during the user's lifetime, either by being placed in a case that no longer survives or by being strung on a cord that passed through the center of the scroll.[29] The Ketef Hinnom scrolls were somewhat smaller than the silver *lamella* for Ina (approximately 1.3 cm smaller in both length and width), but the biggest difference between them is that the extant text on the Ketef Hinnom scrolls is derived entirely from the Hebrew Bible, while only a small fraction of the Tiberias amulet is taken directly from the biblical text. In this regard, the Ketef Hinnom scrolls more closely resemble use of biblical quotations on Samaritan rings and double-sided pendants.

---

[27] The scrolls were originally published in Barkay 1989; Barkay 1992. The date of the Ketef Hinnom texts has been extensively debated since Barkay's original publication; for a discussion of the text's paleography and the stratigraphy surrounding the find, as well as an evaluation of various theories regarding their date, see Barkay et al. 2004. Among the many subsequent publications on these texts, Smoak 2016 is also of note.

[28] With the exception of the vocalization of the divine name, the verses are quoted here in the NRSV translation rather than in the fragmentary versions found on the two Ketef Hinnom scrolls.

[29] Reminiscent of these texts are the *dipinti* inscriptions found on two *pithoi* that marked the gate of a caravanserai at Ḥorvat Teiman (Kuntillet ʿAjrud), which was located a short distance west of the overland trade route between the Red Sea and the Mediterranean. Dated to the late ninth or early eighth century BCE, these inscriptions include the priestly benediction of Deut 6. Fragmentary *dipinti* inscriptions on plaster walls at Deir ʿAlla in the Jordan Valley, dated to approximately the end of the ninth century BCE, also seem to include sacred texts. These inscriptions may offer Iron Age precursors to the later development of placing biblical passages on doorposts in *mezuzot* (*məzûzôt*). See discussion in Barkay 1992, 184; Keel and Uehlinger 1998, 207–9, 25–6. For complete publication of Ḥorvat Teiman, see Meshel 1978; Meshel et al. 2012; for publication of Deir ʿAlla, see Hoftijzer et al. 1976.

The use of biblical quotations

The amuletic use of biblical quotations therefore has a long history in Palestine, extending more than twelve centuries from the Ketef Hinnom scrolls to the examples considered in the present chapter.[30] By late antiquity, noticeable differences in the use of biblical quotations had emerged according to the language in which the amulet was written (see Table 2.2). Among Samaritan amulets, all but one quote biblical material, and there is remarkable consistency in the verses used. In contrast, only eight of twenty-one Aramaic amulets (38.1 percent) and one of eighty-eight Greek amulets (1.2 percent) include biblical material. Somewhat surprisingly, all three of the bilingual amulets from the region, which will be discussed below, likewise contain quotations. Some explanation for the relative absence of biblical excerpts on Greek amulets can be found in the fact that nearly 60 percent of the Greek amulets are gemstones and only a single gemstone

Table 2.2 Biblical quotations on amulets by language

	Samaritan	Aramaic	Greek	Bilingual	Total
Gen 1:6	0	0	0	1	1
Exod 15:3	11	0	0	0	11
Exod 15:26	8	1	0	0	9
Exod 38:8	1	0	0	0	1
Num 10:35–6	9	0	0	0	9
Num 14:14	1	0	0	0	1
Deut 6:4	6	0	0	0	6
Deut 33:26	11	0	0	2	13
Isa 51:15/Jer 31:35[a]	0	1	0	0	1
Amos 4:13	0	1	0	0	1
Ps 46:8/12 (LXX 45:8/12)	0	2	0	0	2
Ps 91:1 (LXX 90:1)	0	0	1	0	1
Ps 94:1 (LXX 93:1)	0	1	0	0	1
Ps 116:6 (LXX 114:6)	0	1	0	0	1
Dan 3:6	0	1	0	0	1
Total with biblical quotations	**17**	**8**	**1**	**3**	**31**

[a] The phrase "who stirs up the sea so that its waves roar – Yahweh of hosts is his name" appears both in Isa 51:15 and Jer 31:35.

[30] Whether this tradition was continuous or not is debated. Gideon Bohak (2008, 136–9; 2014, 248) argued against continuity, while Hanan Eshel and Rivka Leiman (2010, 197) argued for it.

54 CONTESTED CURES

Table 2.3 Biblical quotations on amulets by amulet type

	With quotations	Without quotations	Total
Lamellae	9 (45%)	11 (55%)	20
Gems	1 (2%)	57 (98%)	58
Jewelry	19 (31%)	34 (69%)	53

from Palestine includes a biblical quotation (see Table 2.3). The relative paucity of biblical quotations on gemstones reflects the fact that gems generally do not have lengthy inscriptions, biblical or otherwise. Less than 30 percent (seventeen of fifty-eight) of Palestinian gemstone amulets contain more than two words or twelve letters, and seven of these seventeen came from a single workshop that used softer, local stones that would have been more conducive to inscriptions.[31] The metals used in jewelry amulets and *lamellae* were more malleable and easier to incise than many stones, and the techniques used for carving images on gemstones would have been difficult to adapt to lengthy textual inscriptions. It is therefore likely that practical reasons determined the low rate of biblical inscriptions on gemstones, rather than any ideological motivation.

Beyond the incidence of biblical quotations on amulets in each language, the more interesting revelation of Table 2.2 is a stark difference in the way that biblical material was used in the Samaritan and Aramaic corpora. The biblical quotations from Samaritan amulets were consistently selected from a narrow set of verses, with only one deviation from the norm, while the opposite is true among Aramaic amulets. Only one quotation, the passage from Psalm 46, appears on more than one Aramaic amulet. Furthermore, in most Samaritan examples, the biblical quotations make up the entirety of the amulets' text. This is decidedly not the case among the eight Aramaic *lamellae* with biblical quotations, where the quoted material typically comprises a small fraction of the amulet's total text, much as in the Tiberias amulet for Ina. A further difference pertains to the quantity of citations. Most Samaritan amulets quoted from multiple passages, while no Aramaic amulet quoted more than one verse. A final observation on the use of biblical material pertains to the infrequency with which verses appear in more than one language. In fact, there is only a single verse, Exod 15:26, that appears both on Samaritan amulets (eight times) and on an Aramaic amulet (one time). This quotation gives God's promise not to bring plagues on the Israelites as he had done to the Egyptians.

---

[31] However, many of the "texts" from this workshop are actually pseudo-Greek or pseudo-Hebrew, with the inscription made up of symbols that look vaguely like Greek or Hebrew but that do not actually say anything (Spier 2007, 109–13).

The Aramaic *lamella* that quotes Exod 15:26 is the one found in the apse of the Nirim synagogue, which was quoted at the beginning of Chapter 1. It is also the only extant Aramaic amulet from Israel where a significant portion of the text is comprised of a biblical quotation. The attractiveness of this promise in Exod 15 for a healing amulet is obvious, and its popularity was likely greater than the extant corpus indicates, since it drew the ire of the redactors of the Mishnah. In the Mishnah's deliberation over those who "have no share in the world to come," one type of person included in the list is anyone who "utters charms over a wound and says, 'I will put none of the diseases upon you which I have put upon the Egyptians: for I am the Lord that heals you.'"[32] While this passage deals with a spoken recitation of this verse for healing, it is not much of a stretch to extend its application to a written amulet, especially when the initial application of amulets was likely accompanied by a spoken prayer.

Despite the variety of verses found on Aramaic *lamellae*, the themes represented by these quotations remain fairly consistent, including promises of God's protection (Exod 15:26; Ps 46:8/12, 94:1, 116:6) and his position as master of creation (Amos 4:13; Isa 51:15). In this latter case, the implication is likely that if God created the universe, then he can also control it and bring healing. Only one biblical quotation on an Aramaic amulet does not fit into one of these two categories. A copper *lamella* from Horvat Kanaf threatens the illness-causing demon with Nebuchadnezzar's fiery furnace from Dan 3:6 if he does not cease tormenting the amulet's wearer.[33] While this verse would have served as a demonstration of God's protection of his people, even those in dire straits similar to the ones that the three Hebrew youths found themselves in, this is not its only function. The quotation also acts as a *historiola*, asking God to punish the demons in the same way that he punished the soldiers who tended the fiery furnace and to protect the amulet-wearer just as he protected the young men in the flames.[34] A similar principle seems to be at work in a silver *lamella* from Aleppo in Syria, which used the earthquakes of Job 38:12–13 to demonstrate how God should expel fever- and shiver-causing demons from the body of a woman named 'Aqemu.[35] The similarity between the shaking of earthquakes and the chills that rack the body of someone suffering from malaria make this verse particularly apropos. Beyond specific quotations, Aramaic amulet-writers also drew heavily on the names of God found in the

---

[32] *m. Sanh.* 10:1. All translations of the Mishnah are taken from Danby 1933, with minor changes to update archaic verb tenses and pronouns.

[33] For publication of this amulet, see Naveh and Shaked 1985, 50–5, no. 3; Eshel and Leiman 2010, 191, no. 6.

[34] For a recent treatment of *historiolae*, see Faraone 2018, 229–36.

[35] For publication of the Aleppo *lamella*, see Schwab 1906; Schwabe 1917, 624; Frey 1952, 62–5, no. 819; Testa 1962; Naveh and Shaked 1985, 54–61, no. 4.

Hebrew Bible that reflected his power ("Yahweh Sabaoth"), that highlighted his special relationship with the patriarchs and through them with his chosen people ("God of Jacob" and "God of Israel"), and that emphasized his uniqueness ("I-am-who-I-am").

Some of the same themes found in the Aramaic use of biblical quotations are also found on the Samaritan rings and pendants. Deut 6:4 and Deut 33:26 can be taken as assurances of God's nature and his relationship with the people of Israel, much as in the quotations on the Aramaic amulets. The quotation from Num 10:36, which recalls God's presence with the people of Israel, might be understood as an abbreviated *historiola*, albeit one less clear than the use of Gen 1:6 or Dan 3:6: just as God scattered the Israelites' enemies when they carried the Ark of the Covenant before them, so also he would cause illnesses to flee before the amulet's wearer. Stringing together the quotations that appear on each Samaritan amulet might also create a more extended *historiola* – just as God brought his people out of Egypt and accompanied them to the Promised Land, so too would he be present with the person who wore the amulet. In addition to this potential function of the narrative arc, it is important to recall that the quotations on Samaritan amulets prioritize the divine name, and some may have been chosen expressly for their inclusion of the Tetragrammaton. While that is not to say that quotations on Aramaic amulets do not call attention to God's name, such as the affirmation in Isa 51:15 and Amos 4:13, "Yahweh Sabaoth is his name," these quotations on Aramaic amulets are generally not limited to the Tetragrammaton and another word or two, as on the Samaritan amulets.[36]

As Table 2.2 indicates, there are no quotations of New Testament material on Roman and late antique amulets from Palestine, which is in contrast to the use of New Testament imagery and appeals to Christ (*Christos*) and the Lord (*Kyrios*) on some amulets.[37] This is also a marked departure from Egyptian papyri amulets, which contain many New Testament quotations such as Gospel incipits or the Lord's Prayer.[38] In some examples from Egypt, these quotations comprise the entirety of the amulet's text, much as we saw with the Samaritan amulets or the Ketef Hinnom scrolls. The lack of papyri amulets from Israel invites speculation that such quotations from the New Testament might have

---

[36] This passage can be compared to the frequent Samaritan quotation of Exod 15:3, "Yahweh conquers, Yahweh is his name." However, Samaritan amulets never include *Sabaōth*, as the epithet does not appear in the Pentateuch.

[37] Some of these appeals to Christ and the Lord were seen on the brass rings considered in Chapter 1. Examples of New Testament imagery include two gems showing the raising of Lazarus (Spier 2007, 109, 111, nos. 629, 635), and two more that seem to show Jesus and his disciples (Spier 2007, 111, nos. 636–7).

[38] For example, Daniel and Maltomini 1990, 78–82, no. 29; De Bruyn and Dijkstra 2011; De Bruyn 2017, 143–53.

been used on amulets that are no longer extant. Despite this absence of New Testament textual material, we do find a Hebrew Bible quotation in Greek juxtaposed with obvious Christian iconography on a silver pendant that was excavated in Caesarea. It depicts on the obverse the Holy Rider image discussed in Chapter 1 and on the reverse the archangel Gabriel's annunciation to Mary.[39] Around the edge of the obverse is an inscription in Greek taken from Ps 90:1 (MT 91:1), "He who lives by the help of the Most High, in a shelter of the God of the sky he will lodge."[40] Much as with the assurances offered by biblical quotations on Aramaic amulets, the promise of God's protection in Ps 90:1 likely contributed to its selection. In fact, while this verse only appears once in the present corpus it is commonly found on Greek amulets discovered outside Palestine.[41]

Bilingual amulets

Among the published amulets from Roman and late antique Palestine, three are bilingual.[42] These bilingual amulets offer insight into how ritual techniques might have crossed the notional lines that separated ethnic, cultural, and religious communities. While each of the bilingual amulets is unique, they are united by one trait: all three include biblical quotations. The first bilingual amulet is a copper *lamella* reported as a surface find from 'Evron, in the western Galilee (see Figure 2.3). The amulet's initial four lines are in Hebrew, followed by two small symbols, and finally a longer section in Greek:

> *In Hebrew:* [. . .] HNHHHY, Yahweh and Sabaoth, Yahweh Elohim, I-am-who-I-am, the God Yahweh, the God Elohim, are you Elohim, Yahweh El, and El the El (god) are you. El is your name, El BBL El. YYYYYYY HHHHHHH WWWWWWW HHHHHHH.

> *two symbols*

> *In Greek:* Holy is the Lord! May the God himself who by his Word created all things, by the same Word, grant health [and] salvation for

---

[39] For publication of this amulet, see Frova 1966, 238–40; *CIIP* 2, 574–5, no. 1689.

[40] Translations of the Septuagint are taken from Pietersma and Wright 2007. For examples of similar pendants with the Holy Rider and Ps 90:1 from Syria and Lebanon, see Mouterde 1942–3, 121–3 and pl. VII–IX, nos. 50, 55, 57.

[41] See examples and discussion in De Bruyn and Dijkstra 2011.

[42] In this section, I do not count as bilingual those Aramaic amulets that include Hebrew quotations of biblical texts.

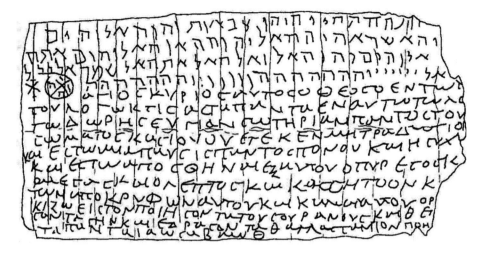

Figure 2.3 A copper *lamella* from 'Evron (Kotansky 1991, with permission of Roy Kotansky)

the whole body of Casius whom Metradotion bore: "And let there be" cessation from every pain, and rest. "And let there be" (that) the fever extinguishes itself from him, [both] the great and the slight (fever). And by (the) names, both his hidden and his excellent, I adjure by the One who made the heavens and founded earth and established sea (and) who made everything, Iaō Sabaoth.[43]

The Hebrew text of the amulet focuses on the identity of God, listing divine names from the Hebrew Bible together with the sevenfold repetition of each letter of the Tetragrammaton. It is only in the Greek text that the name of the amulet's user, Cassius, and the disease from which he suffered are identified. The fever mentioned on this amulet is likely another reference to malaria, just as in the silver *lamella* from Tiberius for Ina. The Greek section begins with the acclamation *hagios kyrios*, "Holy (is the) Lord," reminiscent of the seraphim's hymn in Isaiah's vision (Isa 6:3), before turning to language that emphasizes God's role as creator. The theme of God as creator has already been seen in the Aramaic amulets that quote Amos 4:13 and Isa 51:15, and the reference in the present amulet carries the same implications regarding God's power over creation: if God created the universe, then he must also be able to control it. God is described as "the One who made the heavens and founded earth and

---

[43] Translation is a slightly modified version of that given by Kotansky 1994, 312–25, no 56. Additional discussion of this amulet can be found in Kotansky 1991; Bohak 2008, 231–2; Eshel and Leiman 2010, no. 3.

LAMELLAE AND AMULETS WITH BIBLICAL QUOTATIONS 59

established sea (and) who made everything," using language that is close to, but not exactly the same as Isa 51:13 and Ps 145:6. The amulet's appeal to the God of creation is also found in the request for healing, which twice uses the imperative phrase *kai estō*, "and let there be" from the creation account in Gen 1:6. Just as God created the whole world by speaking it into existence, the amulet uses the same words to ask him to heal Cassius. Although the quotation from the biblical text is minimal, just two words, the creation story would have likely been recognizable, much as with the two-word quotations on Samaritan rings and pendants. The identity of this divine creator is given in the last line: *Iaō Sabaōth*.[44]

The Greek text also refers to the *logos* (word) of God, through whom God created the universe and through whom he could heal Cassius. The idea of God's *logos* participating in creation is known in the Septuagint's translation of the Psalms, in Jewish texts of the Hellenistic period, and in the Gospel of John, but it is not possible to determine which of these sources may have influenced the author of this amulet.[45] In addition to invoking the God of creation and his *logos*, the Greek text adjures (*horkizō*) by the "names, both his hidden and his excellent." The exact names intended by this reference are not specified, but we may see in this phrase a link between the Greek and the Hebrew texts on the amulet. In other words, the hidden and excellent names are found in the Hebrew text, including the Tetragrammaton, whose letters are each repeated a mystical seven times.

Roy Kotansky, who originally published the ʿEvron amulet, considered the text to be "well within the boundaries of acceptable orthodoxy," and likely the product of formal "liturgical incantations among Hellenistic Jews."[46] At the same time he recognized the similarities between the ʿEvron *lamella* and later Christian prayers for the sick. Similarly, Gideon Bohak concluded that the ʿEvron amulet was the product of "Palestinian Jewish authorship."[47] Despite these affirmations of the text's Jewish origin, one of the two symbols found in the space that marks the end of line 4 and the beginning of line 5 – exactly where the language changes from Hebrew to Greek – may complicate this reading. To the right, the Hebrew letters of the Tetragrammaton are arranged from top to bottom and then from right

---

[44] The name *Iaō* appears on many amulets, both in Palestine and elsewhere in the ancient Mediterranean world. In some cases, such as the present one, it should be understood as a simple Greek transliteration of the Tetragrammaton. On other amulets, *Iaō* appears to have been absorbed into the magical *koinē* without any obvious knowledge of Judaism or the Jewish god. See Faraone 2018, 9.

[45] For discussion of the *logos* in this text, see Kotansky 1991, 84–5; Kotansky 1994, 317.

[46] Kotansky 1994, 312–13, 315.

[47] Bohak 2008, 232. See also Bohak 2014, 251.

to left, around which a circle was drawn. Immediately to the left of this circle is a symbol that looks like a Christogram formed out of the superimposed letters iota and chi, the first letters of *Iēsous* and *Christos*, Jesus Christ.[48] Despite the rather unexpected presence of this symbol, Kotansky does not comment on it in either of his publications on this amulet but represents it in his line drawing. Gideon Bohak, on the other hand, considers the symbol briefly and acknowledges that it could be "construed as a Christian sign," although he ultimately rejects this idea in favor of it being a "six-point star."[49] Two anomalies raise questions about Bohak's conclusion that it is a star. First, its vertical bar is decidedly longer than its two crossbars; second, the vertical bar contains two small, horizontal lines or serifs at the ends, which are absent on the crossed lines forming the putative chi. If this symbol was a star, one might expect all six lines to be roughly the same length and for their ends to be decorated in the same way, as is found among some *charaktares* that include small circles at the end of each line. Bohak is undeniably correct that scholars should not place too much significance on simple crosses, with intersected vertical and horizontal lines, when they appear in a text that contains no other apparent Christian influence. However, the symbol on the 'Evron amulet is too detailed for the same principle to apply. While the Jewish origin of the amulet seems clear, ignoring this putative iota-chi obscures a potential point of contact between neighboring communities. Why was this symbol included? That is hard to say. The decision could have been made by either the practitioner or the user. One of them might have seen it on another amulet or heard about it being put on an amulet that later healed someone. In these scenarios, and assuming that it was, in fact, a Christogram, the symbol would reflect Jewish contact with neighboring communities, but the significance of the symbol might have been completely unknown to both the practitioner and the user. As a result, the symbol would tell us nothing about the user's self-identification. However, it is worth pointing out that the two adjacent symbols, the Tetragrammaton circle and the iota-chi, are each comprised of letters that make up a divine name. In other words, there is a certain logic to their juxtaposition that invites speculation about the relationship between the two and what they might have meant to the practitioner and the user.

In contrast to the 'Evron amulet, whose use of biblical material is in keeping with the pattern of Aramaic *lamellae*, the last two bilingual amulets from Palestine are more closely related to the Samaritan examples. Neither of these two Samaritan–Greek amulets was found in the course of controlled

[48] The symbol could also be a poorly preserved example of the more common Christogram chi-rho as an abbreviation for *Christos*.

[49] Bohak 2008, 277.

archaeological excavations, and so our only evidence comes from the objects themselves.[50] The first is a double-sided hematite gemstone reportedly found in the area of Nablus. It has been suggested that the gemstone was originally in a metal setting, which would have enabled it to be worn as a pendant. On one side of the gemstone is the familiar Samaritan inscription, "There is none like God, O Jeshurun," from Deut 33:26. The other side contains a *boēth(e)i* inscription, such as the examples in Chapter 1. Like the *boēth(e)i* ring from Caesarea, this bilingual example also begins with an invocation of the one god, "[There is] one god. Help Markiana."[51] There are plenty of parallels for the Samaritan and Greek inscriptions on their own, but this is the only instance where they are combined on a single amulet. The use of a gemstone for this amulet is also unusual, as it is a medium otherwise unknown for Samaritan amulets from Palestine.

There is no way to determine whether both sides of the Nablus gemstone were designed and executed at the same time. If the two sides were inscribed at different times, the complete lack of other Samaritan gemstone amulets from the region argues for the Greek side as the original one. The same principle is true even if the two sides were composed in tandem: it was likely created within a Greek-speaking community where the use of amuletic gemstones was common. At least two possibilities exist for why the Greek and Samaritan texts could have been combined on this amulet, either at the time of its original creation or at a later date. On the one hand, the user may not have fit neatly into the ethnic and religious categories that certain elites tried to maintain. If this was the case, the Nablus gemstone might have been a natural development of Markiana's exposure to multiple forms of amulets. Alternatively, she could have belonged to a community in which the Samaritan inscription was foreign, but the Greek *heis theos* acclamation was common. As we saw in Chapter 1, this latter description does not necessarily narrow down the community to which she belonged, as *heis theos* had broad appeal. In this case, the inclusion of the Samaritan text might have been similar to the use of *voces magicae, charaktares* and the pseudo-Samaritan inscriptions discussed above: all were powerful elements

---

[50] There are reports of another bilingual Samaritan–Greek amulet from Caesarea, but I have excluded it from consideration since it has not been fully published. It was first mentioned in Ilan 1982, 4, n. 5, and then included by Pummer in his list of known Samaritan amulets (1987, 262–3, no. 14). The ring reportedly quotes from Deut 33:26. Although not stated explicitly, the popularity of this verse on Samaritan amulets (and its absence on either Greek or Aramaic amulets from Palestine) makes it reasonable to surmise that this is the portion of the inscription in the Samaritan script. The ring is also said to include a Greek inscription, although the exact placement and contents of this Greek text have not been published.

[51] Pilcher 1920; Raffaeli 1920–1; Bonner 1950, 299 and pl. XIII, no. 76; Frey 1952, 2.1167; Pummer 1987, 256–7, 260–1, no. 2; Di Segni 1994, 101, no. 19; Spier 2007, 107, no. 624; Magen 2008, 250.

that could enhance the amulet's success, even if their precise meaning was unknown to the user.[52] However, unlike the pseudo-Samaritan inscriptions, where it is likely that the practitioners who carved them could not read the Samaritan script, the inclusion of Deut 33:26, one of the most popular verses on Samaritan amulets, suggests that whoever inscribed the Samaritan text for Markiana was familiar with Samaritan amulets.

The second Samaritan-Greek bilingual amulet is a bronze bracelet, published as a surface find from Caesarea (see Figure 2.4).[53] The surviving part of the bracelet consists of a narrow band (approximately 0.7 cm wide), which widens into a medallion (approximately 1.4 cm in diameter).[54] Other amuletic bracelets from the eastern Mediterranean have several medallions similar to the one on the Caesarea bracelet; since only a small portion of the band survives, we cannot know whether the Caesarea bracelet would have also had additional medallions. On the extant medallion is the Holy Rider image, similar to the one seen on the Gush Halav pendant in Chapter 1. As on that amulet, a Greek inscription encircles the image and reads *heis theos ho nikōn ta kaka* ("One god who conquers evil"). On the band to the right of this medallion a lion is running to the left; that is, the lion runs toward the medallion. To the right of the lion, still on the band, is the beginning of a second *heis theos* inscription. Since the bracelet is incomplete, it cannot be determined whether this was the simple acclamation *heis theos* ("[There is] one god"), or whether the text continued. On the reverse of the Holy Rider medallion,

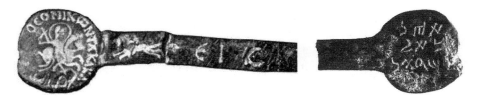

Figure 2.4 A bronze bracelet from Caesarea (Hamburger 1959; Israeli and Mevorah 2000)

---

[52] For a similar discussion on the possible circumstances for the combination of Syriac script and Jewish texts on Babylonian incantation bowls, see discussion in Boustan and Sanzo 2017.

[53] For discussion of this bracelet, see Hamburger 1959; Ben-Zvi 1961, 140; Kippenberg 1971, 155–6; Ringel 1975, 140–1; Ilan 1982, 4; Pummer 1987, 255–6, 260–1, no. 4; Di Segni 1994, 98, no. 7; McLean 1999, 24–5, no. 178; Israeli and Mevorah 2000, 160, 223; Reich 2002, 292, no. 4; Giannobile 2002, 177–82; *CIIP* 2, 571–2, no. 1685; *SEG* 18-625.

[54] The following are found on some of these other bracelets: the Virgin and Child, scenes from the life of Jesus, the Trisagion, and a Greek excerpt from Ps 90:1 (MT 91:1). For examples, see Maspero 1908; Peterson 1926, 91–6; Bonner 1950; Israeli and Mevorah 2000.

that is, the side that would have been touching the skin when the bracelet was worn, there is an inscription in the Samaritan script. Just as in the bilingual hematite from Nablus, the Samaritan text contains the common excerpt from Deut 33:26, "There is none like God, O Jeshurun." The only other published amuletic bracelet from Palestine was reportedly discovered in the vicinity of Jerusalem. Like this Caesarea bracelet, it too contained the Holy Rider and *heis theos ho nikōn ta kaka* on the medallion, but it lacked a Samaritan text on the reverse. On the band of the Jerusalem bracelet an inscription is situated between representations of a lion and a snake: "[There is] one god. Save [and] protect your servant Severina" (*heis theos sōson phylaxon tēn doulēn sou Seuērina*).[55] The extant portion of the Caesarea bracelet does not name the amulet's user.

The combination of the Holy Rider and the acclamation *heis theos ho nikōn ta kaka* is common, including the Caesarea and Jerusalem bracelets and the Gush Halav pendant. In fact, all but one of the amulets from Palestine with *heis theos ho nikōn ta kaka* also contain the Holy Rider; the one example without it, a pendant reportedly from Akko, depicts a scene that might be considered a variant of this image. On the Akko pendant, the nimbate figure is standing, rather than mounted on a horse, and he is holding a whip over the defeated enemy, rather than a spear.[56] On those amulets from Palestine with the full acclamation, the identity of the Holy Rider is not specified; the only ones to include any divine names are the Gush Halav amulet and a second pendant from the same burial complex. In both cases, the pendants' reverse contains the names *Iaō Sabaōth Michaēl* together with additional images.[57] Because these inscriptions are on the amulets' reverse, while the Holy Rider is on the obverse, it is unclear how, if at all, *Iaō Sabaōth Michaēl* should be associated with the Holy Rider.

It is generally assumed that the Greek and Samaritan sides of the Caesarea bracelet were completed by different practitioners, not only because of the

---

[55] Le Blant 1898, 84–6, no. 220; Thomsen 1921, 121–2, no. 207; Di Segni 1994, 103, no. 27; Belayche 2001, 159. Campbell Bonner published two additional amulet bracelets with Holy Rider scenes, but neither has archaeological provenience (1950, 218–19, 306–7, nos. 21–2; see also Bohak 1996, 25, no. 33; Cline 2019, 9).

[56] Dalton 1901, 112, no. 555. Di Segni's listing for this amulet (1994, 97, no. 4) suggests that it is the standard Holy Rider image, but she does not explain the discrepancy between her description and Dalton's, which she cites. See also Faraone 2018, 114, 344, n. 47.

[57] A third bronze pendant from Gush Halav also includes the Greek letters alpha and omega. While not a divine name per se, the letters are typically understood as a reference to the Apocalypse of John, in which God identifies himself several times as the alpha and the omega (Rev 1:8, 21:6, 22:13). See discussion in De Bruyn 2017, 64–5. For the publication of the second and third Gush Halav amulets, see Makhouly 1939, 48–9, kokh 4 and kokh 14, pl. XXXI, no. 5, 7; Di Segni 1994, 95–6, nos. 1a, 1c.

change in language, but also due to the change in technique and quality.[58] Unlike the Nablus gemstone, which seems to be inscribed with care on both the Greek and the Samaritan sides, the bracelet from Caesarea was carefully crafted on the Greek side with stamped decoration, while the Samaritan side was engraved and poorly executed.[59] However, a change in artisans does not necessarily indicate the circumstances of its creation, and there is no way to know whether the Greek and Samaritan texts were executed at the same time. It is possible that the bracelet was not originally commissioned in its present form, but rather purchased from a practitioner who had a supply ready to sell, and that either the original owner or someone who acquired the bracelet later had the Samaritan text inscribed. As with the gemstone, there are no other examples of Samaritan inscriptions on amuletic bracelets from Palestine. The options for why the Greek and Samaritan texts were combined on this bracelet are similar to those for the Nablus gemstone: either it reveals something about the self-identification of the user, or the Samaritan text was believed to augment the bracelet's efficacy.

The identity of this amulet's wearer has been the subject of significant scholarly discussion, but since it was reported as a surface find, archaeological context cannot shed light on this question. The outward-facing Greek text, Greek comparanda for amuletic bracelets, and the superior craftsmanship on the Greek side of the bracelet suggest that it was created by a practitioner skilled in making Greek amulets. Conventional wisdom holds that Samaritans were strictly aniconic in the Roman and late antique periods, and that a Samaritan would have been unlikely to wear a bracelet with the Holy Rider image.[60] While this is no doubt the most probable scenario, this book contains a number of examples where the desire to preserve health and ward off illnesses seems to have been sufficiently pressing that people were willing to transgress the limits imposed on acceptable practice by religious elites if they thought it might help them or their loved ones. In other words, even a member of an aniconic Samaritan community could have been tempted to use a figural amulet if – based on interactions with non-Samaritan neighbors – he or she believed it would be efficacious. While this is unlikely in the present case, the possibility cannot be ruled out.

---

[58] Pummer 1987, 256; *CIIP* 2.

[59] On the Samaritan side of the hematite gemstone, the last word, *Yaśurûn*, is not executed as nicely as the first two lines. This was likely due to space constraints, but it might have implications about the skill and experience of the artisan.

[60] For the idea that Samaritans in the Roman and late antique periods rejected images, see Hamburger 1959, 44–5; Magen 2008, 255. For scholars who are willing to accept the Samaritan use of the Holy Rider image, see Belayche 2001, 159, 199; Faraone 2018, 262.

Amulets and *tefillin*

The beginning of Chapter 1 surveyed the types of textual amulets known in the ancient Mediterranean world. As we saw, there is a significant gap in our knowledge of amulets from Roman and late antique Palestine because one major type of amulets – papyri – does not survive in Israel's climate. That is not to say, however, that all perishable writing materials have disappeared. Arguably the most important archaeological discoveries in Israel in the twentieth century were the texts from the Judaean desert, the Dead Sea Scrolls. Alongside the longer and more famous texts discovered in these caves were more than thirty *tefillin*, slips of parchment with biblical inscriptions that could be worn on the body. Several centuries after the composition of these *tefillin* from the Judaean desert, the *Mekhilta de-Rabbi Ishmael* was redacted and gave the definitive guidelines for the creation of *tefillin*. Prominent among its contents, and also found among the *tefillin* from the Judaean desert, was the passage beginning with Deut 6:4, which was interpreted as a biblical command instituting the *tefillin* ritual.[61] In light of the centrality of Deut 6 in Jewish life by late antiquity, it is interesting that there are no unambiguous examples of Jewish amulets that quote from this passage. The command in Deut 6:7 to repeat these words in the morning and in the evening was fulfilled through twice daily prayer, and the instructions in the following verse to "bind them as a sign on your hand" and to "fix them as an emblem on your forehead" were likewise taken literally.[62] I would suggest that the formalization of the *tefillin* ritual and a concomitant distinction between amulets and *tefillin* is at play in the absence of Deut 6:4 on identifiably Jewish amulets from Palestine.

In biblical Hebrew, *tefillah* (*təpillâ*) simply meant "prayer." An Aramaic papyrus from Edfu, in Upper Egypt, dated to approximately 300 BCE, provides the earliest example of the word being used to refer to a material object when it mentions a "*tefillah* of silver." Bearing a striking resemblance to this "*tefillah* of silver" are also the two small, silver scrolls discovered in the late pre-exilic Ketef Hinnom tomb discussed above. Gabriel Barkay highlighted the continuity that existed between pre-exilic practices in the land of Israel, such as at the Ketef Hinnom tomb, and Persian-period Jewish communities in Upper Egypt, from which the Edfu papyrus originated. He argued that the author of the Edfu papyrus may have been familiar with objects similar to the Ketef

---

[61] For the date of the *Mekhilta de-Rabbi Ishmael*, see discussion in Strack et al. 1996, 253–5. This text does not state the concluding verse of each *tefillin* passage, but most scholars assume the same divisions as those found in the Masoretic text, with the result that this passage would encompass Deut 6:4–9. See discussion in Cohn 2008a, 124–5.

[62] For example, see *Letter of Aristeas* 159–60.

66   CONTESTED CURES

Hinnom scrolls, which had been composed a couple of centuries earlier, and had such items in mind when he referenced a *"tefillah* of silver."[63] The Ketef Hinnom scrolls cite the priestly blessing from Num 6, transforming what had originally been an oral pronouncement into a material object. In the same way, *tefillin* transformed a key component of daily prayers, the *Shema*, into a tangible object. Just as someone who wore the priestly benediction on his or her person would see it as a material expression of the hope that God would "bless you and keep you" (Num 6:24), a person who wore a written version of the *Shema* could see it as embodying God's promise to the obedient that their "days may be long" (Deut 6:2).

Yehuda Cohn has argued persuasively that *tefillin* were an invented tradition of the Second Temple period rather than a "straightforward fulfillment" of a "scriptural obligation" to write out the words of God and physically wear them on one's body. The Jewish encounter with Hellenism, and particularly with its many apotropaic devices, inspired the interpretation of Deut 6 as a command to wear biblical texts as amulets, thereby securing the text's promises for wearers.[64] This may have been facilitated by the growing importance during the Roman Empire of textual components – in contrast to visual elements – on Greek amulets across the Mediterranean. Josephus, for example, is aware of how Deut 6:4–9 was used by his contemporaries, both in daily prayers and as physical reminders of God's protection worn on the body. By remembering past events with physical tokens, Josephus wrote that the Jews expected them to act "as a stimulus for what will be" (*epi de protropē tōn esomenōn*).[65] In other words, these written reminders functioned as amulets to secure similar results for their users. Once Deut 6:4 had taken on this special significance for *tefillin*, it may be that the absence of the verse on identifiably Jewish amulets reflects an effort among some Jews to avoid confusing the boundaries between amulets and *tefillin*. Deut 6:4 was appropriate for Jewish *tefillin*, but not for Jewish amulets.

Cohn's argument that *tefillin* developed at least partially from exposure to Greek amulets, rather than out of an uncomplicated reading of Deut 6, should also be considered in light of the Samaritan rings and pendants discussed in this chapter. Most of the Samaritan examples consist entirely of quotations

[63] Barkay 1992, 184.

[64] Cohn 2008a, 89–91; Cohn 2008b, 42–3. Esther Eshel, Hannan Eshel, and Armin Lange (2010, 213–14) also argue that *tefillin* served an apotropaic purpose, although they reach the conclusion in a different way. Whereas Cohn focuses on the text of *tefillin* from the Judaean desert, and in particular portions of the biblical text that seem to have been deliberately omitted, Eshel et al. focused on the physical characteristics of *tefillin* and point to the fact that the biblical texts were hidden from view as evidence of their apotropaic nature.

[65] Josephus *Ant.* 4.212.

from the Pentateuch, including references to Deut 6. The Samaritan rings would have allowed users to "bind them (i.e. the words) as a sign on your hand" (Deut 6:8). Even the pendants, which we typically imagine as being worn around the neck, where the biblical excerpts would have been on one's heart (cf. Deut 6:6), could have been temporarily affixed to a person's head, as with *tefillin*, further echoing the words of Deut 6:8. While there are no extant Samaritan texts that describe the use of these rings and pendants, Table 1.4 identified a lacuna that may lend support to the idea that they served a similar function to *tefillin*: there are no Aramaic amulets from Palestine that take the form of rings or pendants. If, as I suggest, Jews avoided using Deut 6:4 on amulets because of its significance for *tefillin*, then it is equally possible that they would have avoided rings and pendants if these were perceived as having a significance for Samaritans that was similar to *tefillin*. As we will see in Chapter 7, the rabbis expressed some concern about the use of rings and bracelets as amulets.

While this may explain the absence of Deut 6 on Aramaic amulets and the avoidance of pendants and rings for Jewish amulets, it stands in stark contrast to broader trends that these two chapters on amulets have demonstrated. In general, the people of Roman and late antique Palestine were quite willing to borrow from neighboring ethnic, cultural, and religious traditions in the composition of healing amulets. Divine names, powerful images, *voces magicae*, *charaktares*, and *historiolae*, including biblical quotations, were all common features of amulets across the ancient Mediterranean world and likewise figured prominently in amulets from our region. When faced with illness and injury beyond their ability to treat, people were willing to transgress boundaries if they thought that it would increase their chances of a cure. It was precisely this aspect of amulet use, and ritual healing options more generally, that made them the focus of the elite invective that will be examined in Chapter 7.

PART II

Miraculous Places

CHAPTER 3

In This Holy Place:
Hot Springs as Sites of Ritual Healing

The modern world is no stranger to sites that are sacred to more than one religious tradition. They tend to be places of conflict as each group lays claim to the space as their exclusive domain. The Temple Mount/Haram al-Sharif in Jerusalem and the Ibrahimi Mosque/Cave of the Patriarchs in Hebron are touchstones for conflict between Muslims and Jews, and the brawls among representatives of the various churches that share custody of the Church of the Holy Sepulcher in Jerusalem and the Church of the Nativity in Bethlehem are legendary. Likewise, the sharing of the holy space on Mount Zion, revered by Jews as the tomb of David and by Christians as the site of Jesus' last supper, has met with uneven success. Yet this pattern is not universal, and some shared shrines have allowed multiple traditions to exist alongside one another in relative harmony, such as those where the prophet Elijah, St. George, and Khiḍr are remembered.[1] In Roman and late antique Palestine, one of the most famous shared sites was Mamre, near Hebron, where the coexistence of multiple religious traditions lasted for several centuries. The fifth-century historian Sozomen described Mamre in this way:

> It is recorded that here the Son of God appeared to Abraham, with two angels, who had been sent against Sodom, and foretold the birth of his son. Here the inhabitants of the country and of the regions round Palestine, the Phoenicians, and the Arabians, assemble annually during the summer season to keep a brilliant feast; and many others, both buyers and sellers, gather on account of the fair. Indeed, this feast is diligently frequented by all nations: by the Jews, because they boast of their descent from the patriarch Abraham; by the Greeks (*hellēsi*), because angels there appeared to men; and by Christians, because he who for the

[1] For Elijah, St. George, and Khiḍr, see Ziv 1987; Meri 1999; Laird 2013.

72 CONTESTED CURES

salvation of mankind was born of a virgin, afterwards manifested himself there to a godly man. This place was moreover honored fittingly with religious exercises. Here some prayed to the God of all; some called upon the angels, poured out wine, burnt incense, or offered an ox, or he-goat, a sheep, or a cock . . . [Constantine] rebuked the bishops of Palestine in no measured terms, because they had neglected their duty, and had permitted a holy place to be defiled by impure libations and sacrifices . . .[2]

Sozomen's description highlights two key characteristics of Mamre. First, crowds were drawn to the site for both mundane and ritual activities. Some people visited because of its religious significance while others came to shop or to sell their wares, and – no doubt – many came for both reasons. A second insight gained from Sozomen is that Mamre was noted for its diversity, attracting Jews, Christians, and "Greeks," by which Sozomen meant non-Christians and non-Jews.[3] The last would have included the immediate residents of the region, but the popularity of Mamre was such that it even attracted visitors from further afield – Phoenicia and Arabia. These groups apparently intermingled at Mamre both in its sacred spaces and in areas where the associated market took place. A venerable tree, associated with the story in Gen 18, was located within the Herodian *temenos*, along with an altar on which animal sacrifices took place and a well into which a variety of offerings were thrown. Ultimately a Christian basilica was built within this space in the fourth century.[4] As a direct result of this shared use of sacred space, it was the target of elite criticism.[5] However, even after Constantine ordered that the site be Christianized, it would seem multiple groups continued to coexist there. An anonymous sixth-century pilgrim from Piacenza in northern Italy wrote, "The basilica has four porticoes and no roof over the central court. Down the middle runs a screen; Christians come in on one side and Jews on the other, and they use much incense."[6] Thus, as late as the sixth century, it continued to be a shared space.

The religious situation in Mamre, while not associated with ritual healing, offers a model for the sites discussed in this chapter. I argue that Sozomen's two

---

[2] Sozomen *Hist. Eccl.* 2.4 (translation is a slightly modified version of *NPNF* 2/2:261).

[3] For the diverse character of Mamre, see Taylor 1993, 86–95; Kofsky 1998; Belayche 2001, 96–104; Drbal 2017. For the worship of angels at Mamre, see Cline 2011, 106–18.

[4] For the excavations of Mamre, see Mader 1957; Magen 1991; Ovadiah and Turnheim 2011, 85–9.

[5] Cline (2011, 115–18) argues that the underlying reason for the elite censure of Mamre was that Christians had adopted "pagan" ritual offerings to the angels, so that it was impossible to distinguish between Christian and non-Christian worship.

[6] *Itin. Plac.* 30. All translations of the Piacenza Pilgrim are from Wilkinson 2002, 129–51.

key observations about Mamre also characterized the hot springs of Roman and late antique Palestine: first, both mundane and ritual activities took place at these sites, and second, they drew a diverse crowd of visitors. Since literary references to the hot springs are not as explicit as Sozomen's text on Mamre, examination of the hot springs' patrons and their reasons for visiting extends to epigraphic and archaeological evidence, such as the inscriptions from the *thermae* that begin with the phrase "In this holy place." Most of the evidence discussed in this chapter comes from Hammat Gader and, to a lesser degree, from Hammat Tiberias. Despite this limitation, I would suggest that other hot springs in Palestine functioned in fundamentally similar ways.

Sozomen's account of the situation at Mamre also draws attention to a difference between the ritual healing considered in the present chapter and the amulets of Chapters 1 and 2. At Mamre, as at the hot springs, visitors would have had at least a passing awareness of each other's rituals, as they were focused on the same sites. The same was not necessarily true for amulets. It is indeed possible, and perhaps even likely, that some amulet-users consciously chose amulets that incorporated elements from multiple religious traditions. The bilingual Greek and Samaritan amulets seem to be a clear example of this. If, as I suggested, amulets without the user's name inscribed – such as the reaper gemstones, Holy Rider pendants, or Samaritan rings – were sold or passed on when they were no longer necessary, and if by passing from one hand to the next they also crossed the notional lines dividing ethnic, cultural, and religious communities, it is possible that these users were also conscious of shared rituals. In other cases, such as amulets with *heis theos*, it is not necessarily clear that users would have known that this acclamation was used by a variety of groups in the region. This would also likely be the case for amulets with *voces magicae* and *charaktares*; a user might have had no way to know that the use of such words and symbols extended beyond his or her community. While some amulet-users would have had input into the composition of their amulets, especially for those personalized with the user's name and the specific conditions for which healing was sought, such as the *lamellae* from Nirim and Tiberias, others would have purchased a premade amulet and may have asked few questions about the details it contained. This ignorance would not have been possible at the hot springs. Although preliminary rites would have likely taken place outside the bath complex, in spaces set aside for each community, a certain amount of mixing must have taken place within the bath itself. Thus, as at Mamre, shared ritual space and knowledge of fellow visitors would have underscored this common form of ritual healing.

In their pioneering work on pilgrimage, Victor and Edith Turner centered the concept of "communitas" for understanding pilgrimage experiences across disparate cultures. They argued that the shared experiences of pilgrimage, which remove participants from their daily life, created this "antistructural" communitas

74 CONTESTED CURES

that could transcend societal divisions created by class, power, background, and community affiliations.[7] While it is tempting to see in the Turners' position some explanation of the coexistence of disparate groups at places like Mamre and the hot springs of Palestine, more recent considerations of communitas have questioned the Turners' conclusions. In particular, in their introduction to a 1991 volume John Eade and Michael Sallnow wrote that pilgrimage should be seen as an "arena for competing religious and secular discourses, for both the official co-optation and the non-official recovery of religious meanings, for conflict between orthodoxies, sects, and confessional groups, for drives toward consensus and communitas, *and* for counter-movements toward separateness and division."[8] Thus, while this chapter considers the possibility that the hot springs attracted visitors of diverse ethnic, cultural, and religious groups at the same time, we must not lose sight of the fact that these distinctions persisted, even within the shared space of the baths. Some of this competing discourse, that generated by elite authors, will be considered in Chapter 7. However, differences were likely also perpetuated by visitors to the baths themselves who observed the behavior of people from outside their community; these responses to these shared spaces have been lost to time.

Hot springs as sacred sites

Sites of ritual healing are known throughout the ancient Mediterranean world, particularly those related to the cult of Asklepios, such as at Epidauros, Pergamum, Kos, and Rome, and to those of Serapis and Isis in Egypt. In Palestine, the most popular healing sites were of a markedly different character than these Greek and Egyptian cults, in that they were situated at hot springs. This is not to say that cults at hot springs did not take place elsewhere, but only that they seem to have been particularly prominent in our region.[9] Palestine lies along a geological rift that stretches from eastern Africa to southern Asia Minor. The movement of the tectonic plates produced numerous hot springs, of which seven are known from ancient literary testimonies: Emmaus (Nikopolis), Hammei Ba'arah, Hammat Gader, Hammei Livias, Hammat Pella, Hammat Tiberias, Kallirhoe, and the Waters of Asia. These thermal-mineral springs figured prominently in the ritual landscape of Palestine, where they addressed the universal concerns of sickness and injury. All but the last of these sites have been identified with a fair

---

[7] Turner and Turner 2011 [1978]; see also Turner 1973.
[8] Eade and Sallnow 2013 [1991], 2.
[9] For the question of cult activity at hot springs elsewhere in the ancient world, and the presence of divine healers at these sites, see Croon 1967; Aupert 1991; Ben Abed and Scheid 2003.

degree of confidence, and several have been at least partially excavated.[10] Hammat Gader (Emmatha) was one of the most famous hot springs in antiquity, as well as the only one in Israel to be excavated with a final, published site report. According to Eunapius of Sardis, it was second only to the celebrated thermal-mineral springs of Baiae on the Bay of Naples in Italy.[11] The Decapolis city of Gadara (Umm Qais), to which Hammat Gader belonged, was situated roughly four and a half kilometers away on a steep ridge in modern Jordan. Excavations in the vicinity of the bath complex revealed a synagogue, a church, a theater, and a residential area.[12] A colonnaded street ran from the Yarmuk River to the theater, where it intersected with a wider colonnaded street that went toward the bath complex. The bath was quite large, covering more than 4,600 m² (Figure 3.1).[13] Along the southern side of the complex was a series of hot pools that led up to the hot spring itself in the southeast corner. On the northern side of the complex was a cold-water pool with a number of fountains and niches around its perimeter.

Just as Sozomen recognized that visitors to Mamre came for many reasons, the same was true for Hammat Gader. That people visited the baths for leisure hardly needs stating, as it is easily understood from the ancient sources. This is perhaps best exemplified in Epiphanius' story about the *comes* Josephus who once accompanied the Jewish patriarch's son to Hammat Gader.[14] Epiphanius explained that there was a festival (*panēgyris*) at Hammat Gader every year, using the same word that Sozomen used to describe the annual festival at Mamre. While at the baths, the patriarch's son became infatuated with a Christian woman, who spurned his advances. Epiphanius blamed the opportunity for promiscuity on the fact that men and women bathed together at Hammat Gader, which he called the "deadly nets" (*oletēria diktya*) of the "adversary" (*enantias*).[15] Just as there is no doubt that people visited the hot springs for the leisure they offered, there likewise is little doubt that people came to relax in the hot water for relief from physical conditions. The question, however, is whether the people who came for physical relief saw the hot springs simply as a place where the water would soothe their aches and pains or whether they understood something else to be going on. The answer, almost certainly, is both. In the modern world, people tend to draw a clear line between medical treatments and divine intervention in the form of miracles and faith healing.

---

[10] For the locations of these hot springs and ancient references to each, see Dvorjetski 2007, 162–223. References and bibliography may also be found Avi-Yonah 1976; Tsafrir et al. 1994.

[11] *V. Soph.* 459.

[12] Hirschfeld 1987, 107–16. For the theater's ritual character, see Segal 1994, 45–6.

[13] Hirschfeld 1997, 10.

[14] Epiphanius *Pan.* 30.7–8.

[15] Epiphanius *Pan.* 30.7.

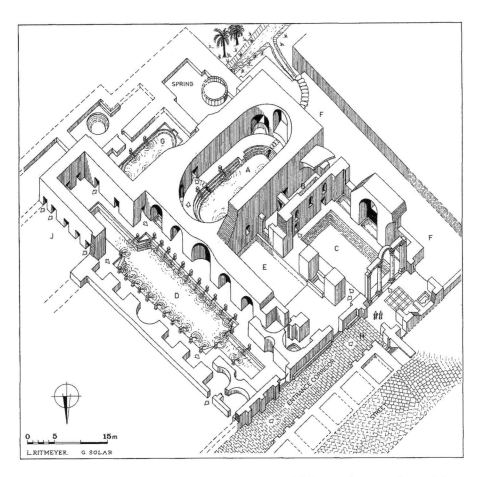

Figure 3.1 Partial reconstruction of Hammat Gader (Hirschfeld 1997, fig. 51; with permission of the Israel Exploration Society)

The distinction was not so sharp in the ancient Mediterranean world, as doctors were frequently found at sanctuaries of the pre-eminent god of medicine, Asklepios, who had according to myth once been a doctor himself. Evidence that at least some visitors understood the hot springs to be sacred and that the healing they experienced was the result of divine intervention can be found in the archaeological remains.

Between sixty and seventy Greek inscriptions from the pavement of the bath complex survive, and these inscriptions unequivocally assert the sacred nature of hot spring.[16] Their language is quite repetitive, frequently including some

---

[16] Di Segni 1997.

variation of "In this holy place be remembered . . ." (*en tō hagiō topō mnēsthē*), a phrase otherwise typically associated with temples, synagogues, and churches.[17] This is quite striking and suggests that at least some visitors came to experience a sacred place rather than, or in addition to, seeking pleasure and relaxation. All of the inscriptions appear to post-date the fifth-century reconstruction of the site following an earthquake.[18] An inscription from the Hall of Piers (Fig. 3.1, Area C) commemorates the 455 CE completion of repairs and renovations, including the new floors into which these Greek inscriptions were set. While there are no surviving inscriptions from before this renovation, votive inscriptions were certainly not a new phenomenon in the fifth century, and there is nothing to preclude the possibility that earlier dedications existed but were damaged and removed during the repairs.[19]

Two additional find categories also attest to the bath's sacred character. One hundred and forty-eight complete oil lamps were discovered along with fragments from roughly two hundred additional lamps. Most of the intact lamps were located in one of two concentrations: sixty were found under a renovated floor in Area B, and another deposit was found an isolated alcove in Area D.[20] These lamps offer somewhat less explicit testimony than the inscriptions, but their deliberate placement reflects a traditional desire to keep votive offerings, or thank-offerings, in the sacred space. Many of these lamps do not contain the soot marks that would have been present if they had been lit even once. This suggested to the excavators that they were deposited as votive offerings, likely related to healing, rather than casually left behind after their use as functional lights. As evidence of ritual healing at Hammat Gader, the lamps antedate the inscriptions, since they were sealed under the fifth-century floors. The earliest lamp dates to the second century and suggests that the practice of leaving votive offerings may have originated at roughly the same time as the construction of the bathhouse.[21] Coins also seem to have been left

---

[17] For references to synagogues as "holy places," see Levine 2000, 238; cf. Fine 1997.

[18] In 363 CE, a major earthquake struck Palestine, causing extensive damage that stretched from the Galilee to Petra. A letter attributed to Cyril of Jerusalem names Hammat Gader among the sites damaged by the earthquake. See Brock 1977, 276.

[19] An engraved pair of hands and feet in the pavement of the Hall of Inscriptions might suggest that some visitors continued to offer votive offerings after the Muslim conquest. The hands and feet were inscribed on top of an earlier Greek inscription, which means that they post-date it, although their precise date cannot be determined. See discussion in Amitai-Preiss 1997, 273–46; Dauphin 2000, 73; Belayche 2017, 674. For a votive foot found at the Pool of Bethesda in Jerusalem, see Chapter 4.

[20] Uzzielli 1997, 319.

[21] Uzzielli 1997, 320. Belayche points to the date of these lamps as one of several indications that Hammat Gader did not acquire its sanctity only in the Byzantine period. See 2017, 677–80.

78 CONTESTED CURES

at Hammat Gader as votives.[22] The corrosive mineral waters mean that many of the smallest coins cannot be dated precisely, although in general they come from the Byzantine rather than Roman period.

The idea that hot springs were seen as sacred has been regularly observed by scholars, but the way that visitors encountered them as sacred spaces and the form that associated rituals took is poorly understood. Only one straight-forward account exists. A detailed entry on Hammat Gader by the Piacenza Pilgrim describes the late sixth-century ritual that took place there:

> We went to a city called Gadara, which is Gibeon, and there, three miles from the city, there are hot springs called the Baths of Elijah (*termas Heliae*). Lepers are cleansed there, and have their meals from the inn (*xenodochium*) there at public expense. The baths fill in the evening. In front of the furnace (*clibanum*)[23] is a large tank. When it is full, all the gates are closed, and they are sent in through a small door with lights (*luminaria*) and incense, and sit in the tank all night. They fall asleep, and the person who is going to be cured sees a vision. When he has told it the springs do not flow for a week. In one week he is cleansed.[24]

The Piacenza Pilgrim describes a night-time ritual, with supplicants entering the pool carrying *luminaria*. While in the bath, the supplicants fall asleep in the expectation of a vision. Who or what they see in this vision is not speci-fied. A week after the vision, the individual is miraculously cured. The role of *luminaria*, lighting the way in the dark as visitors enter the bath, could explain the preference for lamps as votive offerings at Hammat Gader. One concen-tration of votive lamps was discovered under the floor in Area B, and Yizhar Hirschfeld and Giora Solar proposed that the ritual described by the Piacenza Pilgrim took place there, as it is close to the source of the hot spring and con-tains the only pool that had doors that could be completely closed off, as the passage describes.[25] Since both Area B and the earliest lamp fragments from the ritual deposits date to the second century, when the complex was first built, it is possible that some sort of incubation ritual took place in this space from the site's early years. However, some scholars have suggested that Area B was

---

[22] Barkay 1997, 300. For similarities between the coins at Hammat Gader and those at 'Ein Tzur (discussed in Chapter 4), see Barkay 2000a, 855–8; Barkay 2000b, 416. For coins as votive offerings in the ancient word, see discussion in Sauer 2005, 91–121; de Cazanove 2015, 190–1.

[23] Wilkinson uses the word "basin" for *clibanus*, but I prefer Judith Green and Yorum Tsafrir's choice of "furnace." For discussion of the *clibanus* (or *klibanos* in Greek) as the source of the hot water, see Green and Tsafrir 1982, 84.

[24] *Itin. Plac.* 7. For difficulties in the manuscript tradition of this text, see Renberg 2016, 2:810, n. 3.

[25] Hirschfeld and Solar 1981, 208–11; see also Dauphin 1996–7, 61.

renovated following the fifth-century earthquake and that by the time of the Piacenza Pilgrim's visit, the ritual must have taken place elsewhere.[26]

Some may object to my use of the word "incubation" to refer to the healing ritual described by the Piacenza Pilgrim.[27] These objections center around the question of whether "incubation" can rightly be attached to any Christian practices, including the sixth-century account regarding Hammat Gader.[28] Arguments against labeling this as incubation are based on several factors, including a chronological break separating Christian incubation from earlier practices, Christian distrust of dreams, and structural differences between the earlier forms of incubation and Christian rites. Despite these objections, I maintain that the term is warranted to describe what took place at Hammat Gader.[29] Concerns about a chronological break between Greco-Roman incubation and Christian incubation need not necessarily apply at Hammat Gader. Hammat Gader seems to have been in continuous use from the baths' construction in the second century until after the arrival of Islam. Incubation was common in Greek healing cults, and if incubation began while the site was controlled by the Greek city of Gadara, there is no reason to suggest an interruption in this practice before the Christianization of the region. It could have been adopted and modified by Jewish and Christian visitors early on. The absence of a literary description of incubation before the Piacenza Pilgrim in this case does not necessarily need to be taken as evidence of absence. As Hedvig von Ehrenheim argued, local memories of incubation may have been retained around sites with a history of incubation, even if formal cultic support for the practice had disappeared.[30] The second objection, Christian distrust of dreams, gets to the heart of what this book is about – the tension between what actually took place and the rhetoric

[26] Nicole Belayche (2001, 272; 2017, 674–5) proposes that the incubation ritual took place in Area A, the Oval Hall, while Gil Renberg (2016, 2:813) prefers Area G.

[27] Fritz Graf (2015, 242–3) offers a notable exception to the general consensus that this was a healing ritual. While he recognizes that healing was involved, he claims that the bathers' primary objective was "to be purified by divine grace."

[28] For example, Graf 2014; Graf 2015; Renberg 2016, 2:792–807. Scholars who do use the term "incubation" to describe Christian practices include Alice-Mary Talbot (2002), Ildikó Csepregi (2012), Hedvig von Ehrenheim (2016), and Nicole Belayche (2017).

[29] Until recently, Ludwig (Ludovicus) Deubner's examination (1900) of incubation in the Greek and Roman worlds remained a standard text, alongside a number of more specialized collections and the indispensable compilation of Asklepios testimonies by Edelstein and Edelstein (1998, particularly T. 414–42). Gil Renberg's new, two-volume treatment of incubation (2016) in the ancient Near East, Egypt, Greece, and Rome has significantly advanced the scholarly discussion of both therapeutic and divinatory incubation. Additional studies worth noting are Oppenheim 1956; Flannery-Dailey 2004; Harrisson 2014. Recent work on sanctuaries of Asklepios also considers incubation, including Steger 2004; Riethmüller 2005; Melfi 2007; Steger 2016.

[30] Ehrenheim 2016, 85.

of elite authors about what *should* take place. In other words, just because elite Christian authors had a negative opinion of dreams, this does not mean that all Christians held them in a similar light, and in fact this rhetoric might have been a reaction to the fact that dreams *were* highly regarded by some Christians. The final objection, differences in form between Christian and non-Christian rites, is certainly to be expected; nevertheless, the anonymous pilgrim's account still meets most definitions of incubation.

Kimberly Patton articulated three criteria of incubation, all of which the Hammat Gader ritual had in common with other cults throughout the ancient Mediterranean world – intentionality, locality, and epiphany.[31] Patton observed that the "theology of incubation highly localizes the god," which likely hindered the initial adoption of this ritual technique among Jews and Christians, to whom it seemed uncomfortably close to polytheistic practices.[32] The question of incubation is intimately connected to that of sacred sites, as it is the place, not a temple official or charismatic healer, that is understood to facilitate cures.[33] Sacred places have taken a variety of forms from antiquity to the present, but J. Z. Smith argued that what makes something sacred – in this case a site – is the presence of ritual activity.[34] Despite early opposition to the concept of sacred sites, Christian authorities eventually recognized and accommodated their popular veneration, including places that were previously the focus of non-Christian cult.[35] I would suggest that the Piacenza Pilgrim's description of lepers at Hammat Gader represents a true incubation ritual, meeting all three of Patton's criteria. Furthermore, as Smith argued, ritual reifies sanctity, and thus it is through the practice of an incubation ritual that the hot springs can be recognized as sacred sites, confirming the testimony of the "holy place" (*hagios topos*) inscriptions found at Hammat Gader.

Visitors to the hot springs

The population of Palestine in the second to the sixth centuries CE was diverse, which as is argued throughout the book facilitated borrowing of rituals, particularly in popular practices related to healing. For some groups of visitors, the evidence of their presence at the hot springs is straightforward. The earliest reference to the hot spring at Hammat Gader comes from Strabo in the

---

[31] Patton 2004, 202–27.

[32] Patton 2004, 216.

[33] Csepregi 2015, 49–50.

[34] Smith 1987, 105. For a discussion of Smith's definition as it relates to the development of holy sites in fourth-century Palestine, see Markus 1994, 264–6.

[35] Csepregi 2015, 51, 53–5. For the gradual recognition of sacred sites, see Markus 1994; Safrai 1998b.

first century BCE, and the construction of the bath complex itself dates to the second century CE.[36] The original excavators, lacking clear evidence of the circumstances surrounding the spring's monumentalization, concluded that it was built by the local, Semitic population of Gadara following Greco-Roman models.[37] Estée Dvorjetski offered an alternative proposal that Roman soldiers, rather than local inhabitants, were responsible for the construction. The Roman army patronized local healing cults throughout the Mediterranean in large numbers, due in part to the harsh realities of life on a military campaign, and Dvorjetski argued that the army allocated "considerable military resources" to the development of therapeutic facilities.[38] The probability of the army's involvement at Hammat Gader, she contended, is augmented by numismatic and epigraphic evidence that places *Legio X Fretensis* in the area.[39] Furthermore, Dvorjetski offered a story in the medieval rabbinic compilation *Midrash ha-Gadol* (Deut 26:19), which describes Emperor Hadrian meeting a girl covered in sores as he made his way from Hammat Gader to Gadara, as additional evidence for an official Roman presence at the site. In response to Dvorjetski, the excavators of Hammat Gader concurred that the army was stationed in the region of Gadara and that there could have been Roman influence on the bath alongside the efforts of the local population, but they questioned her conclusion that the army's presence alone proves that it was responsible for the bath's construction.[40] Regardless of who actually built the bath complex, there can be no question that in its early years the hot spring was dominated by the local, polytheistic inhabitants, including the Roman army stationed nearby. Although the evidence is circumstantial at best, the fact that the earliest lamps from Hammat Gader date to the second century could suggest that an incubation ritual, with subsequent votive offerings, began at roughly the same time.

For Christian visitors to Hammat Gader, the Piacenza Pilgrim offers definitive proof, which is reinforced by archaeological evidence. Most of the votive

---

[36] Strabo *Geographica* 16.2.45.

[37] Hirschfeld and Solar 1984, 39.

[38] Dvorjetski 2007, 106. See also Ploeg 2018, 166–262.

[39] An inscription from Gadara records the legion's dedication to Hadrian on the occasion of his visit to Syria-Palestine in 130 CE. Numismatic evidence also confirms this. Coins in honor of the emperor's visit were issued by cities where the Tenth Legion was known to be quartered, and so the fact that Gadara issued a coin would suggest an army presence in the city. Coins from Gadara also appear with countermarks of the Tenth Legion, offering further evidence that some of the soldiers were camped in the area. See discussion in Dvorjetski 2007, 367–9. In addition to this evidence for the Tenth Legion, a recently discovered Latin inscription from Hammat Gader indicates that the Sixth Legion was also at Hammat Gader. I return to this inscription in greater detail below.

[40] Hirschfeld 1997, 478.

82   CONTESTED CURES

lamps lack distinguishing iconographic motifs or inscriptions that would indicate the religious self-understanding of their dedicators, but some are decorated with crosses, making their dedication by Christians likely.[41] The votive inscriptions also offer conclusive proof for the presence of Christians among the dedicators, through the inclusion of crosses or distinctly Christian language.[42] However, the presence of Christians among these inscriptions is unsurprising, since they post-date the fifth-century renovation, and any non-Christian who installed an inscription may have chosen not to draw attention to their identity.

Jewish presence at Hammat Gader cannot be confirmed on the basis of votive offerings alone. Names that could be Jewish appear on a few inscriptions, but the onomastics are insufficient to prove that Jews patronized the site in search of miraculous cures.[43] However, rabbinic texts do confirm that Jews visited the hot springs, including prominent rabbis, and their attitude toward travel to Hammat Gader on the Sabbath may hint at the site's ritual character.[44] I would suggest that the impressive synagogues built near Hammat Gader and Hammat Tiberias offer more substantial proof that Jews visited the hot springs for ritual healing.[45] Hammat Tiberias was located on the west side of the Sea of Galilee, roughly 18 km northwest of Hammat Gader. Unlike Hammat Gader,

[41] In general, the lamps conform to the typologies known from Palestine and Transjordan, mostly their northern regions. See Uzzielli 1997. For the Semitic use of ritual lamps, see Belayche 2001, 97–9.

[42] Crosses appear on Di Segni 1997, nos. 2, 11, 13, 20–3, 27, 30–1, 35, 37, 40, 44, 49, 52–4, 58, 63. Christ is invoked on nos. 26 and 71.

[43] Names from two inscriptions (Di Segni 1997, nos. 2 and 21) suggest that the family had recently become Christian, perhaps to maintain their administrative positions. In general, individuals in these inscriptions with military, administrative, and honorific titles should be identified as Christians, given the political climate of the fifth century. Several names (Di Segni 1997, nos. 6, 8, 10–11, and 36) appear to be Greek transliterations from Armenian, Egyptian, Germanic, and Semitic languages, but family origins alone cannot prove an individual's religious identity. A relatively unattested name that could be Jewish appears on no. 35. Di Segni also argued that no. 32 presents a covert message of Jewishness, on the basis of the individual's name and the multiple possible meanings for the chi-mu-gamma acronym. A final inscription that could be Jewish is Di Segni's no. 38, on the basis of Semitic names and the use of a slightly different formula to introduce the inscription.

[44] See discussion of Rabbi Judah ha-Nasi in Chapter 7.

[45] Patton's criteria for incubation have been applied to passages from the Hebrew Bible and later Jewish literature. Juliette Harrison (2014) argues that stories from the Hebrew Bible describe divine revelations or epiphanies in the form of a dream, but that many are missing one of the three constituent elements of incubation. Patton (2004, 218–19) suggests that the biblical authors deliberately suppressed elements of incubation, such as in Jacob's dream at Bethel in Gen 28. In Jewish literature from the Hellenistic and Roman periods, knowledge of contemporary incubation rituals is easier to detect (Gnuse 1993; Flannery-Dailey 2004, 153–64). Johannes Lindblom (1961, 103–6) argued that some of the Psalms were intended for use in incubation rituals, which is of interest in the context of a site where Roman and late antique Jews sought healing alongside their non-Jewish neighbors.

where substantial architectural elements of the bath complex have been uncovered, little remains of the Hammat Tiberias baths. However, at both Hammat Gader and Hammat Tiberias, evidence for Jewish patronage of the hot springs can be seen in the construction of nearby synagogues. The key detail about these synagogues is that they were located in the immediate vicinity of the hot springs, rather than in the larger towns of Gadara or Tiberias.[46] The towns were located at some distance from their respective hot springs, two and a half kilometers away in the case of Tiberias, and four and a half kilometers away in the case of Gadara, making it impractical for their Jewish inhabitants to attend the synagogues near the hot springs on a routine basis. While small settlements did spring up around both bath complexes, it seems unlikely that the impressive synagogues at Hammat Gader and Hammat Tiberias were built only for the people who dwelled there. Instead, it is probable that these synagogues were built to accommodate Jewish visitors to the *thermae*.

Inscriptions from these synagogues substantiate the presence of Jews among the visitors to the hot springs. The synagogue at Hammat Gader underwent major renovations in the fifth century to repair damage caused by the same earthquake that affected the bath complex, and its inscriptions consequently post-date this restoration. Four Aramaic inscriptions are extant in the synagogue's mosaic pavement, each of which begins with the phrase "And be remembered for good . . ."[47] The names found in these inscriptions indicate that the synagogue attracted patrons not merely from Hammat Gader or Gadara, but from around the Galilee and the Golan.[48] In addition, the presence of Roman and Greek names, female donors, and civic titles highlights the distinctiveness of this synagogue when compared to others in the region.[49]

---

[46] Tiberias was reported to have thirteen synagogues of its own (*b. Ber.* 8a). Tiberias and Hammatha (Hammat Tiberias) started out as two separate towns, but the Tosefta indicates that by the time of its composition, the two had merged to form one town (*t. 'Erub.* 5:2).

[47] Sukenik 1935, 39–55.

[48] Benefactors are identified from Sussita, Sepphoris, Kefar Aqavia, Capernaum, and Arbel. See Dauphin 2000, 72–3.

[49] Dvorjetski 2007, 310–11. Based on the unique character of these inscriptions, Dvorjetski (2007, 311) argued that some of the synagogue's benefactors may not have been Jewish, but rather gentile patrons of the *thermae* who thought their financial contributions to the synagogue would facilitate a cure at Hammat Gader. There is no doubt that people of many cultural and religious traditions visited the *thermae*, but neither onomastics nor other details included in the inscriptions offer conclusive proof that gentiles patronized the synagogue while visiting the baths. Female patrons, Greek and Roman names, and Jewish participation in civic offices are attested in other Jewish communities, even if they are relatively uncommon in the immediate vicinity of Hammat Gader. For example, inscriptions from Acmonia and Sardis demonstrate that the Jewish community participated in civic life and held official positions, while inscriptions from Apamea indicate that Jewish women were quite visible in their community. See discussion in Trebilco 1991, 37–126.

84   CONTESTED CURES

The diverse nature of these inscriptions can best be understood as the product of non-local visitors to the bath complex, who commemorated their quest for healing by making dedications at the nearby synagogue.

The relationship between synagogue and bath complex is more visible at Hammat Tiberias. Some of the inscriptions from this synagogue are similar to those found in the bath complex at Hammat Gader. For example, the inscription from the west aisle reads, "May he be remembered for good and for blessing (*mnēsthē eis agathon kai eis eulogian*). Profotouros the elder built this stoa of the holy place (*tou hagiou topou*). A blessing on him. Amen. Shalom."[50] The request that the dedicator be remembered (*mnēsthē*) recalls inscriptions from the Hammat Gader baths, but a second shared phrase is more striking. Both the bath complex and the synagogue are called a "holy place" (*hagios topos*). In other words, visitors to the thermal baths described them in the same language that Jews used to describe their synagogue. A second characteristic of the synagogue inscriptions is also important. Eight inscriptions were placed at the north end of the center aisle of the Hammat Tiberias synagogue; in six of them, the patrons linked their gifts to the fulfillment of a vow or prayer. For example, Maximos commemorated his visit with these words: "Maximos made [this dedication] because he vowed [it] (*Maximos euchomenos epoiēsen*). May he live [long]."[51] Of these eight inscriptions, only the two longer ones do not contain this reference to a vow, likely due to the space constraints. The substance of the patron's vow is not known. However, the promise of a physical offering, in this case an inscription, to express thanks for a miraculous cure was common in the ancient Mediterranean world. These are votive offerings. Given the location of this synagogue in the immediate vicinity of the hot springs, it is quite possible that the vows memorialized in the inscriptions were related to healing experiences at the *thermae*. In fact, by the fifth century CE, it might have seemed more appropriate to Jews that they commemorate their visit to the hot spring at the synagogue rather than inside the bath complex itself, which by that point was dominated by Christian patrons such as Empress Eudokia, whose inscription will be considered below.

Divine healers at the hot springs

In the absence of dedications that explicitly name the divine healers credited with miracles experienced in the *thermae*, we can only speculate about their identity. Greek and Roman visitors may have identified the divine healer as

---

[50] Dothan 1983, 60–2.
[51] Dothan 1983, 55–6.

Asklepios, as he was the healing god par excellence in the Greek world. The most persuasive evidence in Palestine for the link between Asklepios and the hot springs can be found in coins issued by the city of Tiberias that depict Hygieia, the daughter of Asklepios and the goddess of health, sitting on a rock from which a stream emerges, holding a serpent in her right hand and feeding it from a *phialē* in her left hand.[52] The stream depicted on these coins is meant to represent Hammat Tiberias, and the snake invoked Asklepios, to whom the animal was sacred. Hygieia's link to Asklepios was made more explicit in a variation of this type produced in the third century that depicted Hygieia, still with serpent and *phialē*, standing opposite her father Asklepios.[53] Circumstantial evidence from the region of Hammat Gader can perhaps be found in an inscription set up by a man named Asklepios and in carved gemstones depicting Asklepios and Hygieia found in Umm Qais (ancient Gadara), which could reflect the god's popularity in the region.[54] Serapis, who was also known as a healer and who was likely associated with Asklepios at a cult site in Jerusalem beginning in the second century CE, was popular on gemstones from Umm Qais and could have been another divine healer to whom visitors to the hot springs appealed.[55]

While we cannot rule out that Christian visitors might have expected to see Jesus during an incubation dream, the Piacenza Pilgrim's description of Hammat Gader mentions another potential divine healer who would have resonated with both Jews and Christians. The pilgrimage diary describes Hammat Gader as a place with "hot springs called the Baths of Elijah (*termas Heliae*). Lepers are cleansed there . . ."[56] This tells us two things: first, that in the sixth century the baths were named for the prophet Elijah, and second, that healing at this time was particularly associated with lepers, although this does not mean people did not visit the site for other types of cures too.

---

[52] Rosenberger 1977, 64, nos. 6–7; Meshorer 1985, 24, no. 78. For a similar coin minted later under Commodus, see Rosenberger 1977, 16. For the city coins issued in Roman Palestine, including those issued by Tiberias, and their implications for understanding the local Jewish population, see Schwartz 2001, 136–42.

[53] Rosenberger 1977, 67, no. 19; Meshorer 1985, 35, no. 86. Asklepios and Hygieia also appear on coins from Neapolis (McCasland 1939b, 225; Rosenberger 1977, 6, no. 6; 17, no. 74; 21, nos. 98 and 102; Meshorer 1985, 49, nos. 127–8). Among the coins from Gadara are some that depict the Three Graces and Herakles, which Dvorjetski (2007, 355–9) suggests were associated with the bath complex in its early days. While Herakles was sometimes seen as a patron of hot springs, there is no evidence either he or the Three Graces were said to have appeared in incubation dreams. For the patronage of hot springs by Herakles and Asklepios, see Croon 1967.

[54] Di Segni 1997, no. 5; Henig et al. 1987, 21, nos. 185–91.

[55] Henig et al. 1987, 9–10, nos. 26–38.

[56] *Itin. Plac.* 7.

86 CONTESTED CURES

The association between lepers and Elijah was likely based on the story of Na'aman, who in the Hebrew Bible was healed from this disease after immersing himself seven times in the Jordan River.[57] While it was not actually the prophet Elijah who performed this miracle, but rather his student Elisha, it would seem that in the region surrounding Hammat Gader, Elisha's deed was assimilated to the reputation of the far more popular Elijah.[58] Indeed, already in the fourth century, pilgrims such as Egeria were being shown the cave of Elijah on the east side of the Jordan River in the region of Gilead, not far from the hot springs.[59]

Elijah was also associated with Hammat Gader in the century before the Piacenza Pilgrim wrote his account. When Empress Eudokia visited the site in the middle of the fifth century, she composed a poetic inscription that was set into the pavement of the Hall of Fountains (Figure 3.1, area D). Her inscription lists sixteen parts of the bath complex, one of which she calls "pure Elijah" (*Ēlias hagnos*):

> Of the Empress Eudokia
> In my life many and infinite wonders have I seen
> But who, however many his mouths, could proclaim, O noble Clibanus
> By your strength, having been born a worthless mortal? But rather
> It is just that you be called a new fiery ocean.   5
> Paean and life source, provider of sweet streams.
> From you is born the infinite swell, here, once there another.
> On this side boiling, but there in turn cold and tepid.
> You pour forth your beauty into four tetrads of springs.
> An Indian woman and a matron; Repentinus; pure Elijah;   10
> Good Antoninus; dewy Galatia and

---

[57] 2 Kgs 5:1–14. The "leprosy" mentioned by the Piacenza Pilgrim and in 2 Kgs 5 was likely not the disease known today as "leprosy" or Hansen's disease, but rather a generic term used to refer to a number of skin ailments. See discussion in Hulse 1975. The story from the medieval *Midrash ha-Gadol* (Deut 26:19), mentioned earlier, describes Hadrian meeting a girl covered in sores as he made his way from Hammat Gader to Gadara. If this account preserves a historical memory, it suggests that Hammat Gader held special appeal for those with skin conditions back to the second century CE. It is worth noting that the *Life of Hadrian* in the *HA* also describes the emperor as having suffered from a skin condition (*De vita Hadriani* 26). Although material from the *HA* must be treated with healthy skepticism, Epiphanius also attributes "leprosy" to the emperor (*On Measures and Weights* 14). In addition to Hammat Gader, the Piacenza Pilgrim notes three other sites in Palestine where lepers bathed and received healing: Hammei Livias and the Baths of Moses (10) and the Pool of Siloam (24).

[58] Hirschfeld 1997, 5. Shimon Gibson argues that confusion between Elijah and Elisha arose among the followers of John the Baptist, and that this caused the two figures to be merged in later tradition, such as seen at Hammat Gader. For John the Baptist as the disciple and forerunner of Elijah *redivivus*, see Gibson 2004, 142–4.

[59] *Itin. Eger.* 16.1, 3.

Hygieia herself; the large warm (baths) and the small warm (baths);
The Pearl; the old Clibanus; an Indian woman and also another
Matron; the strong (woman) and the nun, and the (spring) of the Patriarch.
For those in pain your mighty strength (is ever constant).   15
But (I will sing) of god, famous for wisdom . . .
For the benefit of men and . . .[60]

Eudokia's inscription confirms that Elijah was connected with the hot spring by
the fifth century CE, but I would suggest that it also allows for the possibility of
a much earlier association. Efforts have been made to associate the "four tetrads
of springs" found in the inscription's second column with a set of sixteen fountains or pools in the archaeological remains. While this has not been possible, Di
Segni must nevertheless be correct that the names corresponded in some way to
"individual parts of the baths or elements of the water system" that Eudokia saw
as she toured the site.[61] Our inability to locate the features does not negate the
fact that the inscription presents them as identifiable elements within the bath
complex. Among the eponymous names given to these "springs" are two that
date to the second century CE. The oldest identifiable name in the inscription
is in line 11, *Antōninos eus* ("good Antoninus"), a shortened form of *Antōninos
eusebēs*, the name by which the emperor Antoninus Pius was known in the
East. As the successor of Hadrian, whom we saw a late rabbinic tradition placed
at Hammat Gader, Antoninus Pius may have also visited the site and contributed to its beautification.[62] Another early patron, Repentinus, is found in line
10. Since the original excavations at Hammat Gader, a new Latin inscription
was uncovered that sheds light on this Repentius. The inscription mentions a
vexillatio of the Sixth Legion and ascribes some or all of the site's construction
to it at the end of the second century. Sex. Cornelius Repentinus is named as
the *leg(ato) Aug(usti) pr(o) pr(aetore)*, under whose command a *vexillatio* of *Legio
VI Ferratae* completed a building project.[63] The name Repentinus is otherwise not attested in this region, making it highly probable that the Repentinus
mentioned in Eudokia's inscription was this same governor.[64] According to
Werner Eck, enough is known about the career of Cornelius Repentinus that
the legion's dedicatory inscription must be dated to between 189 and 192 CE.[65]

---

[60] This translation is a slightly modified version of the one published by Green and Tsafrir 1982,
77–91.

[61] Di Segni 1997, 230.

[62] Werner Eck argues that Commodus, not Antoninus Pius, was the emperor for whom part of
the bath complex was named. Since both emperors had the name Antoninus, he suggests that
Eudokia was simply confused when she composed this text (2014, 214).

[63] Eck 2014, 212–14.

[64] Green and Tsafrir 1982, 87–8.

[65] Eck 2014, 213.

88 CONTESTED CURES

Antoninus Pius and Repentinus, therefore, were likely both associated with the *thermae* from its early years, and it may be that the "springs" named for the two were in an older part of the bath complex. Sandwiched between these two second-century names is Elijah. If Elijah was also associated with an older part of the building, as his appearance with Antoninus Pius and Repentinus might indicate, then we could have evidence for a long-standing association between Elijah and the hot springs. Thus, as a famed local wonderworker from the Hebrew Bible, Elijah's name was given to part of the baths, alongside the names of important benefactors and figures from Greek myth, such as Hygieia and the nymph Galatea.

A story from the Yerushalmi that attributes a miraculous cure to Elijah may also suggest a connection between the prophet and Hammat Gader. This episode concerns R. Judah ha-Nasi, who was considered one of the most important teachers of the Tannaitic era and who was credited with the compilation of the Mishnah. He was plagued with numerous physical ailments, and it has been observed that of all the sages identified in the Talmudic writings, we know more about R. Judah's health, or to be more precise his ill health, than we do about any other.[66] Details about his symptoms, remedies, and personal physician are numerous, and scholars have expended considerable effort trying to diagnose his underlying conditions.[67] Among the many medical complaints that rabbinic texts attributed to R. Judah was a prolonged toothache:

> Jehudah lived in Sepphoris seventeen years. Of these he suffered from toothache for thirteen years . . . At the end of thirteen years and thirty days, Elijah visited him [Rebbi] in the likeness of the older Rebbi Hiyya. He said to him, how does my lord feel? He said to him, one tooth hurts me. He said to him, show it to me. He showed it to him, he put his finger on it and it was healed. The next day, the older Rebbi Hiyya came to him and asked him, how does Rebbi feel, what is with that tooth? He said to him, from the moment that you put your finger on it, it was healed.[68]

The appearance of the prophet Elijah in this passage marks a significant departure from accounts of him in the Hebrew Bible and rabbinic texts. In biblical stories, Elijah was known for his prophecies and for his ability to bend the laws of nature. For example, Elijah orchestrated a three-year drought and later caused it to rain (1 Kgs 17–18), and he brought about the spontaneous

---

[66] Dvorjetski 2002, 39.

[67] For investigations of R. Judah's medical diagnosis, see Guttmann 1954; Shoshan 1977; Dvorjetski 2000; Dvorjetski 2002.

[68] *y. Ketub.* 12:3 (34d–35b). All translations of the Yerushalmi are from Guggenheimer 2000.

combustion of a water-laden altar (1 Kgs 18:36–40). While Elijah did perform a healing miracle in the raising of the widow's son (1 Kgs 17:17–23), such cures were not commonly ascribed to him in the Hebrew Bible. Talmudic accounts of Elijah likewise credit him with miracles, but Kristen Lindbeck demonstrated that most of these miracles do not relate to illnesses or physical ailments.[69] Rather, they revolve around a disguised Elijah rescuing a Jewish protagonist from a dangerous predicament. In fact, the episode in which Elijah heals R. Judah's toothache is one of only two stories in the Talmud when the prophet was said to have healed someone.[70] The general lack of miraculous cures credited to Elijah in both biblical and rabbinic literature becomes more prominent in light of his association with Hammat Gader.

I propose that the story of R. Judah's thirteen-year toothache and his vision of Elijah as the agent of his cure were not informed by the accounts of Elijah found in the Hebrew Bible or elsewhere in the Talmud, where the prophet rarely performed miraculous cures. Rather, by the time that the Yerushalmi with its story of R. Judah's toothache was redacted, a long-standing link between Elijah and Hammat Gader may have conditioned rabbinic authors to see the prophet as a source of healing, a connection that manifested itself in the story about the rabbi's toothache. Furthermore, the Yerushalmi says that R. Judah's pain was relieved through a dream or vision, the effects of which persisted in the waking world. Epiphanies of this sort are precisely the way that healing frequently occurred through incubation, according to the well-known testimonies from the cult of Asklepios. This detail underscores the likelihood that the rituals practiced at Hammat Gader were a form of incubation and that these rituals informed the story about R. Judah's toothache. The possibility that Asklepios and Elijah coexisted at Hammat Gader as divine healers for different groups of visitors has a certain logic, as Elijah's miracles and fiery chariot to heaven (2 Kgs 2) parallel Asklepios' wondrous cures and divine ascent in Greek myth.

* * *

It is hard to conceptualize how a site such as Hammat Gader could have been so many things to so many different people. How do leisure and ritual activities

---

[69] Lindbeck 2010, 95–135.

[70] The other rabbinic story in which Elijah heals someone has a comedic element and may have been intended as a lesson to readers. Elijah appeared to Rav Shimi bar Ashi, who had swallowed a snake. To get rid of the snake, Elijah instructed him to eat a gourd with salt and to commence running; over the course of a three-mile run, the snake was expelled (b. Šabb. 109b). There is a nearly identical story in which Rav Shimi is not the patient, but rather the miracle-worker, and it is unclear which version is older. See discussion in Lindbeck 2010, 107.

coexist in the same space? How do Jews and Christians pursue ritual healing alongside devotees of Asklepios? It is tempting to see in the Piacenza Pilgrim's description a way to relieve the first of these tensions – that is, between the ritual and leisurely uses of the bath complex. Antoninus described an incubation ritual that took place at night and specified that the doors were closed, perhaps to prevent access by anyone not participating in the ritual. It might be inferred that by the sixth century the hot spring was open to everyone during the day, while those expressly seeking healing came at night. From a purely practical perspective, the absence of crowds of pleasure-seekers in the baths might produce a setting that would be more conducive for incubation dreams. This suggestion does not preclude the possibility that visitors to the baths during the day might have also experienced divine epiphanies to which they attributed miraculous cures, but it nevertheless offers a plausible explanation for how the hot springs were able to accommodate the different reasons that people had for visiting them.

In response to the second question, about the coexistence of multiple traditions, nothing more than conjecture can be offered. Seth Schwartz has argued that the religious behavior of Jews living in Greco-Roman cities may have been largely indistinguishable from their non-Jewish neighbors, and I suggest that Jewish incubation at the hot springs would support this contention.[71] The preliminary rites that Jews, Christians, and supplicants of Asklepios completed – including offerings and purifications such as known from the cult of Asklepios or prayer and reception of the Eucharist among Christians – would have distinguished these groups.[72] The synagogue and church excavated at Hammat Gader near the *thermae* would have accommodated these preliminary prayers for their respective communities.[73] An observation that Nicole Belayche made on the ability of multiple religious traditions to coexist in the Galilee perfectly accounts for the situation at the hot springs:

> The nature of the religions (pagan and monotheistic) present in the region largely explains what historically appears to be informed cohabitation but without intermingling. It is impossible to speak here of 'syncretism'; . . . Rather, we find a successful integration without religious acculturation.[74]

[71] Schwartz 1998, 207.
[72] For Christian preparatory rites, see Ehrenheim 2009, 269.
[73] It has been suggested that a temple was located on or near the site of this church, which could have accommodated preparatory rituals of some visitors. See discussion in Sukenik 1935, 30; Hirschfeld 1987, 113; Belayche 2001, 271; cf. Graf 2015, 244; Renberg 2016, 2:812, n. 7.
[74] Belayche 2001, 86.

At the hot springs, separation of preparatory rites from the incubation could have facilitated this "cohabitation." Inside the bath complex itself, in contrast, visitors may have been indistinguishable from each other, since the encounter with the divine healer was a private religious experience. A dream epiphany offered direct and personal contact between the supplicant and the divine.

In the end, I would suggest that the primary difference between the incubation experiences among visitors to the hot springs was the identity of the divine healer whom visitors expected to see. On any given night, one person might dream of Asklepios while his or her neighbors saw Elijah, Jesus, or Serapis. This coexistence of ritual traditions within the same space recalls the situation at Mamre, with which this chapter began. In his introduction to Mamre and other shared ritual sites, Rangar Cline made the following observation that resonates with our discussion of the thermal-mineral springs:

> . . . prior to the fourth century many of the participants in rituals at these sites may not have thought much about worshipping alongside those of different religious traditions, because they believed that the presence of those belonging to different religious traditions could not impugn the ritual power of the site.[75]

---

[75] Cline 2011, 105.

CHAPTER 4

In Which Many Miracles Are Worked: Ritual Continuity at Healing Sites

A site sometimes grouped with the hot springs discussed in the previous chapter is Emmaus. Located a short distance west of Jerusalem, along the road between Jerusalem and Jaffa, Emmaus was renamed Nikopolis in 223 to mark its new civic status. At Emmaus is the intersection of two kinds of sacred sites in Palestine. First, its Greek name "Emmaus" derives from the Hebrew "Ḥammat" and suggests that the site was named for a local hot spring.[1] To the inherent sacredness of the spring, a second characteristic was added: an association with the life of Jesus. An account given by Sozomen adds a detail to the story about the post-resurrection appearance of Jesus not found in the canonical version in Luke 24:13–34:

> Just beyond the city where three roads meet, is the spot where Christ, after His resurrection, said farewell to Cleopas and his companion, as if he were going to another village; and here is a healing fountain in which men and other living creatures afflicted with different diseases wash away their sufferings; for it is said that when Christ together with His disciples came from a journey to this fountain, they bathed their feet therein, and, from that time the water became a cure for disorders.[2]

[1] While its name indicates the presence of a hot spring, archaeological excavations have not identified a thermal-mineral spring in the area. Mordechai Gichon (1979, 102) pointed out that the absence of modern hot springs in the area does not preclude their presence in antiquity, as the water could have been stopped by one of several significant seismic events. For the possibility that the name could designate a spring understood to be miraculous, regardless of the water's temperature, see discussion in Dvorjetski 2007, 208, 216.

[2] Sozomen *Hist. Eccl.* 5.21 (*NPNF* 2/2:561–2). For additional references to Emmaus, see Avi-Yonah 1976, 55; Baldi 1982, 706–18; Tsafrir et al. 1994, 119–20; Dvorjetski 2007, 208–23. Dvorjetski (1997, 567–71) proposed that the spring at Emmaus was already known to be therapeutic in the first century CE and that Vespasian situated the *Legio V Macedonia* camp at Emmaus in part to enable him to make use of the spring. See also Belayche 2001, 65.

As in Chapter 3, water is again the central feature of this story. However, Sozomen omits any reference to a hot spring, and it is not clear whether he knew anything about the water's properties. The salient detail for Sozomen was the extra-biblical tradition about Jesus washing in a fountain. According to Sozomen, Jesus' unremarkable use of the fountain to wash dirty feet transformed it into a source of healing, not just for every sort of human ailment, but also for animals.

Emmaus thus became a destination for Christian visitors, drawn both to a site from the life of Jesus and to a place that promised miraculous cures. In this regard, Emmaus was not unique. This chapter focuses on two healing sites that similarly became stops on the pilgrimage route of early Christians: the Pool of Bethesda in Jerusalem and Shuni/'Ein Tzur, located northeast of Caesarea. In the former case, abundant literary evidence confirms the continuity of ritual healing as the site changed hands, with an event from the life of Jesus solidifying its significance for Christians. Pilgrims flocked to the Pool of Bethesda, and many miracles were reported as taking place within its precincts. The situation at Shuni/'Ein Tzur is very different. A single sentence in a pilgrimage text puts it on the map as a therapeutic site, but no connection to Jesus' life is known. That is not to say definitively that no such tradition ever existed, but only that if it did, it has long since been lost to time. Lacking detailed literary accounts, it is on the basis of archaeological evidence alone that the continuity of ritual practice can be posited for Shuni/'Ein Tzur.

At both the Pool of Bethesda and Shuni/'Ein Tzur, therefore, we have examples of the continuity of cult. The Christian transformation of earlier healing sites, with the modification of old rituals or the introductions of new ones, enabled miraculous cures to persist in a way that transcended the shifts in the cultural or religious self-identification of the site's visitors.[3] This is somewhat different than the argument made in Chapter 3. There is no doubt that the hot springs of Palestine changed hands, with the initial development of the sites taking place under the auspices of non-Jewish and non-Christian elites before eventually coming under the control of Christians in late antiquity. Yet the argument in Chapter 3 focused on the possibility of the coexistence of cult, with visitors from multiple communities using the hot springs at the same time. No such argument is being made for the Pool of Bethesda and Shuni/'Ein Tzur. As a result, they do not warrant the disapproval of the patristic authors who will be considered in Chapter 7, and since there is no evidence of incubation at these sites, they likewise do not fall under elite censure of this

---

[3] For a classic treatment of similar phenomena, whereby earlier cult sites are incorporated into later ones belonging to new religious communities, see the discussion of "archaic" pilgrimage in Turner and Turner 2011 [1978]. In the Christian context, this calls to mind the famous letter of Gregory the Great to Abbot Mellitus, instructing him to Christianize the temples and festivals of the people whom he encountered in Britain in order to facilitate their conversion to Christianity (Bede *Hist. Eccl.* 1.30; cf. Gregory the Great *Ep.* 76.

94 CONTESTED CURES

practice. In fact, the Pool of Bethesda was normalized within the liturgical life of Jerusalem, suggesting that Christian authorities approved of, and perhaps even managed, the healing rites that took place there.

There is something about the conversion of earlier sacred sites into new ones that serve the needs of a conquering people or a newly ascendant religion that captures the imagination, both in antiquity and today. In a region as fraught with religious significance and conflict as Palestine, there is considerable interest in these processes. As a result, scholars have, from time to time, proposed that additional healing sites similarly maintained a reputation for cures amid the political and religious transformations of ancient Palestine. In the concluding pages of this chapter, three such sites will be examined briefly to sketch additional options for ritual healing and to re-examine the evidence needed to demonstrate continuity at any given site.

The Pool of Bethesda

The Pool of Bethesda in Jerusalem enjoyed a long tradition of ritual healing that persisted despite the region's political transformations. The New Testament locates a miracle of Jesus there, narrated only in the Gospel of John, and this episode would have lasting implications for the site's association with ritual cures:

> Now in Jerusalem by the Sheep Gate there is a pool,[4] called in Hebrew Bethzatha, which has five porticoes (*stoas*). In these lay many invalids – blind, lame, and paralyzed.[5] One man was there who had been ill for thirty-eight years. When Jesus saw him lying there and knew that he had been there a long time, he said to him, "Do you want to be made well?" The sick man answered him, "Sir, I have no one to put me into the pool when the water is stirred up; and while I am making my way, someone else steps down ahead of me." Jesus said to him, "Stand up, take your mat and walk." At once the man was made well, and he took up his mat and began to walk.[6]

The author of John implies that in the late Second Temple period, the Pool of Bethesda attracted visitors for its healing properties. The paralytic in this story

[4] The site is sometimes referred to as the Probatic (*probatikos*) Pool, for the reference in John to its location at the Sheep Gate.

[5] John 5:3b–4 is not found in the earliest manuscripts but is inserted at this point in later manuscripts.

[6] John 5:2–3a, 5–9. For textual difficulties in verse 2, alternate spellings, etymologies of the pool's name, and the use of the dual in the Copper Scroll, perhaps reflecting the two pools, see Jeremias 1966, 9–12, 34–6; Wilkinson 1978, 95–6; Küchler 1994, 130–8; Wahlde 2006b, 559–62; Charlesworth 2011, 1–3.

describes a custom in which people attempted to enter the pool before others, either by descending into it on their own or by being put in by someone else, with the expectation that the first person into the water would be healed. The signal that people were to enter the pool was the water being "stirred up." The oldest papyri copies of the pericope and the earliest uncial manuscripts include no additional details explaining these circumstances. However, beginning in the fifth century, copies of John include the following between the list of visitors' physical afflictions in verse 3 and the introduction of the man who would be healed in verse 5:

> . . . waiting for the stirring of the water; for an angel of the Lord went down at certain seasons into the pool and stirred up the water; whoever stepped in first after the stirring of the water was made well from whatever disease that person had. (John 5:3b–4)

Due to the absence of these verses in the earliest copies of John 5, most scholars assume that they constitute a later gloss included to supplement the otherwise imprecise details about the nature of the tradition.[7] Even without the added text, the author of this story would have readers believe that a healing cult existed at the Pool of Bethesda in the first century CE and that Jews were numbered among its patrons.

Widespread consensus now holds that the Pool of Bethesda described in John 5 is located on the grounds of the Church of St. Anne, situated just inside the Old City of Jerusalem near the Lion's Gate (St. Stephen's Gate).[8] Explorations of the site began in the mid-nineteenth century, after it was gifted to the French government in recognition of its contributions during the Crimean War.[9]

---

[7] For the manuscript tradition and textual analyses of John 5 see, for example, Brown 1966, 207; Duprez 1970, 129–30; Schnackenburg 1990, 94–5.

[8] Among those who see the site at the Church of St. Anne as the setting for the John 5 narrative are Jeremias 1966, 36–8; Wahlde 2009, 132–5; Gibson 2011, 25–7.

[9] For the history of the site in the nineteenth and twentieth centuries, see Jeremias 1966, 25–32; Duprez 1970, 28–33; Gibson 2011, 17–20; Dauphin 2011a; Wahlde 2013, 268–72. Today it is held by the Pères Blancs, who maintain a monastery on the site and who have a French academic team to advise them. Although a number of short studies and articles have been published, a comprehensive site report has not yet been produced. The politics of archaeological excavation and publication have complicated the situation, and while today the site is open to the general public, the finds themselves are generally inaccessible. For the details about the French acquisition of the site and subsequent excavations, see Dauphin 2011a. For the archaeological remains, see Mauss 1888; Masterman 1905; Vincent 1926, 669–73, 685–98; Vliet 1938, 139–55; Jeremias 1966; Benoit 1967; Duprez 1970; Mackowski and Nalbandian 1980, 79–83; Pierre and Rousée 1981; Devillers 1999; Belayche 2001, 160–7; Baert 2005; Dauphin 2005; Gibson 2005; Gibson 2009, 59–80; Wahlde 2009; Abed Rabbo 2011; Arnould-Béhar 2011; Berman 2011; Dauphin 2011b; Dauphin 2011c; Gibson 2011; Kingsley 2011.

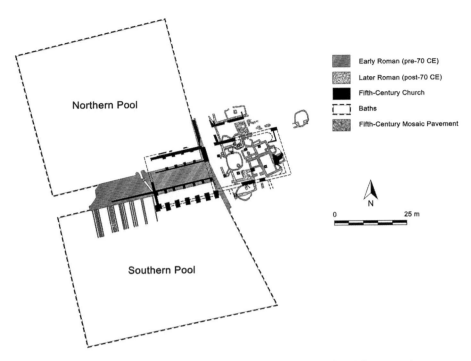

Figure 4.1 Plan of the Pool of Bethesda (Drawing by D. Weiss, after Gibson 2011)

Excavations have revealed complex remains, whose western and eastern portions seem to have developed along different lines (see Figure 4.1). The relationship between the two parts of the site, at least until the fifth century CE, and the precise nature of the construction in the eastern part have been the subject of significant scholarly disagreement. Shimon Gibson argued persuasively in 2005 that the two large pools on the western side of the site functioned as a *miqveh* and an *ostar*, an interpretation that is now fairly well accepted.[10] A *miqveh* is a Jewish ritual bath; immersion in it rendered the bather ritually pure. Given the pool's large size and proximity to the Temple Mount, located a short distance to its south, it was a natural stopping place for pilgrims and would have accommodated crowds who arrived in Jerusalem for annual festivals. These visitors could immerse before proceeding to the temple courts.[11]

The southern of the two pools was the *miqveh*, identifiable by the steps hewn into the rock on the west side, which facilitated ritual immersion. The

---

[10] Gibson 2005. Yoel Elitzur (2008) dissented from this consensus, claiming instead that the pools of Siloam and Bethesda were swimming pools.

[11] For the use of water by pilgrims to Jerusalem in the late Second Temple period, see Gurevich 2017, 119–29.

ostar was located immediately to its north and collected rainwater, which was used to replenish the water in the *miqveh*. A tunnel in the wall that separated the two pools allowed water from the northern pool to flow into the southern one when a gate was lifted. Replenishing the *miqveh*'s water in this way reflects the requirements for a *miqveh* that would later be codified in the Mishnah.[12] Opinion is divided as to whether the two pools were constructed at the same time or whether the northern pool preceded the southern. Given the challenges of dating rock-cut features such as the pools, suggestions for the original construction of the northern pool range from the Iron Age to the building program of Herod the Great. Those who think that the northern pool predated the southern suppose that it functioned originally as a reservoir, before being converted into an *ostar*.[13]

The earliest reference to the site after the New Testament is Origen's third-century *Commentary on John*, which describes the arrangement of the five stoas mentioned in John 5:2. According to Origen, four of the porticoes surrounded the pools and a fifth was situated between them.[14] In the fourth century, Cyril of Jerusalem gave the same arrangement of the five stoas and added that it was in the fifth one that the sick gathered to await healing.[15] Correlating Origen's and Cyril's testimonies to what we know of the archaeological remains, this would suggest that the fifth stoa was built on the wall that separated the *miqveh* from the *ostar*. Given the destruction inflicted on Jerusalem in 70 CE and the mixed testimony as to whether the five stoas were still standing in subsequent centuries, some scholars have questioned whether Origen and Cyril could be certain of the site's original layout.[16] Jerome Murphy-O'Connor further noted

---

[12] For discussion of rabbinic regulations for *miqva'ot* in light of the Pool of Bethesda, see Gibson 2005.

[13] For the argument that the northern pool was earlier than the southern, see Pierre and Rousée 1981, 24–5; Wahlde 2009, 121–3; Wahlde 2013, 269–72; cf. Wahlde 2006a. Wahlde (2013, 277–9) argues that the conversion of earlier reservoirs to accommodate ritual immersion at the Pool of Bethesda and at the Pool of Siloam should both be dated the second century BCE and reflect increased attention to ritual purity. For the argument that the northern and southern pools were constructed at the same time, see Jeremias 1966, 33; Gibson 2011, 23–5.

[14] Preuschen 1903, 532–3, fragment 61.

[15] Cyril of Jerusalem *Homily on the Paralytic* 2. Theodore of Mopsuestia also repeats this information about the arrangement of the stoas in his *Commentary on the Gospel of John*. For text and translation, see Jeremias 1966, 18, n. 39.

[16] Wilkinson (1978, 103) suggested that Origen's description of the arrangement of the five porticoes around the pools and across the wall that separated them was an attempt to accommodate the biblical text to what he could see at the site in his own time, and seemed to expect that some other arrangement of stoas was more likely, "What the five porches were like or where they were can therefore be known only by further archaeological work – if indeed anything of them has survived." This would open the possibility that the five stoas known to the author of John were much smaller components of the eastern part of the site, making the absence of first-century columns among the archaeological excavations somewhat less problematic.

98   CONTESTED CURES

that, given the very large size of the two pools revealed in the excavations, such a plan would have required between one and two hundred columns. However, not a single column dating to the correct period has been found at the site.[17] The surviving column fragments are too late to support a stoa that would have been known by the author of John. The absence of this archaeological evidence is one reason that some scholars have sought the setting for the story in John 5 in the remains on the eastern part of the site.[18]

The first-century CE architectural remains to the east of the *miqveh-ostar* have been interpreted alternatively as a healing site or the basement of a building. The underground spaces consist of a large cistern, a number of plastered basins, and several small pools or baths. Antoine Duprez determined that these underground rooms underwent two distinct periods of use, one before the destruction of the Jerusalem temple and one after it. While Duprez would ultimately argue that the space had a ritual function in both phases, he recognized that there was no evidence for ritual activity in the grottos prior to the destruction of the Temple, that is, while the *miqveh* was still used for its intended purpose immediately to the west. The argument for these underground chambers being used for healing rituals in the first century CE rests on two factors: first, the continuity of sacred space – if it was a cult site after the foundation of Aelia Capitolina, it was probably a cult site before the destruction too – and second, the presumed ritual character of the water installations.[19] In contrast, Shimon Gibson re-examined the archaeological remains and concluded that while the subterranean grottos did in fact undergo these two different phases of use, they had no ritual function during either phase. Gibson argued that they were simply the basement of an adjacent building, and that the cistern and baths played no role in healing rituals.[20]

The establishment of the Roman colony of Aelia Capitolina following the Bar Kokhba revolt brought many changes to Jerusalem, among them a healing cult in the eastern section of the St. Anne site. Votive offerings confirm

[17] Murphy-O'Connor 2012, 430; see also Benoit 1967, 56. Given the frequency with which ancient building material has been reused, modified, and moved in the intervening two thousand years, Wahlde does not find the absence of these columns to be persuasive evidence that the five stoas were not laid out as described and suggests that some of the surviving columns may have been Herodian but were reworked into their present form in the Byzantine period (2009, 123–5).

[18] Among those who see the healing of John 5 situated in the eastern part of the site are Benoit 1967, 55; Duprez 1970, 38; Wilkinson 1978, 102–4; Pierre and Rousée 1981, 26; Ovadiah and Turnheim 2011, 82.

[19] Duprez 1970, 38–43; see also Wilkinson 1978, 102–4; Pierre and Rousée 1981, 26–7. There seem to have been periods in which the site fell out of regular use, such as between the destruction of the Jerusalem temple in 70 CE and the founding of Aelia Capitolina in 135 CE, but the memory of this site's association with healing may have persisted despite these gaps.

[20] Gibson 2011.

the presence of a therapeutic site, but the exact location of its temple remains unclear. Some have speculated that it stood on the foundations uncovered between the Crusader church of St. Anne and the *miqveh*. Adding weight to this suggestion is the presence of a large quantity of ashes, including pig bones, in a *favissa* immediately to the north of these foundations.[21] Pig bones in a previously Jewish city point to a non-Jewish presence, and the burial of the bones in a pit to keep them within the sanctuary may indicate that animal sacrifice had become part of the ritual activity at the site.[22]

Unlike the rather fragmentary architectural evidence, the votive offerings are more straightforward. Two dedications show female supplicants. The first is a marble relief of a reclining, naked woman with the hand of an unknown person extended to her, in a pose reminiscent of fifth-century BCE Attic reliefs of Asklepios and Amphiaraos. The second is a terracotta figurine of a woman who seems to be dressing or indicating a place on her body that was healed. Both make sense as votive offerings in a healing cult. A third votive can also be understood as expressing thanks to the god for healing. It is in the shape of a foot and carries the inscription *Ponpēia Loukilia anethēken*, "Pompeia Lucilia dedicated (this)."[23] Although the dedicatory inscription was written in Greek, the woman's name is Latin. Votive feet are particularly common dedications to Serapis, and a fourth votive relief seems to identify Serapis as the god worshipped in this sanctuary. Two non-contiguous fragments of a third-century relief depict a god with a serpent body and a bearded, human head wearing a *modius*, which scholars have interpreted as Serapis.[24] The deity is pictured along with two ears of wheat, situated in the middle of four columns surmounted by a pediment.[25] The remaining two votive dedications, models of merchant ships, are somewhat more unusual in the context of a healing shrine. However, Duprez argued that they further support the identification of Serapis as the god of this shrine, as he was known for protecting those

---

[21] Duprez (1970, 54 and pl. III) labeled these foundations as no. 12 and the area where the ashes and pig bones were found as no. 13. Pierre and Rousée labeled this latter area as a *favissa*. See also Pierre and Rousée 1981; Belayche 2001, 164.

[22] It should be noted that pork was regularly consumed by the Roman army and that pig bones are therefore a regular component of the faunal deposit wherever the Roman army was present, as it was in Aelia Capitolina. See Weksler-Bdolah 2014, 55–6.

[23] For other examples of feet as votive dedications at shrines of Serapis, see Dow and Upson 1944; Le Glay 1978.

[24] It can be expected that at a healing sanctuary such as this in the Greek East, Serapis would have been assimilated to Asklepios, and so this installation at the Pool of Bethesda site is often referred to as a cult of Serapis-Asklepios. For the assimilation of Serapis to Asklepios in Palestine and elsewhere in the Greco-Roman world, see Duprez 1970; Pearcy 1988, 377–8.

[25] Duprez 1970, 49–50; Arnould-Béhar 2011. It should be noted that some do not see these two fragments as belonging to the same relief. For example, see Eliav 2005, 113–14, especially fig. 12.

who traveled by sea.[26] This collection of votives offers a few insights into the sanctuary's clientele. First, it is clear that the site was popular among women, as three of the six published votives can be attributed to female supplicants. Second, the only name preserved on these votives is a Latin one, even though the inscription was written in Greek. This likely reflects the cult's status among the households of the Roman residents of Aelia Capitolina who filled military and administrative roles. We may also speculate that the two ship votives were dedications of merchants visiting the city.

It is likely that the zenith of the site as a sanctuary dedicated to Serapis, or possibly Serapis-Asklepios, was the period between the creation of Aelia Capitolina and the departure of *Legio X Fretensis* for Aila (modern Aqaba) in the late third century CE.[27] The third century also marks the first post-biblical Christian reference, that of Origen, to the Pool of Bethesda, permitting the possibility that Christians visited it to commemorate the Gospel story while it still functioned as a Roman healing sanctuary. Writers from the third century to the first half of the fifth century – including Origen, Eusebius (and Jerome's translation of Eusebius), the Bordeaux Pilgrim, Cyril of Jerusalem, Eucherius, and Theodore of Mopsuestia – regularly included it among the key sites to see in Jerusalem.[28] These descriptions draw on the biblical text, but also introduce details that were likely told to pilgrims visiting the site – storytelling that anyone who has visited Jerusalem today can easily imagine.[29] Some particulars were intended to explain the conditions that pilgrims observed on the ground, such as the tradition that one of the pools had red water because sacrificial animals had been washed in it. Others may have reflected theological concerns or attempts to inscribe Christian superiority onto the religious topography of Jerusalem. For example, the Bordeaux Pilgrim situates a description of the Pool of Bethesda between two references to Solomon; the first reference was to pools that Solomon was said to have built, and the second to a crypt where he was said to have tortured demons. As we will see in Chapter 5, Solomon was known in late antiquity as someone who possessed superior power to control demons and thereby expel sicknesses. Oded Irshai argues that the juxtaposition of Solomon and the Pool of Bethesda was a deliberate move by the

---

[26] Duprez 1970, 52–3. See also Belayche 2001, 166–7.

[27] Belayche 2001, 163, cf. 10.

[28] Eusebius *Onom.* 240; *Bordeaux Pilgrim* 589; Eucherius *Letter to Faustus* 127.8. Ancient testimonies about pilgrimage sites have been collected in Baldi 1982; Wilkinson 1999; Wilkinson 2002. For the suggestion that some traits ascribed to the Pool of Bethesda in these sources are the result of authors transposing features from the Pool of Siloam in the southern portion of the city to the Pool of Bethesda on the north side of the Temple Mount and vice versa, see Jeremias 1966, 14–16; Wahlde 2006a, 243; Wahlde 2009, 125–7.

[29] For the types of stories told about these sites, see discussion by Wilkinson 2002, 64–5.

Bordeaux Pilgrim to prove that Jesus' miracles were superior to Solomon's healing powers and to highlight Jesus' "acts of salvation."[30]

Sometime in the fifth century a church was built at the Pool of Bethesda; John Rufus mentioned it in the *Life of Peter the Iberian* as the "church of the Paralytic" and in *Plerophoria* as the "church of the Probatic Pool."[31] It soon came to be associated not only with Jesus' raising of the paralytic but also with the birth of Mary.[32] This latter commemoration explains the name of the Crusader church that still stands today: St. Anne, the mother of Mary.[33] The Byzantine basilica on the site was built to the east of the *miqveh-ostar*, with the nave covering the portion of the site where the cult of Serapis-Asklepios seems to have been located.[34] The arches and piers that supported the basilica's atrium, to the west of the nave, are still visible today, rising from the floor of the *miqveh*. That this was an important church in Jerusalem is reflected not only by the literary testimonies that count it among Jerusalem's key sites, by also by the Madaba map, where it appears to the left of the eastern gate of the city.[35]

With the Christianization of Palestine and the growth of pilgrimage, churches were built to commemorate events from the Hebrew Bible and from the birth, ministry, and passion of Jesus. While it is easy to see the church at the Pool of Bethesda as just one more example of this phenomenon, and one that did double duty by commemorating both the paralytic and Mary's birth, it is not this simple. Around the turn of the fifth century, Jerome translated Eusebius' *Onomasticon* into Latin, inserting some of his own observations as he went. Among Jerome's additions to Eusebius' text is this observation regarding one of the two pools: "the other (pool) reddens in a remarkable fashion, as if with bloody waters, and bears witness to the miracles of the ancient work (wrought) in it" (*alter mirum in modum rubens quasi cruentis aquis antiqui in se operis signa testatur*).[36] This red water was seen as confirmation of the site's sacred

---

[30] Irshai 2009, 477–80.

[31] John Rufus *V. Petr. Ib.* 134; John Rufus *Plerophoria* 18.

[32] Theodosius *Topography of the Holy Land* 8; *Itin. Plac.* 27; Sophronius *Anacreonticon* 20.81–94. In addition to these texts that mention Mary alongside the healing of the paralytic are a few that focus only on the New Testament miracle, such as Pseudo-Athanasius' *Homily on the Sower* 15. For how the site became associated with Mary's life, see discussion in Baert 2005, 3–7.

[33] For the mosaic pavement to the north of the fifth-century basilica and roughly contemporary to it, see Dauphin 2011c, who argues that the botanical elements depicted in the mosaic floor reflect a liturgical cycle commemorating the life of Mary.

[34] See discussion in Gibson 2011, 32–3.

[35] Tsafrir 1999, 160.

[36] Jerome *Eusebii Onomasticon* s.v. Bethesda. The fourth-century Bordeaux Pilgrim also referred to the sick being cured at the Pool of Bethesda in language that is ambiguous as to whether it is simply describing the account in John 5 or whether the sick continued to be cured there. The key verb is in the imperfect: *Ibi aegri multorum annorum sanabantur.*

102 CONTESTED CURES

character, not only in the distant past when Jesus performed his miracle, but also in the world of Jerome and his contemporaries. In time, visitors to the site would come in expectation of being healed. Writing more than a century and a half after Jerome, the Piacenza Pilgrim located these cures in the Basilica of Mary, "in which many miracles are worked." The Piacenza Pilgrim says that the basilica was built out of one of the original five stoas around the pool (*Revertentibus nobis in civitatem venimus ad piscina natatoria, que habet quinque porticus ex quibus una habet basilicam sanctae Mariae, in qua multae fiunt virtutes*).[37]

It would seem, then, that a local tradition held that just as Jesus had healed the paralytic in this place, he would continue to heal those who visited the Pool of Bethesda in search of their own miraculous cures. This made the miracle of John 5 not simply an event from the distant past, but a living reality in which visitors could participate. As Edith Turner wrote in her preface to the paperback edition of her and Victor Turner's *Image and Pilgrimage in Christian Culture,*

> The search for *illud tempus* is not a search for a fusty, dead past, or nostalgia: in pilgrimage it is the journey to the actual place containing the actual objects of the past, whose very stones seem to emit the never obliterated power of the first event – a certain shadowy aura.[38]

This combination of pilgrimage and healing is not unique, and a number of sites associated with miracles appear in the pilgrimage literature, including Hammat Gader, as we saw in the previous chapter. While it is true, as John Wilkinson observed more than forty years ago, that obtaining cures was probably not the primary reason for travel to the Holy Land, the expectation that miracles could be experienced at certain sites would have been woven into the fabric of pilgrimage.[39] It is likely that the report of miracles at certain sites would have influenced the inclusion of these places in popular pilgrimage itineraries and enabled the continuity of these healing traditions into late antiquity.

In sum, the location occupied today by the Church of St. Anne underwent at least two, and possibly three, phases as a healing site. Votive offerings indicate that it functioned as a sanctuary for Serapis or Serapis-Asklepios after the Romans established the colony of Aelia Capitolina on the remains of Jerusalem. Christian appropriation of the site later turned it into both a pilgrimage destination and a site of ritual healing. The veracity of John's association of the *miqveh* with ritual healing in the first century CE, prior to the destruction

---

[37] *Itin. Plac.* 27 (CCSL 175:143).
[38] Turner and Turner 2011, xv.
[39] Wilkinson 2002, 74, n. 136. See discussion in Talbot 2002, especially 153–4.

of the Temple, is less certain. John's testimony must certainly be taken with a grain of salt, since his aim in part must have been to demonstrate the superiority of Jesus to other healing traditions.[40] Nevertheless, the results of the archaeological excavations on the grounds of St. Anne's are suggestive. Why was the cult of Serapis-Asklepios established in the immediate vicinity of the *miqveh*? Was it simply a convenient location immediately outside a secondary gate into the city? Or was there a prior practice of ritual cures at the site that made it a logical location for the new cult? If the latter was true, it is unlikely that such a tradition would have been officially sanctioned by any of the leading Jewish factions in the city, but a popular belief that immersion at specified times could result in healing cannot be ruled out. Ildikó Csepregi, in her discussion of a Greek sanctuary that was reborn as a Christian one reputed for incubation and miracles, observed that the non-Christian past of sacred sites was not completely obliterated, but rather transformed and subordinated to the new Christian narrative of the site: "[they] provided the background against which the new saints' power grew more visible and which legitimized their role as the new patrons of the site, its function or the thaumaturgic and miracle-working qualities associated with the place."[41] I would suggest that this is essentially what took place at the Pool of Bethesda. The fact that the cult to Serapis-Asklepios was destroyed and that Jews abandoned the *miqveh* as a site for ritual immersion highlights Christian superiority in the new ritual landscape of Jerusalem. The miracle performed by Jesus at the Pool of Bethesda in the Book of John was not simply commemorated there, but was, in a way, relived by people who experienced healing for themselves.

Shuni/'Ein Tzur

Like the Pool of Bethesda, Shuni/'Ein Tzur combined Christian pilgrimage and healing, but two traits set it apart from its far more famous counterpart. First, only a single literary testimony regarding the site's healing tradition survives. This means that our understanding of it must come largely from archaeological evidence. Second, the sole reference does not connect it to a tradition about Jesus, as we saw at the Pool of Bethesda and at Emmaus. Despite the scarcity of evidence, I would suggest that the continuity of ritual healing as the site changed hands can again be observed. Furthermore, as with the Pool of Bethesda and the hot springs, water continues to be a defining element at this therapeutic site.

---

[40] Maureen Yeung (2002, 64–97) situates the healing at the Pool of Bethesda amid the competition between belief in Jesus and in Asklepios as savior–healers.

[41] Csepregi 2015, 55.

The fourth-century Bordeaux Pilgrim's itinerary gives the following description: "At the third milestone (from Caesarea) is Mount Syna, where there is a spring in which, if a woman bathes, she becomes pregnant."[42] This is the totality of our literary evidence. Two alternative sites, both northeast of Caesarea and separated by approximately 2 km, have been associated with this passage (See Figure 4.2). The first is Shuni, whose local Arabic place name into the nineteenth century preserved the memory of the Maioumas festival that took place there.[43] Most scholars see this as the location described by the Bordeaux Pilgrim, due to similarities between "Mount Syna" and "Shuni."[44] Much of the literary evidence for the Maioumas festival and its

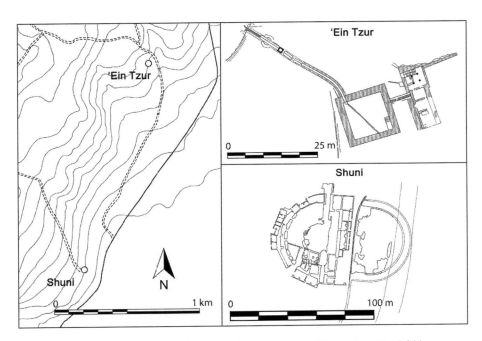

Figure 4.2 Plan of the Shuni and 'Ein Tzur (Drawing by D. Weiss, after Hirschfeld 1995 and Shenhav 1997)

[42] *Itin. Burd.* 585. The Bordeaux Pilgrim points to a second spring that is associated with fertility, the spring of Elisha (*fons Helisaei*) a short distance from Jericho (*Itin. Burd.* 596). The pilgrim explains how in 2 Kgs 2:19–22, Elisha miraculously transformed this spring that had once been known to induce miscarriage into one where now any woman who drinks its water is assured children.

[43] For the various testimonies to the Arabic place name, see Henderson 1992, 24; Dvorjetski 2012, 103, 109–13. For the Maioumas festival, particularly in Palestine, see Segal 1994, 11, n. 33; Belayche 2001, 249–55; Dvorjetski 2001; Dvorjetski 2012.

[44] For example, Shenhav 1993, 1382; Belayche 2001, 197–8; Friedheim and Dar 2010, 405; Dvorjetski 2012, 104.

association with fertility comes from elite Christian and Jewish authors who were highly critical of the cult and its popularity.[45] According to the sixth-century chronicler John Malalas, the celebration took place every three years and was accompanied by night-time revelry.[46] The excavated remains of a theater and adjacent semicircular pool concur with what we know about the Maioumas festival's water rites.[47] In addition to the Maioumas' emphasis on fertility, which was shared by the Bordeaux Pilgrim's Mount Syna, the excavator of Shuni proposed that a cult of Asklepios also existed at Shuni. Evidence for the cult of Asklepios includes a statue, dated on stylistic grounds to the late second or early third century, and medical instruments.[48] A temple and building that could have served as a hostel for those visiting the sanctuary were also uncovered. Water installations and theaters, such as those found at Shuni, were also typical in Asklepieia. If the Maioumas festival only took place every three years, the water installations and theater may have also been used at other times by the cult of Asklepios.[49]

The alternative site for the Bordeaux Pilgrim's Mount Syna is a spring named 'Ein Tzur, which is located a short distance away at Ramat Hanadiv. Yizhar Hirschfeld and the others who worked with him on the site report identified 'Ein Tzur as the Bordeaux Pilgrim's Mount Syna.[50] During the Herodian period, the spring fed an aqueduct, pool, and bathhouse, all of which belonged to a large, fortified compound located at the top of the adjacent hill.[51] The hilltop settlement was destroyed during the Jewish revolt, but in the third century CE the area around the spring was renovated and the pool replastered.[52] By this point, 'Ein Tzur had come under the control of

---

[45] See discussion in Belayche 2001, 252; Dvorjetski 2012, 101–3.

[46] John Malalas *Chronographia* 12.3 (Dindorf edition pp. 284–5). For translation, see Jeffreys et al. 1986.

[47] For excavations at Shuni, see Shenhav 1990a; Shenhav 1990b; Shenhav 1993; Wolff 1993.

[48] For the statue, see Shenhav 1990a, 61; Shenhav 1993, 1383; Wolff 1993, 158; Shenhav 1999; Weingarten 1999, 292, n. 4; Fischer 2008, 489. Belayche (2001, 197) sees this statue as confirmation of the site's "therapeutic nature," since she observes that depictions of Asklepios are "more or less absent" in Caesarea other than on gemstones. The identification of this statue as Asklepios has been doubted by Rivka Gersht (1996, 435, n. 4) and Dvorjetski (2012, 108–9), who prefer to see it as Poseidon. For the medical instruments, see Weingarten 1999, 292, n. 4. The coexistence of medical practitioners and healing cults is well known throughout the ancient Mediterranean world; see discussion in Wickkiser 2006, 33–7.

[49] Shenhav 1990a, 61.

[50] Hirschfeld 2000a, 721–2. Hirschfeld's (1995, 43) earlier report on his excavations at 'Ein Tzur suggested that Shuni, rather than the spring, was the subject of the Bordeaux Pilgrim's comment, but he seems to have changed his mind later. He also referred to the coins as evidence that 'Ein Tzur was a "wishing well" (Hirschfeld 2000c, 336), and Barkay called it a "wishing spring" (2000a) or a "wishing well" (2000b, 417).

[51] For the excavation of 'Ein Tzur, see Hirschfeld 1995; Hirschfeld 1998; Hirschfeld 2000a.

[52] Hirschfeld 1995, 43; Barkay 2000a, 855.

nearby Shuni, and a new aqueduct was built to convey water to the pools in Shuni.[53] The suggestion that 'Ein Tzur be identified with the Bordeaux Pilgrim's Mount Syna finds support in the cache of more than two thousand, mostly low-denomination, coins found in the pool near where it was filled by the spring. As discussed in Chapter 3, coins could be used as a votive offering in thanks for – or possibly in anticipation of – a miracle. The earliest coins at 'Ein Tzur date to the fourth century, coinciding with the Bordeaux Pilgrim's testimony about Mount Syna. The greatest percentage of coins come from the sixth century, and the latest coins are from the seventh. However, Rachel Barkay noted that these coins were discovered in "a natural small socket in the pool's floor," and she suggested that they may have been left behind when additional coins were gathered by the people who administered the site.[54] If Barkay's hypothesis is correct, it allows the possibility that the spring was also quite popular in the fourth and fifth centuries, but that most of those coins had been removed as part of its periodic upkeep.

In sum, the evidence points to a constellation of three different sets of ritual practices in the area northeast of Caesarea. Two were located at Shuni, where the Maioumas and the Asklepios cults seem to have existed side by side. The third was 2 km away, where the deposit of coins at 'Ein Tzur suggests the existence of additional rituals related to health or healing.[55] Is it possible to determine which of these forms the backdrop to the ritual described by the Bordeaux Pilgrim? I would argue that all are pertinent. In order to offer a Christian alternative to the Maioumas and Asklepios cults in Shuni, the Christian ritual described by the anonymous pilgrim may have developed at the nearby Ramat Hanadiv pool, which like the pools in Shuni was filled with water from 'Ein Tzur.[56] Strictly speaking, this is neither the coexistence of cult that we saw at Hammat Gader nor the continuity of cult that we saw at the Pool of Bethesda, but a slightly different scenario. The key is the water of 'Ein Tzur. Since the water used in rituals at Shuni came from 'Ein Tzur, then water from the same source – the pool at Ramat Hanadiv – may have been seen as a viable alternative for rituals in Shuni. In other words, Christian pilgrims did

---

[53] Hirschfeld 2000b, 720; Friedheim and Dar 2010, 405–6.

[54] Barkay 2000a, 856.

[55] For comparable sites where coins are left as votive offerings for health or healing, see Barkay 2000a, 856–7.

[56] Susan Weingarten wrote that the excavator of Shuni, Eli Shenhav, suggested that the Bordeaux Pilgrim reflects the Christianization of Shuni's earlier cults (1999, 292, n. 4). In contrast, Yizhar Hirschfeld (1998, 115–16) argued that the deposition of coins at 'Ein Tzur was connected to the Maioumas cult in Shuni and demonstrates that the Maioumas cult continued through the end of the Byzantine period, despite Christian attempts to forbid it. See also Friedheim 2006, 87–8; Friedheim and Dar 2010, 405.

not need to visit Shuni to participate in ceremonies related to health or fertility. They could avoid the "pagan" taint of Shuni yet still benefit from the water used in its rituals. Ultimately, 'Ein Tzur would outlive Shuni as a site of ritual activity. By the end of the sixth century, the theater at Shuni had ceased its ritual function and the orchestra was converted into an olive press.[57] In contrast, the deposit of coins at 'Ein Tzur continued into the seventh century, with its zenith in the sixth.

The Asklepios and Maioumas cults would have attracted visitors from the local polytheistic populations and, based on epigraphic evidence, likely those from further afield as well.[58] We can also be certain of Christians' participation in local rituals, based on the Bordeaux Pilgrim's description. While it is reasonable to suggest that non-Christians patronized Shuni and Christians visited 'Ein Tzur, the ferocity of Christian denunciations of the Maioumas festival may indicate that it had a broad appeal. If Christians had not been tempted by the Maioumas, there would have been little need for such invective. As has already been discussed, nearby Caesarea was the Roman provincial capital, with a diverse population including devotees of Greek and Roman cults, Jews, Samaritans, and Christians. Both literary and epigraphic evidence attest to Jews' presence in the region of Shuni but do not indicate whether Jews participated in its rites.[59] We have equally scant evidence about the patrons at 'Ein Tzur, as the votive coins cannot be used to determine the religious or cultural self-understanding of the people who deposited them.

If there was indeed an attempt to create at 'Ein Tzur a Christian alternative to Shuni, this raises the question of the Christian ritual's intended purpose. The Bordeaux Pilgrim's description is very brief, and while it does indicate that fertility was an important concern, it does not mean that this was the only reason that visitors came to the site. In fact, Laurie Douglass has argued that this anonymous pilgrim was in general concerned with matters related to women, and that the text may have even been written by a woman, which could offer some context for why fertility was highlighted in this passage.[60] Just because a healing site was especially known to attract those with a particular condition, in this case fertility concerns, it does not mean that they were its exclusive patrons. If 'Ein Tzur gave a Christian alternative to the rituals at Shuni, including its cult of Asklepios, then we might expect that 'Ein Tzur also attracted a broader range of visitors.

---

[57] Shenhav 1993, 1384.

[58] Shenhav 1999, xvii, 127–33.

[59] See Kefar Shuni entries in Avi-Yonah 1976, 73; Tsafrir et al. 1994, 165. For the inscription with the Hebrew word *shalôm* ("peace"), see Shenhav 1990a, 59.

[60] Douglass 1996; cf. Weingarten 1999. For more on the Bordeaux Pilgrim, see Elsner 2000.

108   CONTESTED CURES

Ritual continuity at other sites

The phenomenon of a site perceived to be sacred by multiple groups or traditions, whether simultaneously or diachronically, holds a certain fascination. Given our evidence across the ancient Mediterranean world for examples of this sort, it is not surprising that this possibility has been proposed for additional locations in Palestine. The pages that follow will briefly consider three of these additional sites: the Pool of Siloam in Jerusalem, the basilica of Dora (Dor) on the Mediterranean coast, and an area just south of the sanctuary of Pan at Paneas (also known as Banias or Caesarea Philippi) in the northern Golan. In the first two cases, there is no proof of continuity with earlier healing cults at the site. At Paneas, the evidence is so fragmentary that only the most tentative hypothesis is possible. Although I ultimately do not see evidence for continuity of therapeutic cults at the first two, their position on Christian pilgrimage routes underscores the role of healing in the late antique ritual landscape of Palestine.

Pool of Siloam

Like the Pool of Bethesda, the Pool of Siloam was the site of a New Testament miracle attested only in John:

> As [Jesus] walked along, he saw a man blind from birth. His disciples asked him, "Rabbi, who sinned, this man or his parents, that he was born blind?" Jesus answered, "Neither this man nor his parents sinned; he was born blind so that God's works might be revealed in him . . ." When he had said this, he spat on the ground and made mud with the saliva and spread the mud on the man's eyes, saying to him, "Go, wash in the pool of Siloam" (which means Sent). Then he went and washed and came back able to see.[61]

Excavations south of the Temple Mount, near the Gihon spring, have revealed another large, public *miqveh*, which has been identified as the setting for the Johannine miracle of the man born blind.[62] While the Pool of Bethesda was ideally situated as a *miqveh* for pilgrims approaching the temple from the north, the Pool of Siloam fulfilled a similar function for those coming from the south. During the annual pilgrimage festivals, the pool was likely busy as people flocked to Jerusalem. The author of John does not include any details

---

[61] John 9:1–3, 6–7.
[62] Gibson 2005, 283–5; Reich and Shukron 2011, 248–50; Wahlde 2013, 274–7.

in 9:1–7 that suggest a pre-existing healing cult, such as in John 5 at the Pool of Bethesda. The setting of both miracles at large *miqva'ot*, however, contributed to the author's intention to show Jesus' superiority to Jewish law, particularly with regards to ritual purity.[63] To commemorate the miracle at the Pool of Siloam, a late antique church was built so that the south aisle extended over the pool believed at the time to be the site of the miracle in John 9.[64] Evidence for the church's significance can be seen in the fifth-century extension of Jerusalem's city wall to the south to include the Pool of Siloam along with the area known today as the City of David.[65] In the sixth century, the Piacenza Pilgrim reported that the pool was known as a site of miracles: "In these waters many miracles take place, and lepers are cleansed" (*In quibus aquis multae virtutes ostenduntur, immo et leprosi mundantur*).[66] Sophronius also mentioned that cures took place at the Pool of Siloam: two men were healed of their blindness after traveling to Jerusalem to wash in the Pool of Siloam, following instructions that they received at the martyrion of Sts. Cyrus and John in Egypt.[67]

The Christian healing site at the Pool of Siloam therefore developed from the commemoration of Jesus' healing of the man born blind in John 9. The

---

[63] Wahlde 2013, 279–80.

[64] For excavations at the Pool of Siloam, see Bliss and Dickie 1898, 178–210; Reich and Shukron 2005; Reich et al. 2007, 163–7; Reich and Shukron 2011. It should be noted that the Byzantine Pool of Siloam was near, but not actually the same as the pool known to the author of John 9. For an overview of the development of pools on the south side of the City of David and at the Gihon spring, see Wahlde 2013, 274–6.

[65] For the extension of the walls of Jerusalem, see Bliss and Dickie 1898, 307–9, cf. 193–5, 209–10; Mitchell 1919, 38. According to the Piacenza Pilgrim (*Itin. Plac.* 25), the person responsible for this expansion of the city walls was the Empress Eudokia, whose poetic inscription at Hammat Gader we saw in Chapter 3. She is understood to have also been responsible for the construction of the church at the Pool of Siloam. The empress seems to have had an interest in ritual healing, especially during the final years of her life, which she spent in Palestine. In addition to her attention to the Pool of Siloam and Hammat Gader, she was also particularly devoted to Stephen, whose martyrdom is described in Acts 7:54–60. She built a church in Jerusalem dedicated to St. Stephen, located today on the grounds of the École biblique, perhaps out of gratitude for a miraculous cure that she attributed to Stephen's relics. See *Vita Melaniae* 59; cf. Hunt 1982, 223; Clark 1986, 103–5; Sowers 2008, 46. It is possible that this interest in ritual healing is also manifested in the multi-volume poetic account that she wrote about Cyprian, a magician who converted to Christianity and who later became Bishop of Antioch. According to Eudokia's description of Cyprian's life, he performed healings and exorcisms both as a "pagan" practitioner and later as a Christian specialist. See discussion and translation of text in Sowers 2008, 134–204.

[66] *Itin. Plac.* 24.

[67] Sophronius *Miracles of Cyrus and John* 46. Sophronius writes that one of the two men, a tribune from Alexandria, received the instructions to wash at the Pool of Siloam in a dream. The other, a Pachmonian monk, is simply said to have heard the command while at the shrine.

idea that there was a pre-Christian tradition of healing at the Pool of Siloam is much more tenuous. Some scholars have suggested that the Gihon spring, which fed the Pool of Siloam, had for centuries been understood to possess special qualities. Ya'akov Meshorer surveyed references to the pool beginning in the Hebrew Bible and proposed that it was known by residents of Jerusalem for its "magical powers."[68] Others have tried to locate a Roman healing shrine at the Pool of Siloam after the city was refounded as Aelia Capitolina, much as the cult of Serapis developed at the Pool of Bethesda. However, the evidence for such a cult is unpersuasive. This argument is based on depictions of Hygieia, and possibly the nymphs, on coins from Jerusalem, and on a brief reference to "a shrine of the nymphs" in a later rabbinic text.[69] Neither the coins nor the rabbinic evidence indicates where this shrine to Hygieia or the nymphs should be located. Indeed, the Hygieia coins could have been minted in connection to the cult of Serapis at the Pool of Bethesda, where Serapis may have been assimilated to Asklepios. Hygieia, the goddess of health, often appeared in connection to sanctuaries of her father, Asklepios, as we saw in Chapter 3 on the coins issued by the city of Tiberias. The lack of any convincing evidence for a Roman or Jewish cult at the Pool of Siloam means that neither continuity nor coexistence of cult should be understood at this site. Nevertheless, the presence of Christian healing rituals, and their importance in late antiquity, is certain.

Dora

The Byzantine church at Dora also seems to have offered visitors an opportunity for healing.[70] There was a tomb in the south aisle of the basilica that contained two bodies, whose names have not been preserved. A pipe allowed oil to pass over the saints' remains and then be collected by the faithful and used to anoint the sick.[71] Relics of saints and encounters with living holy men were part of the ritual fabric of pilgrimage in the region, alongside visits to sites associated with the Hebrew Bible and the life of Jesus. Claudine Dauphin's conclusion that the cult of these saints at Dora attracted Holy Land pilgrims is

[68] Meshorer 1982, 18; Meshorer 1989, 57.

[69] See discussion in Meshorer 1982; Meshorer 1985, 63, no. 178; Meshorer 1989, 29, 56–7, 74–5, 114–17, nos. 29, 75, 84; Belayche 2001, 168–9; Gibson 2005; Gibson 2009, 59–80. Although Meshorer associated these coins with the Pool of Siloam when he originally published them, Yaron Eliav (2005, 113 and 273, n. 87) pointed out that these coins could equally be in reference to the healing sanctuary at the Pool of Bethesda.

[70] Dauphin 1979, 236; Dauphin 1986; Dauphin 1993; Dauphin and Gibson 1994–5, 26–7; Dauphin 1997, 152–63; Dauphin 1999.

[71] For the *ampullae* that held oils such as this, and for the practice more generally, see discussion in Vikan 1995, 384–5; Vikan 2010, 33–40; Elsner 2018, 19–22.

persuasive, but the same does not hold true for her proposal that incubation was practiced in the basilica. Incubation certainly did occur at some saints' tombs, as the examples provided by Dauphin demonstrate, but it was by no means a universal phenomenon, nor was it a required component of ritual healing. For example, there is no evidence of incubation at either the Pool of Bethesda or 'Ein Tzur, even though both were associated with healing. Neither epigraphic evidence nor literary texts refer to incubation in this church, and architecture alone cannot be used to prove the practice.[72]

As at the Pool of Siloam, the evidence for Christian healing rituals at Dora is certain, but the suggestion that this is a continuation of an earlier, Greek practice of incubation is not. Excavations at the basilica revealed an earlier building below the church, which Dauphin reasonably identified as a temple. A "partially rock-cut adyton" was found in this earlier construction, in the area that would later become the basilica's peristyle court. By analogy to rock-cut features in the temples of Apollo at Didyma and Claros, Dauphin proposed that the temple was dedicated to Apollo. She reads a difficult section of Josephus' *Against Apion* 2.10 as confirmation of this identification.[73] Dauphin presents no evidence of Asklepios at the site but assumes that worship of him must have eclipsed that of his father, Apollo, by the third century BCE. Dauphin seems to have made this proposal to advance her conclusion regarding the continuity of incubation at Dora and because within the Greek pantheon Asklepios is most commonly associated with the practice.[74] Unfortunately, the idea that Apollo was the original deity worshipped here is less than fully persuasive, and the proposal of an Asklepios cult is conjecture.[75] We are left with a Christian healing site, but no continuity of cult.

Paneas

A short passage by Eusebius mentions an image of Jesus that he saw in Paneas. Eusebius reported that it depicted Jesus and the woman whom he healed in Matt 9:20–2:

---

[72] Gil Renberg (2016, 1:34) cautions against the use of architecture alone as evidence for incubation: "there has been too great a willingness to identify stoas as incubation dormitories at sites not otherwise associated with incubation." Even in the cult of Asklepios, with which incubation is particularly associated, Renberg argues that it cannot be assumed at every site (2016, 1:124). For the difficulties in identifying spaces used for incubation on the basis of architecture alone, see also Ehrenheim 2009.

[73] Dauphin 1999, 406–7, 416–17.

[74] Dauphin 1999, 418.

[75] In the absence of additional epigraphic or textual evidence, some scholars have more or less accepted Dauphin's arguments (e.g. Markschies 2006, 200–4; Markschies 2007, 108–84; Ovadiah and Turnheim 2011, 50; Csepregi 2015), while others have rejected them (e.g. Graf 2015, 255–6; Renberg 2016, 2:540–2).

112 CONTESTED CURES

The woman with a hemorrhage, who as we learn from the holy gospels was cured of her trouble by our Savior, was stated to have come from here. Her house was pointed out in the city, and a wonderful memorial of the benefit the Savior conferred upon her was still there. On a tall stone base at the gates of her house stood a bronze statue of a woman, resting on one knee and resembling a suppliant with arms outstretched. Facing this was another of the same material, an upright figure of a man with a double cloak neatly draped over his shoulders and his hand stretched out to the woman. Near his feet on the stone slab grew an exotic plant, which climbed up to the hem of the bronze cloak and served as a remedy for illnesses of every kind. This statue, which was said to resemble the features of Jesus, was still there in my own time, so that I saw it with my own eyes when I resided in the city.[76]

The New Testament does not specify where this woman lived, and the setting of Matthew 9, where the story is found, seems to be Capernaum, on the Sea of Galilee. Eusebius' story about Paneas being the hometown of this woman points to a local community there with some lasting interest in the woman, in healing, or in both. Eusebius' additional detail about the local plant that could produce cures, regardless of the illness that a person had, may suggest that the area's inhabitants were interested in healing more broadly.

These pieces of information are certainly not conclusive proof of a healing sanctuary at Paneas. However, a couple of scholars have tentatively suggested that a sanctuary may indeed have existed here, with the potential for both non-Christian and Christian phases. Immediately following his description of the statues, Eusebius says that Gentiles (*tous ex ethnōn*) were in the habit of setting up images, which we call votive offerings, to Jesus as part of their "Gentile custom" (*ethnikē synētheia*).[77] In this passage, Eusebius may be offering both a general observation about votive offerings and commenting on the specific images that he saw in Paneas. Lee Jefferson, in considering the possibility that the statue group seen by Eusebius originally represented Asklepios and was only later repurposed as a statue of Jesus and the hemorrhaging woman, observed: "The local population at Paneas obviously interpreted the statue as a healer, which influenced the Christian population to model it after a Christian healing story."[78] This interpretation of the Paneas statue is particularly suggestive in light of Asher Ovadiah and Yehudit Turnheim's argument that

---

[76] Eusebius *Eccl. Hist.* 7.18. Translations of Eusebius' *Ecclesiastical History* are taken from Louth 1989. Both Sozomen (*Eccl. Hist.* 5.21) and Philostorgius (*Eccl. Hist.* 7.3) also take note of this statue.

[77] Eusebius *Eccl. Hist.* 7.18.4.

[78] Jefferson 2014, 89. See also Hauck 1880, 45–6; Harnack 1962, 118–19.

a sanctuary of Asklepios existed at Paneas alongside its more famous cults of Pan, Zeus Heliopolitanus, and Augustus.[79] While the evidence is very limited, they called attention to three discoveries. First, a statue base found at the site contained a dedicatory inscription to Asklepios.[80] Second, a life-size marble head that depicted either Asklepios or Zeus, dated to the Antonine or Severan periods, was also discovered in the precinct.[81] Finally, a series of structures south of the sanctuary of Pan included monumental buildings, a *cryptoporticus* and water system. The importance of water in the cult of Asklepios and the potential of the *cryptoporticus* to function as an incubation chamber contributed to the hypothesis that an Asklepieion may have been established here in the first century CE.[82] Ovadiah and Turnheim concluded that Eusebius' description of the votive offering at Paneas "corroborates the continuation of the pagan healing tradition at Paneas/Banias in the Early Christian period."[83]

The evidence from Paneas is extremely fragmentary, both for the identification of a cult to Asklepios and even more so for a later Christian phase. Nevertheless, of the three proposed sites, it is the most provocative. At the very least, I would suggest that the Christian residents of Paneas had an interest in healing. This interest might reflect the presence of an older healing cult, whose remnants they attempted to Christianize with traditions about Jesus.

* * *

Localized healing cults in Palestine were not limited to the sites discussed in Chapters 3 and 4. Additional sites associated with ritual healing are, for the most part, poorly understood, with only isolated pieces of archaeological evidence or a brief comment in an ancient text. For example, two additional sanctuaries of Asklepios are known. Evidence for the first, on Mount Gerizim, is limited to numismatics, including a spring clearly depicted as part of the sacred space.[84] Likewise, a single reference to the Neoplatonist philosopher Proclus' lost hymn to Asklepios Leontouchos attests to the presence of this cult in Ascalon (Ashkelon). Although scholars have tried to connect this reference

---

[79] Ovadiah and Turnheim 2011, 3–19. This idea has also been entertained by Belayche (2001, 163; see also 288, 302, n. 165).

[80] Maʿoz 1996, 4; Friedland 1997, 95.

[81] Friedland 1997, 126–30; Maʿoz 1998, 23–4; Ovadiah and Turnheim 2011, 11, 17 n. 62.

[82] Ovadiah and Turnheim 2011, 11–14. As noted above, the practice of incubation cannot be determined on the basis of architecture alone, but the potential for an Asklepieion at Paneas remains even without interpreting the *cryptoporticus* as a space for incubation. See discussion in Tzaferis and Israeli 1996, 6; Tzaferis and Israeli 1997, 12–13; Ovadiah and Turnheim 2011, 18, n. 112.

[83] Ovadiah and Turnheim 2011, 14.

[84] Meshorer 1985, no. 143; Belayche 2001, 203–5; Ovadiah and Turnheim 2011, 79.

to visual representations on coins and gemstones, the cult of Asklepios Leon-touchos largely remains a mystery.[85] It is likely that other places associated with healing also existed. When Sozomen recounted the details about the plant at the foot of the statue in Paneas, together with the story about Jesus visiting Emmaus with which we began this chapter, he made the following observation: "It appears that innumerable other miracles were wrought in different cities and villages; accounts have been accurately preserved by the inhabitants of these places only, because they learned them from ancestral tradition."[86] Given how little we know about the healing tradition at places like Emmaus and the Bordeaux Pilgrim's Mount Syna, it is not difficult to imagine that additional sites, associated with healing in late antiquity, are absent from the literary record.

As we have seen, healing sites in Palestine have a particularly close association with water. In the most popular category of therapeutic sites – the hot springs – water was the central element around which the site was developed. Likewise, traditions about Jesus' miracle at the Pool of Bethesda involved a large ritual bath, where water was the necessary characteristic for ritual purity. Even at Shuni/'Ein Tzur, where we have limited knowledge of the rituals, it was a spring where votive coins were left, and it was the same spring that connected the earlier rituals at Shuni to what was probably a Christian rite at 'Ein Tzur. Broadly speaking, the presence of water is not unusual and is in fact expected at Greco-Roman healing sanctuaries, but the situation in Palestine goes beyond such associations.[87] Here, water seems to define many sites, rather than forming one of several constituent parts. Even more striking than the presence of water was the potential for the continuity or even coexistence of healing rituals in the same location across more than one ethnic, cultural, or religious tradition.

---

[85] Marinus of Neapolis *V. Procli* 19. See discussion in Belayche 2001, 231–2; Finkielsztejn 1986; Mastrocinque 2011; Geiger 2012.

[86] Sozomen *Hist. Eccl.* 5.21 (*NPNF* 2/2:343).

[87] For the distinction between the water necessary for a sanctuary's regular functions and water as a source of healing, see Scheid 1991; Aupert 1991; Ben Abed and Scheid 2003; de Cazanove 2015.

PART III

Miraculous People

CHAPTER 5

In the Name of Jesus of Nazareth the Crucified: Ritual Practitioners Who Offered Cures

Throughout this book, the phrase "ritual healing" has been used to refer collectively to options for seeking divine intervention to relieve physical ailments. People visited sacred sites, often associated with water, in the expectation of a dream or vision that would heal them. Others affixed amulets with powerful texts and images on their body to heal infirmities or to ward off diseases. In many situations, there would have been ceremonies or rituals that accompanied these forms of healing, such as preliminary sacrifices at local healing shrines or prayers recited when an amulet was first put on. In other cases, the process associated with these cures was informal, personal, and supplemented by no special rites. In this chapter, we turn to the words and actions believed to bring about a cure without the need for an inscribed amulet or a sacred site. In other words, the ceremonies themselves were the cures.[1]

Some of the rituals discussed in this chapter may have been conducted by the individual in need of healing him- or herself, but more frequently we can imagine that the words and actions were performed by another. Although these rituals required someone to perform them, the identity of that person was somewhat irrelevant as long as they possessed the necessary knowledge and skills. This is in contrast to Chapter 6, which also considers people as agents of healing, but whose healers were understood to possess some sort of special quality that enabled them to work miracles. Among the healers of Chapter 5, two broad categories can be identified. The first are ritual practitioners who performed healing rites within Jewish and Christian communities. Typically, these individuals held some sort of an official role that gave them the requisite knowledge and authority. The second category of ritual practitioners are those

---

[1] Although I use "ritual healing" to describe all of the healing options explored in this book, others could restrict this phrase to the healings considered in this chapter (e.g. Theissen 2010, 51–2).

whom we can call freelancers.[2] While some of these freelancers may have held positions within the hierarchy of cults or religious communities, the healing rituals that they performed were not officially sanctioned.[3] These practitioners used their specialized knowledge to work with clients in need of healing and were likely paid for their services.[4] These two broad categories of practitioners relate to the context in which each worked and can be mapped onto the responses to their cures found among elite authors. Those performing rites prescribed by a community would have faced no censure by their coreligionists, and in fact their cures were seen by some as the only legitimate method of seeking divine healing. Freelancers, on the other hand, were frequently denounced as magicians, as will be shown in Chapter 7. Despite this rhetorical dichotomy maintained by elite authors, I argue that there was no functional difference between these two broad categories of practitioners, regardless of whether they operated with or without the approval of a religious community.[5] For both, it was the spoken word, sometimes accompanied by ritual actions, that was believed to bring cures, either by addressing an illness-causing demon directly or by invoking a higher power for protection against the same.[6] While the identity of the person saying these ritual words was generally not a key factor in their efficacy, a recurring characteristic, as we will see, was the appeal to an earlier authority as the author or source of the ritual.

Unlike the forms of healing discussed in the first four chapters, it will be more difficult in Chapters 5 and 6 to narrow the discussion of healing to Palestine. The reason for this is simple – there is little archaeological evidence from the region to shed light on these practices, and Palestinian provenance cannot be assigned for many of the literary sources under consideration. The texts from the Judaean desert are the one notable exception to the lack of local archaeological evidence, and while they will be considered here, they predate much of the material discussed in the book. Also pertinent to this discussion are the *Greek Magical Papyri* (*PGM*) discovered in Egypt. While they originate outside Palestine, the lack of comparable evidence from our region means that they will be used with caution to give some sense for what might have existed. Literary texts, which must therefore form the bulk of our evidence for Chapters 5 and 6, offer rich sources. Even

---

[2] My use of "freelance" to describe some of the ritual specialists of this chapter is modeled on Heidi Wendt's use of "freelance experts" to describe a range of individuals in the Roman world (2016).

[3] For examples from Egypt, see Frankfurter 1997.

[4] See, for example, Matthew Dickie (2001, 216–34) on "itinerant magicians."

[5] Fritz Graf (1991) made an analogous argument with regard to the nature of prayer. He concluded that on the basis of the prayer alone, there was no significant difference between texts labeled as magical or religious.

[6] For a similar distinction between liturgical and freelance practitioners among the Dead Sea Scrolls, see discussion in Eshel 2003a.

RITUAL PRACTITIONERS   119

if they originated elsewhere, such texts were copied and moved around, and may well have circulated in Palestine.

Ritual practitioners

We begin with two anecdotes, one about an exorcism ritual and the other about a baptism that resulted in a cure. These stories underscore the importance of ritual words and actions for healing. Unlike the miracles by charismatic healers considered in Chapter 6, the key to the healings of this chapter lies in specific words and actions and not in the identity of the person performing them. Epiphanius tells a story in the *Panarion* about the conversion of Josephus, an influential Jewish official in the court of Patriarch Hillel II whom we first met in connection to Hammat Gader in Chapter 3. After experiencing a number of visions that credited his recovery from assorted illnesses to the Christian God, a reluctant Josephus decided to test the veracity of his visions. He accomplished this by performing a ritual on a local "madman" (*mainomenos*) who lived in Tiberias.[7] Epiphanius narrated the encounter:

> So he (Josephus) brought the man inside, shut the door, took water, made the sign of the cross over it, and sprinkled it on the madman with the words, "In the name of Jesus of Nazareth the crucified be gone from him, demon, and let him be made whole!" Falling down with a loud cry, the man lay motionless for a long time foaming profusely and retching, and Josephus supposed that he had died. But after a while he rubbed his forehead and got up and, once on his feet and seeing his own nakedness, he hid himself . . .[8]

The key detail here is an invocation of Jesus. Josephus issued a direct command to the demon, using Jesus' name; according to Epiphanius, this was the reason that the afflicted man recovered. After witnessing the miraculous cure of the demon-possessed man, Josephus concluded that the healing he had himself experienced was also the work of the Christian God. He proceeded to renounce Judaism and accept baptism for himself.[9]

A second story can be found in the *Spiritual Meadow* of John Moschos, a sixth- to seventh-century monk from Syria who traveled widely throughout

---

[7] Epiphanius' details about the man being naked and unable to wear clothes call to mind the Gerasene demoniacs in the New Testament. The story of the Gerasene (Gadarene) demoniac(s) can be found in Matt 8:28–34, Mark 5:1–20, and Luke 8:26–39.

[8] Epiphanius *Pan.* 30.10. This translation is from Williams 2009.

[9] See discussion in Jacobs 2012, 42–3.

120 CONTESTED CURES

the Holy Land and Egypt. John Moschos related an episode in which several men journeyed from Alexandria to Palestine, and along the way, one of them, a Jew, became deathly ill. Although the sick man's companions carried him in turns, the group was too far from any town and too short on resources to find help for him. As they prepared to leave the dying man in the desert and to continue without him, he made one final request. He wished to die a Christian and asked his Christian companions to administer baptism to him. At first, his companions demurred: "Truly, brother, it is impossible for us to do anything of the sort. We are laymen and baptizing is the bishops' work and priests'."[10] In the end, however, one of the group took charge and pronounced the trinitarian formula of baptism while the others responded "Amen." Since there was no water present, they performed the baptism by pouring sand over the initiate's head. John Moschos reported that at the conclusion of this baptismal ceremony the man immediately made a full recovery, and the group continued their journey to Ashkelon, where they presented themselves to the bishop with news of the miracle.[11]

The stories told by Epiphanius and John Moschos are about unconventional rituals. In neither case are they performed by the specialists, Christian clergy, whose job it normally was to do such things. The lack of water in John Moschos' account further illustrates its unorthodox nature. Nevertheless, they reflect a milieu that attributed apotropaic power, and even miraculous cures, to ritual words and actions. These are what J. L. Austin called "performative utterances" or "speech acts," whereby something is accomplished through spoken words:

> to utter the sentence (in, of course, the appropriate circumstances) is not to *describe* [italics in the original] my doing of what I should be said in so uttering to be doing or to state that I am doing it: it is to do it.[12]

Josephus does not describe an exorcism in Epiphanius' narrative, he actually performs it through a speech act. His command to the demon with the invocation

---

[10] John Moschos *Prat.* 176. Translations of John Moschos are taken from Wortley 1992.

[11] Two other conversion stories are of note. According to Epiphanius, Josephus witnessed the Jewish Patriarch Hillel II being baptized on his deathbed. Although Hillel died several days later, this story could be read as suggesting that Hillel's health rallied somewhat after his baptism, giving him enough time to receive instruction from the bishop (*Pan.* 30.4, 6). The second conversion story, told by Socrates Scholasticus, takes place in Constantinople. The early fifth-century archbishop of the city, Atticus, encountered a paralyzed Jew who asked to be baptized. Before this encounter, the man had sought out medical treatment and Jewish prayer but found no cure. After a brief period of instruction, Atticus baptized him, and the man was immediately healed (Socrates Scholasticus *Hist. Eccl.* 7.4).

[12] Austin 1962, 6. For the application of Austin's work to ritual contexts and so-called "magical" texts, see discussion in Tambiah 1973, 218–29; Kropp 2010; Frankfurter 2019b.

"In the name of Jesus of Nazareth the crucified" effects a real change in the world, in this case a miraculous cure.[13] The efficacy of these two rituals appears undiminished by the absence of the individuals typically charged with such ceremonies. In fact, in the story of Josephus, the person performing the ritual is not even a Christian. He is a Jew whose goal is to test the Christian God. Put simply, these stories underscore the belief that ritual words can be effective even, as with Josephus, in the absence of the speaker's belief in them.

In contrast to these stories by Epiphanius and John Moschos, much of the evidence for healing of the type considered in this chapter comes from sources that illustrate the institutional authority of the person charged with performing the rituals. It is of note, though, that the individuals themselves are largely anonymous. Outside the unusual stories just considered, most references to this sort of healing come from handbooks or manuals that contain the words to be used in given situations; personal stories about people using the rituals are few. This relative anonymity differs from the stories about charismatic healers who attracted crowds of sick in search of cures, which will be considered in Chapter 6.

An early example of a religious functionary performing protective rituals can be found among the texts discovered in the Judaean desert in the vicinity of Qumran. A leading figure in the Qumran community, the Maskil, had liturgical and educational responsibilities.[14] At official gatherings the Maskil played a public role, both in the fight against demons and in the recitation of standard blessings over the community.[15] The longest and best preserved of the ritual texts assigned to the Maskil survives in two partial copies, 4Q510 and 4Q511, and often goes by the title *Songs of the Maskil.* It seems to have contained a series of prayers or songs, all of which were intended to protect the community against demons. We will return to the texts of these prayers below; for now, the key point is that the Qumran community delegated these protective rituals to the holder of a particular office.

Evidence for the oral recitation of healing and exorcistic texts in corporate settings is lacking for Roman and late antique Judaism. Certainly, the private use of psalms continued. The Yerushalmi calls Ps 91 the "song of the afflicted," recited by people in times of need.[16] Elsewhere, as will be seen in Chapter 7, the rabbis' rejection of the practice of saying a prayer over a wound indicates that it did not have the same standing as a communal ritual within rabbinic Judaism as the Maskil's protective rituals had at Qumran. Yet this

---

[13] Austin 1962, 14.

[14] For an overview of the Maskil's educational and liturgical roles in the Qumran community, see Newsom 1990.

[15] For example, 1QS III.13, IX.12, 1QH^a XX.11, 1QSb, 4QS^b IX.1.

[16] y. ʿErub. 10:11 (26c); y. Šabb. 6:2 (8a–b).

does not necessarily mean that Jews uniformly had a poor opinion of such rituals. Rabbinic control of Jewish life in late antiquity was in many ways more aspirational than actual, and it is possible that the recitation of exorcistic psalms continued to be practiced within Jewish communities over which the rabbis did not exercise control. Gideon Bohak, in fact, argues that synagogues continued to be seen as places of healing, citing evidence from New Testament miracle stories and from the condemnation of John Chrysostom.[17] He also points to the preservation of an exorcistic psalm in a handbook from the Cairo Genizah that is almost identical to one found in cave 11 at Qumran as further evidence of their continued ritual use.[18] Thus, while Roman and late antique evidence is missing for the communal recitation of psalms for healing and protection, there are some hints that the practice persisted.

Early Christian texts also assign the task of healing and protecting against demons to community members who held particular offices. The earliest evidence for a Christian healing rite comes from the Book of James in the New Testament, where the sick are to summon "elders (*presbyteroi*) of the church" to pray and anoint them with oil (Jas 5:14).[19] The *Apostolic Tradition* and *Apostolic Constitutions*, dated to the third and fourth centuries respectively, likewise assign the task of performing rituals that heal and protect to bishops and *presbyteroi*.

For the Maskil and Christian clergy, then, there seems to be a twofold qualification to perform these rituals, one explicit and the other implicit. First, the individual must hold the position tasked with performing the ritual. Second, while not stated, it is implied that the individual must also know the correct form that these rituals are to take. Indeed, the correct performance of speech acts is seen by Austin as a necessary component for their efficacy.[20] Yet the stories by Epiphanius and John Moschos reveal that in some circumstances, the rituals may be performed by anyone who knows their correct form, regardless of whether they hold the designated office. In such situations, ritual knowledge trumps institutional authority. Among freelance practitioners, this knowledge and ability to perform the rituals seems to be the only required characteristic. For example, a ritual from the *Sepher ha-Razim*, a late third- or early fourth-century Jewish text, instructs the practitioner to recite "I, N the son of N, beseech you that you will give me success in healing N the

---

[17] Bohak 2008, 314–15.
[18] Bohak 2008, 303–4; Bohak 2012.
[19] Although the exact date and provenance of James are difficult to determine, there are some factors that suggest it originated in the early Christian community of Palestine. For a detailed analysis and review of the literature regarding these questions, see Allison 2013, 3–32, 94–8.
[20] Austin 1962, 14–15.

son of N."[21] Although texts such as this one instruct the practitioner to provide his name during the ritual, the individual's identity itself is immaterial. There is no indication that the ritual was restricted to certain practitioners; the only requirement is that they know the proper form, including in this case the correct point to insert their own name.

Ritual authority

While the identity of the person who performed these rituals seems to have been of little importance, the person credited with creating them was significant. This appeal to an earlier authority presumably offered proof of the ritual's efficacy and advertised the fact that it could be traced back to a figure who was widely recognized as a ritual expert. This can already be seen, for example, among the Dead Sea Scrolls. 11Q5 (11QPsalms^a) calls four psalms by the biblical king David "songs to perform over the possessed."[22] Another find from the Judaean desert, 11QApocryphal Psalms (11Q11), seems to be a handbook with texts for combating demons, and some scholars have suggested that the psalms found in it were the Davidic psalms known to the author of 11Q5.[23] For example, David is identified as the author of a psalm that begins on line 4 of the fifth column, and, at the beginning of the second column, his son Solomon is charged with invoking God's help against demons. The appearance of David and Solomon in 11QApocryphal Psalms reflects a popular belief that the two biblical kings had special knowledge of diseases and demons, and that this knowledge had been passed down through the generations.

The conviction that David knew how to combat demons was not limited to the author of 11QApocryphal Psalms. Josephus' retelling of the initial meeting between Saul and David in 1 Sam attests to similar perspective by casting David in the role of a ritual practitioner. In the Hebrew Bible, 1 Sam explains that following David's anointing by Samuel, the "Spirit of the LORD" had departed from the reigning king, Saul, and that "an evil spirit from the LORD tormented" him.[24] Seeking relief, Saul ordered that a skilled lyre-player be found to ease his spirits. David was known to someone in the royal household and was summoned to perform this service. The chapter concludes with the following observation: "And whenever the evil spirit from God came upon Saul, David

---

[21] *Sepher ha-Razim*, the first firmament, lines 31–4. Translations of the *Sepher ha-Razim* are from Morgan 1983. For the text, see Margalioth 1966.

[22] 11QPsalms^a XXVII.9–10. Translations from the Dead Sea Scrolls are taken from García Martínez and Tigchelaar 1997.

[23] For example, Nitzan 1992, 53–4; Puech 1992, 78–9; Alexander 1997, 325–6; Eshel 2003b, 83.

[24] 1 Sam 16:14.

124   CONTESTED CURES

took the lyre and played it with his hand, and Saul would be relieved and feel better, and the evil spirit would depart from him."[25] Josephus' version of this story follows the biblical narrative, but his description of David's activities may reflect healing practices that would have been recognizable to his audience in the first century CE. Josephus expanded on the biblical account in his description of Saul's ailment:

> he was beset by strange disorders and evil spirits which caused him such suffocation and strangling that the physicians could devise no other remedy save to order search to be made for one with power to charm away (*exadein*) spirits and to play upon the harp.[26]

Josephus adds a detail about doctors being consulted first about Saul's condition, and it was at their suggestion that Saul searched for someone who was skilled in combating these spirits. Josephus wrote that Saul "had no other physician than David, who, by singing his songs (*hymnous*) and playing upon the harp, restored Saul to himself."[27] Whereas in the Hebrew Bible, David's expertise was limited to instrumental music, in Josephus' version it has been expanded to include the recitation of hymns. Several observations about Josephus' retelling of the story of Saul and David are worth noting. While it is possible the hymns that Josephus attributed to David were simply understood as soothing, like the instrumental music mentioned both in the Hebrew Bible and by Josephus, there is good reason to suspect that Josephus' audience would have understood David to be acting as a ritual practitioner with knowledge of the damage that demons could inflict and the correct hymns to expel them, since the verb used by Josephus to describe David's performance (*exadein*) can be used of a ritual text intended to effect a cure. Josephus did not identify the hymns that David sang over Saul, but the attribution of exorcistic hymns to David in the texts from the Judaean desert suggests that in the Second Temple period there may have been collections of hymns attributed to the biblical king and that the readers of Josephus might have understood these to be what David performed for Saul.

By the Roman period, Josephus could also repeat popular, extra-biblical traditions that God had given David's son Solomon knowledge of demons, illnesses, and the means for expelling them.[28] One of the most famous examples

---

[25] I Sam 16:23.

[26] Josephus *Ant.* 6.166 (Thackeray 1956). See also *Ant.* 6.213–14 and discussion in Bohak 2008, 99–100.

[27] Josephus *Ant.* 6.168 (Thackeray 1956).

[28] There is a *baraita* in the Bavli that also refers to an ancient formulary, one associated with King Hezekiah. *b. Ber.* 10b records a tradition that Hezekiah hid away the "book of cures" during his religious reforms in Judah at the end of the eighth century BCE, an action for which the rabbis commended him.

is the story of Eleazar, who performed exorcisms for Vespasian while the latter was campaigning in Palestine. The Eleazar episode was offered by Josephus to demonstrate the veracity of these Solomonic legends and to prove that his wonderworking legacy survived among contemporary exorcists. Josephus reported that Eleazar successfully expelled demons in front of an audience that included not only Vespasian himself, but also his sons, his officers, and his entire army. The account begins with Josephus' explanation of Solomon's expertise at dealing with demons and his assurance that the ritual performed by Eleazar could be traced back to the biblical king:

> And God granted him (Solomon) knowledge of the art used against demons (*daimonōn*) for the benefit and healing of men. He also composed incantations (*epōdas*) by which illnesses are relieved, and left behind forms of exorcisms (*exorkōseōn*) with which those possessed by demons drive them out, never to return. And this kind of cure is of very great power among us to this day, for I have seen a certain Eleazar, a countryman of mine, in the presence of Vespasian, his sons, tribunes and a number of other soldiers, free men possessed by demons, and this was the manner of the cure: he put to the nose of the possessed man a ring which had under its seal one of the roots prescribed by Solomon, and then, as the man smelled it, drew out the demon through his nostrils, and, when the man at once fell down, adjured the demon never to come back into him, speaking Solomon's name and reciting the incantations (*epōdas*) which he had composed.[29]

This exorcism uses a natural material that was thought to possess an inherent exorcistic property – the root embedded in Eleazar's ring.[30] After the exorcism, Eleazar pronounced spoken "incantations" (*epōdas*) to prevent the demon from returning to his victim. Josephus mentioned that the root was placed under the ring's seal, but gives no indication as to what was inscribed on the seal and whether this seal was believed to contribute to the ritual's efficacy. The story concludes by explaining that its purpose was to ensure that Solomon's "surpassing virtue of every kind" be known to everyone.[31] In this

---

[29] Josephus *Ant.* 8.45–7 (Thackeray 1956).

[30] The use of natural substances to force demons away, in this case a root that had been encased in a ring, is not unique to Josephus. Additional examples occur in the deuterocanonical Book of Tobit, in the *PGM*, and in the *Testament of Solomon*. Justin Martyr is also aware that fumigation was one method of exorcism (*Dial.* 85.3). For the use of fumigation to ward off demons, see Bohak 2008, 88–94; for a discussion of similar treatments used for the wandering womb, see Faraone 2011. As is true of all the rituals discussed in this chapter, the identity of the person who conducted the fumigation was generally less important than the accuracy with which it was performed.

[31] Josephus *Ant.* 8.49 (Thackeray 1956).

126   CONTESTED CURES

way, Josephus bookended the story about Eleazar's successful demonstration by referencing the pivotal role of Solomon.

The biblical king is likewise given significance as a purveyor of specialized ritual knowledge in the *Testament of Solomon*, a literary book of Christian "magic" from late antiquity whose precise date and provenance are unknown. The author, in the voice of Solomon, identifies the purpose of the text:

> at my death I wrote this testament to the sons of Israel and I gave (it) to them so that (they) might know the powers of the demons and their forms, as well as the names of the angels by which they are thwarted.[32]

Like Josephus' story about the exorcist Eleazar, this text also includes a story about Solomon using a ring to gain control over *daimones*, in this case to help him construct the Temple in Jerusalem.[33] Over the course of the text, Solomon questions a series of *daimones*, who tell him of their powers and the means by which they are controlled.

Jubilees, a second-century BCE Hebrew text, credits the biblical Noah with the composition of ritual texts. Written by a Palestinian Jew, *Jubilees* retells the events of Genesis to harmonize them with a new, 364-day calendar.[34] It was popular among members of the Dead Sea Scrolls sect, as indicated by the fifteen fragmentary copies found in the Qumran caves. *Jubilees* mentions a book containing divine cures that Noah composed at the direction of an angel. According to the angelic narrator, God commanded an angel to teach Noah remedies that could combat demonic attacks:

> And he told one of us to teach Noah all of their healing because he knew that they would not walk uprightly and would not strive righteously. And we acted in accord with all of his words. All of the evil ones, who were cruel, we bound in the place of judgment, but a tenth of them we let remain so that they might be subject to Satan upon the earth. And the healing of all their illnesses together with their seductions we told Noah so that he might heal by means of herbs of the earth. And Noah wrote everything in a book just as we taught him according to every kind of healing. And the evil spirits were restrained from following the sons of

---

[32] *T. Sol.* 15.14. For the development of Solomonic traditions in Christianity and Judaism, see Boustan and Beshay 2015.

[33] *T. Sol.* 1.5–7.

[34] For the interpretation that the calendar of *Jubilees* was a solar one that replaced an older, lunar calendar, see Jaubert 1953; Jaubert 1957. A re-evaluation of this hypothesis is offered in Ravid 2003. For the date, provenance, and language of *Jubilees*, see Wintermute 1983, 43–5.

Noah. And he gave everything which he wrote to Shem, his oldest son, because he loved him much more than all of his sons.[35]

Since one in ten of the "evil ones" would be permitted to stay on earth, rather than to be "bound in the place of judgment," God knew that they would antagonize Noah and his descendants with physical ailments. The angels educate Noah about how the demons attack and reveal instructions for how he can negate their effects, using both natural remedies and "every kind of healing" taught by the angels. The author of *Jubilees* underscored the enduring significance of this episode by saying that Noah transcribed the angelic remedies exactly as he was instructed and that he bequeathed this written repository of knowledge to his descendants. This identification of Noah as the author of powerful texts used for exorcisms and healing persisted into late antiquity. *Sepher ha-Razim*, the late third- or early fourth-century text mentioned above, is a so-called "magical" book attributed to Noah. The opening lines of its preface establish its *bona fides* and attest to Noah as a skilled ritual practitioner:

This is a book, from the Book of the Mysteries, which was given to Noah, the son of Lamech . . . by Raziel the angel in the year when he came into the ark (but) before his entrance . . . And he learned from it how to do wondrous deeds, and (he learned) secrets of knowledge, and categories of understanding . . . to declare the names of the overseers of each and every firmament and the realms of their authority, and by what means they (can be made) to cause success in each thing (asked of them) . . .[36]

Listed among the many beneficiaries of this book are Moses and Solomon, both of whom were remembered in the Roman and late antique periods for their ability to perform wonderous feats.[37]

A couple of centuries after *Sepher ha-Razim* was composed, a slightly different version of this appeal to authority can be found in Cyril of Scythopolis' accounts of several monks from the Judaean desert. As we will see in Chapter 6, these monks were primarily known as charismatic healers who were able to work cures through their own innate power or their close connection to God. Alongside these charismatic cures, however, Cyril mentioned the monks healing through the use of oil. In these stories, Cyril did not portray the monks as performing any sort of personal miracle, drawing on their own special abilities. Instead, they seem to be performing a ritual such as those found in the

---

[35] *Jub.* 10:7–14. This translation from Wintermute 1983.
[36] Translations of the *Sepher ha-Razim* are from Morgan 1983.
[37] For more on Moses, see Chapter 6.

128 CONTESTED CURES

early church orders, to which we will turn shortly. What makes these stories relevant here is the authority that they invoke. Rather than calling on the reputation of Noah, David, or Solomon, the monks in Cyril's stories call on the power of Jesus' cross. None of the early church orders describing the use of oil for healing include any information about the procurement of this oil, but all of the examples from Cyril specify this detail. In Cyril's lives, the oil used for healing was associated with Jesus' cross. The fact that each of the monks described by Cyril lived in the Judaean desert, and thus in close proximity to Jerusalem and its chief relic, would have made this seem to be a viable option. According to Cyril, the monk Sabas used this oil to heal injuries resulting from a bad fall,[38] Sabas and another monk, John the Hesychast, both made use of this oil to expel demons,[39] and yet a third monk, Cyriacus, used oil from the cross to cure a boy suffering from epilepsy.[40] I would suggest that using oil from Jesus' cross would have been understood as imbuing these anointings with particular potency. Just as the attribution of hymns or prayers to Noah, David, or Solomon would have strengthened the ritual's perceived power, so attributing the origin of anointing oil to the cross of Jesus would have had the same effect.

Ritual words

As we have already seen, the central components of the ritual cures in this chapter are the words spoken by the practitioner. This was true in Epiphanius' story about Josephus and in John Moschos' story about the unusual baptism. These ritual words can largely be divided into two categories: those spoken directly to the demon believed to be afflicting an individual, and those directed at a higher power requesting help on behalf of an induvial or group. In both categories, *historiolae* may be employed. As we saw in Chapter 2 on amulets, *historiolae* invoke past events to produce similar outcomes in the present. Most

---

[38] Cyril Scyth. *V. Sab.* 45.

[39] Cyril Scyth. *V. Sab.* 63 and *V. Jo. Hes.* 21.

[40] Cyril Scyth. *V. Cyriac.* 9. These stories can be contrasted with another one that Cyril told about Sabas (*V. Sab.* 46). While entertaining a guest, Sabas discovered that there was no wine available and turned a gourd full of vinegar into wine. Sabas gave this gourd to his visitor when he departed, and the gourd remained in his family. The visitor's son later related the following about the gourd: "We had this gourd in our house for many years and, when any-one was unwell, the people of the house filled it with water and sprinkled the patient. This mere sprinkling relieved the sick person of all bodily illness." While the application of water as an agent of healing recalls what we have seen in the church orders, its use here seems to be directly connected to the personal miracle-working power of Sabas rather than with any sort of liturgical rite. The holy man's charismatic miracle endowed an object with long-lasting healing powers.

of the texts considered here are manuals or handbooks that preserve the words used by practitioners in various settings, but to start, I turn to a couple of literary accounts that describe anonymous practitioners using ritual words.

Lucian of Samosata, a regular critic of traditional Greek religion, reflected on the common image of the Palestinian wonderworker, with which he evidently expected his readers to be familiar. In *Lover of Lies*, Lucian tells the tale of how the skeptic Tychiades was schooled by Ion on the efficacy of various ritual cures, including those offered by exorcists from the Levant:

> But you do not need to take my word for it – everybody knows the Syrian from Palestine who is such an expert at this. He takes anyone who falls down at the sight of the moon and twists their eyes and foams at the mouth and sets them back on their feet and sends them off again sound in mind, delivering them from their affliction for a large fee. Whenever he stands over them as they lie afflicted and asks them whence they have come into the body, the sick man himself makes no response, but the demon answers, speaking in Greek or in the language of its country of origin, and explains how and when it entered the person. The Syrian adjures it to leave, and if it does not obey, he drives it out with threats. I saw one leaving: it was black and smoky in color.[41]

Lucian, writing in the second century CE, does not identify the religious community to which these exorcists belonged, and Celsus, a Greek philosopher also writing in the second century, suggests that such techniques were not the purview of any one group. In his critique of Christian wonderworkers, Celsus wrote: "Christians get the power which they seem to possess by pronouncing the names of certain *daimones* and incantations (*kataklēsesi*), hinting I suppose at those who subdue *daimones* by enchantments (*katepadontōn*) and drive them out."[42] Celsus took issue with Christian doctrine and with its claims of exclusivity. In this passage, he argued that Christians, beginning with Jesus, use the names of demons to expel them. The New Testament certainly portrays Jesus talking directly to demons, and in the case of the Gerasene demoniac(s) learns that the demon's name is Legion.[43] However, conversing with a demon while trying to expel it was not unique to the Christian tradition. Acts describes non-Christians doing the same thing:

---

[41] Lucian *Lover of Lies* 16. This translation is a slightly modified version of the one given by Ogden 2007.

[42] Origen *C. Cels.* 1.6. Translations of *C. Cels.* are from Chadwick 1953.

[43] Mark 5:1–20 and Luke 8:26–39; cf. Matt 8:28–34, which includes Jesus' conversation but omits the demon's name. Other examples where Jesus addresses the demon directly during the course of the exorcism include Mark 1:21–6, 9:14–29; Luke 4:31–6.

Then some itinerant Jewish exorcists tried to use the name of the Lord Jesus over those who had evil spirits, saying, "I adjure you by the Jesus whom Paul proclaims." Seven sons of a Jewish high priest named Sceva were doing this. But the evil spirit said to them in reply, "Jesus I know, and Paul I know; but who are you?"[44]

Underpinning this passage lies the assumption that spoken formulae could be effective, even if the person using them lacked faith. This is implied by the author of Acts, who identified these unsuccessful exorcists as Jewish, rather than followers of Jesus. This is similar to the assumptions that inform the story told by Epiphanius about Josephus successfully performing a Christian healing ritual. However, unlike Epiphanius, the identity of the practitioner did in fact matter in Acts 19.

Celsus' critique of the exceptionality of Christian exorcism resonates with the rest of the material presented in this book. He essentially claimed that what Christians were doing was no different than what other contemporary wonderworkers were doing. Two of the words that Celsus used, however, are more complicated: incantations (*kataklēsesi*) and enchantments (*katepadontōn*). Contention over these words was rooted in their implications concerning the source of the wonderworker's power. Origen, a Christian scholar and apologist who responded to Celsus, took issue with his use of *kataklēsis* ("summoning" or "incantation"). Origen did not define what constituted a *kataklēsis* and what made him reject the term, but he did give a fairly concise description of the method that his Christian contemporaries used to expel demons:

> For they do not get the power which they seem to possess by any incantations (*kataklēsesin*) but by the name of Jesus with the recital of the histories (*historiōn*) about him. For when these are pronounced they have often made *daimones* to be driven out of men, and especially when those who utter them speak with real sincerity and genuine belief.[45]

Despite Origen's insistence on the distinctiveness of Christian miracles, what he is describing here is no different than what is seen in other sources. Christians were calling on the name of a divine figure whom they believed could perform the miracle, in this case Jesus, and using stories from his life – *historiolae* – to ensure the ritual's effectiveness. A few lines after the passage quoted above, Origen repeated these two central elements, the name of Jesus and *historiolae*, and added a third possibility: "with other words which are believed

[44] Acts 19: 13–15.
[45] Origen *C. Cels.* 1.6.

RITUAL PRACTITIONERS   131

to be effective, taken from the divine scripture."[46] Origen suggested that "real sincerity and genuine belief" made the ritual especially successful, but the implication is that the words themselves could be powerful, even in the absence of perfect faith, as we saw in Epiphanius' story about Josephus.

Turning now to manuals that preserve ritual words, we revisit the Judaean Desert and the *Songs of the Maskil*. Throughout the *Songs of the Maskil*, the tone alternates between intimidating warnings directed at the demons and descriptive praise of God. The juxtaposition of warning and praise is not accidental, as the speaker explicitly states that he praises God in this way "in order to frighten and terrify" the demons and to make them "forlorn" (lines 4–5). The act of performing these songs was understood as sufficient to repel the demons and to protect the community against further attacks. [47] In addition to speech intended to terrify demons, it may be that the text originally included *historiolae* which are not preserved in the extant scroll: "I shall recount your marvels and engrave them (as) the laws of praise of your glory."[48] While these "marvels" could simply be the words of praise found throughout 4Q510–11, it is also possible that brief narratives of God's past deeds – *historiolae* – were used to invoke the power of these events and apply it to the present.

11QApocryphal Psalms, whose invocation of David and Solomon was considered above, also includes a combination of praise directed to God and warnings to demons beginning in its third column. Although fragmentary, the first two columns seem to include words for adjuring and a cure. Demons are adjured to force them from their victims; when the demon has departed, the sick person is healed. This would make 11QApocryphal Psalms an appropriate text for use with those who are sick or tormented by demons. The extant portion of 11QApocryphal Psalms concludes with a version of Ps 91:

> [He that lives] in the shelter of [the Most High, in the shadow of] the Almighty [he stays.] He who says [to YHWH: My refuge] and [my] fortress, [my God] is the safety in which [I trust.] [For h]e will save you from the [net of the fow]ler, from the dead[ly] pestilence.[49]

Among the things which the psalm promises that the people protected by God will not fear are "the plague that rages at [n]oon, or the pestilence that [in dar]kness proceeds." The psalm indicates that safety from diseases and other ills is guaranteed by the angels that God sends to protect his people. In light of these assurances, it is fitting that the apotropaic use of this psalm was

[46] Origen *C. Cels.* 1.6.
[47] For the appearance of some of these evil forces in *Enoch* and *Jubilees*, see Nitzan 1994, 237.
[48] Lines 2–3 of fragments 63–4.
[49] 11Q11 VI3–14. The text found on 11QApocryphal Psalms is not identical to that found in the Masoretic text.

132   CONTESTED CURES

not limited to this manuscript. It would continue to be popular in the centuries that followed, appearing both on amulets and in the Yerushalmi as the "song of the afflicted."[50]

A third text from the Judaean desert, 4QExorcism ar (4Q560), seems to be part of a handbook containing rituals for use in various circumstances, perhaps collected by a skilled practitioner who knew the dangers of various demons.[51] 4QExorcism ar is fragmentary and difficult to translate, but it addresses itself to both male and female demons and seems to mention "fever and chills" and tooth pain.[52] There are no indications that this text was used in communal settings like the *Songs of the Maskil*, which has led some to conclude that it was a handbook used by a freelance practitioner. In II.5–6, the speaker says "And I, O spirit, adjure [. . .] I enchant you, O spirit [. . .]." This direct address to the demon uses speech to combat demons, a pattern also present in the *Songs of the Maskil*.[53]

In contrast to these Jewish texts from the Judaean desert, those found in the Egyptian desert are several centuries later and reflect influence from a variety of Egyptian, Jewish, and Christian traditions. One such example, *PGM* IV.3007–86, is attributed to a legendary Egyptian wonderworker, much as we have already seen with appeals to the authority of Noah, David, and Solomon.[54] The long text to be spoken by the practitioner begins by addressing the demon directly: "I conjure you by the god of the Hebrews, Jesus."[55] Along with extended *voces magicae*, the spoken text references the seal of Solomon and the exodus story and is peppered with allusions to the Hebrew Bible. The direct address to the demon continues throughout, concluding "I conjure you, every daimonic spirit, by the one who oversees the earth and makes its foundations tremble, [the one] who made all things which are not into that which is." The implication seems to be that if God created all things, he can also control them. This is precisely the sentiment expressed in some of the biblical quotations found in Aramaic *lamellae* and in the Hebrew–Greek *lamella* from 'Evron discussed in Chapter 2.

---

[50] *y. 'Erub.* 10:11 (26c). Ps 3 is also mentioned in this passage as a psalm that was commonly used for "the afflicted," although it is found neither among the exorcistic and apotropaic prayers of the Dead Sea Scrolls nor on amulets from the region.

[51] See discussion in Penney and Wise 1994; Naveh 1998; Bohak 2008, 111–12; Reed 2020, 206–7, 214–16.

[52] Penney and Wise (1994, 640–2) also suggest that the final two words in this line designate a physical pain in the chest, rather than figurative heartache. For "fever and shivering" on formularies, see *PGM* VII lines 211–14, 218–21, CXIXb; cf. *SM* vol. 1, no. 13, which just includes "shivering" but does not mention fever.

[53] Other exorcistic texts from the Judaean desert include 4Q444 (4QIncantation), 6Q18 (6QHymn), 8Q5 (8QHymn). For more on these texts, see Wacholder and Abegg 1995, 335–6; Eshel 2003a; Eshel 2003b.

[54] Betz 1992, 96, n. 386.

[55] Translations of the *PGM* are from Betz 1992.

Another ritual for expelling *daimones*, found earlier in the same handbook, blends Christian elements into a ritual that is heavily influenced by the Hebrew Bible. The instructions in *PGM* IV.1227–64 are preceded by a title that advertises the ritual's effectiveness, "Excellent rite for driving out *daimones*." The text continues with the words to be spoken by the practitioner:

> *Hail, God of Abraham; hail, God of Isaac; hail, God of Jacob; Jesus Chrestos, the Holy Spirit, the Son of the Father, who is above the Seven, who is within the Seven. Bring Iaō Sabaoth; may your power issue forth* from him, NN, *until you drive away this unclean daimōn Satan, who is in him.* I conjure you, *daimōn*, whoever you are, by this god, SABARBARBATHIŌTH SABARBARBATHIOUTH SABARBARBATHIŌNĒTH SABAR-BARBAPHAI. Come out, *daimōn*, whoever you are, and stay away from him, NN, now, now; immediately, immediately. Come out, *daimōn*, since I bind you with unbreakable adamantine fetters, and I deliver you into the black chaos in perdition.[56]

This ritual would have been performed by the specialist on behalf of a client, who was named in two separate places in the text, as well as in the amulet to be made following the text's recitation. Roy Kotansky argued that the Coptic sections of the text, indicated in italics above, likely had their origins in Jewish liturgical formulae to which Christian elements were added.[57] Invoking divine power with names from the Hebrew Bible and New Testament, along with *voces magicae*, the practitioner addresses the *daimōn* directly and instructs it to depart. Illustrating Austin's theory of performative speech, the text suggests a shared belief by the practitioner and client that by saying "I bind you" and "I deliver you," the words effect a real change. In Austin's argument, this ritual is an example of "an accepted conventional procedure having a certain conventional effect, that procedure to include the uttering of certain words by certain persons in certain circumstances," provided that it "be executed by all participants both correctly and completely."[58]

The technique of addressing a demon directly can also be found in early Christian liturgical texts, where exorcisms are typically associated with baptism.[59]

---

[56] The portions of this text in italics were written in Coptic rather than in Greek.

[57] Kotansky 1994, 178–80.

[58] Austin 1962, 14–15.

[59] This Christian link between exorcism and initiation into the community recalls what we saw earlier in 4QSongs of the Maskil. If the exorcistic texts in 4QSongs of the Maskil were sung during the sectarians' annual ceremony to mark the renewal of the covenant, then initiation into both the Qumran community and the Christian community required apotropaic rites intended to protect members from demonic attacks and, presumably, from the illnesses that these demons inflicted. See discussion Eshel 2003a, 410.

134 CONTESTED CURES

The *Apostolic Tradition* gives detailed instructions on the acceptance of new Christians into the community. In the final preparation of catechumens for baptism, each is exorcised on a daily basis up to and including on the eve of their baptism.[60] At the appointed time, candidates disrobe and approach the water:

> And when the presbyter takes hold of each one of those who are to be baptized, let him bid him renounce saying: "I renounce you, Satan, and all your service and all your works." And when he has said this let him anoint him with the Oil of Exorcism saying: "Let all evil spirits depart from you."[61]

As already seen in other examples, this text reflects a consensus that when these words are spoken, "Let all evil spirits depart from you," these spirits do indeed depart. The *Apostolic Tradition* was attributed to Hippolytus of Rome in the first part of the third century, and, although the text originated in the West, it is known to have circulated in Syria already in the fourth century and possibly even in the third.[62] Egeria, a pilgrim who wrote extensively about both the holy places and the rites that were celebrated there, confirmed that these pre-baptismal exorcisms were practiced in the fourth-century Jerusalem church. She described how those preparing for baptism were exorcized daily, following the morning service, throughout the weeks of Lent.[63]

The spoken words considered up to this point have been directed at a demon. Others were directed instead toward a higher power whose help was sought for healing and exorcism. These two forms of address are not mutually exclusive. The *Apostolic Tradition*, for example, contains both. It instructs that oil be prepared prior to being administered to the sick, who would either consume it or be anointed with it. The officiant is to "render thanks" for the oil:

> O God, who sanctifies this oil as you do grant unto all who are anointed and receive of it the hollowing wherewith you did anoint kings (and) priests and prophets, so (grant that) it may give strength to all that taste of it and health to all that use it.[64]

This prayer calls to mind the anointing of figures in the Hebrew Bible to set them apart for God's work, such as in the stories of Aaron (Exod 30:30), David

---

[60] *Trad. ap.* 20.3–8.

[61] *Trad. ap.* 21.9–10. Translations of the *Apostolic Tradition* are slightly modified versions of those found in Chadwick and Dix 1992, with modernized verb forms and pronouns.

[62] Chadwick and Dix 1992, xliv–xlvi.

[63] *Itin. Eger.* 46.1. See also Cyril Hier. *Catech.* 1.9, 13–14.

[64] *Trad. ap.* 5.2.

(1 Sam 16:12–13), and Elisha (1 Kgs 19:16). Just as God used oil to designate and empower these biblical heroes, here he can use oil to work miracles in the present. The *Apostolic Constitutions*, a Syrian church order, contains a more detailed prayer to consecrate water and oil for healing purposes. The bishop, or in his absence the *presbyteros*, is to perform the following blessing:

> O Lord Sabaoth, the God of powers, the creator of the waters, and the supplier of oil, who are compassionate, and a lover of mankind, who has given water for drink and for cleansing, and oil to give man a cheerful and joyful countenance; do you now also sanctify this water and oil through your Christ, in the name of him or her that has offered them, and grant them a power to restore health, to drive away diseases, to banish demons, and to disperse all snares through Christ our hope . . .[65]

This is another example of a text that calls on a divine healer to intervene, rather than addressing the demon directly. The first words of this prayer use one of the names for God found regularly in the Hebrew Bible. The phrase *Kyrios Sabaōth*, or Lord Sabaoth, is found commonly in the Septuagint where the Hebrew originally read *Yahweh Ṣĕbā'ôt*. Sabaoth is usually just transliterated from the original Hebrew into Greek, but in this prayer from the *Apostolic Constitutions* the transliteration is followed by a gloss of the Hebrew term, "God of the powers." These powers are the heavenly hosts over which God is master. As we have already seen in Chapters 1 and 2, *Sabaōth* appeared commonly on amulets, where it seems to have become a powerful name that may have had little or nothing to do with its use in the Hebrew Bible. Here, the pairing of the transliteration and its translation into Greek suggests that the author of this prayer is well versed in the names for God found in the Hebrew Bible. The next phrase continues these biblical allusions with a reference to the creation story. As in *PGM* IV.3007–86 and in the *lamella* from 'Evron for Casius, the text suggests that since God created all things, he can also manipulate them for healing purposes. This hints at more developed *historiolae*: just as you, God, did something in the past – in this case create water and oil – so also you can use water and oil to produce cures today.

Sepher ha-Razim, the late third- or early fourth-century Jewish handbook, also contains examples of invoking higher powers to heal. This so-called "magical" book addresses all aspects of the human condition, such as securing favor from authorities, predicting the future, speaking to the dead, causing harm to one's enemies, and making someone fall in love. Alongside these other issues are instructions for healing and protection. The text contains a description of the seven firmaments that comprise the heavens. In each of the

---

[65] *Const. ap.* 8.29. This translation is a slightly modified version of *ANF* 7:494.

136 CONTESTED CURES

first six are a series of angels who can be called upon to accomplish various tasks; the seventh is occupied by God, who sits on his throne. This complex cosmology is not unique to the *Sepher ha-Razim*, with examples beginning in the Hellenistic period. The very first encampment of the first firmament pertains to healing. Following a list of seventy-two angelic names the reader is instructed to recite "the name of the angel who rules over the first encampment, who is called 'WRPNY'L, and say there, seven times, (the names of the) seventy-two angels who serve before him."[66] This passage details several additional parameters pertaining to the timing of the ritual, lighting an incense fire, and maintaining purity. However, the focus of the *Sepher ha-Razim* is its long lists of angelic names, which form the centerpiece of this healing ritual.

A similar situation is present in the *Testament of Solomon*. Unlike *Sepher ha-Razim*, which can be assigned to a Jewish milieu, the *Testament of Solomon* is a Christian text, albeit with the possibility that the Christian author reworked earlier Jewish material. The text includes healing and apotropaic rituals, such as that found in a speech by a demon named Lix Tetrax:

> I was assigned to draw out the fever which strikes for a day and a half. As a result, many men, when they see [a particular star], pray about the day-and-a-half fever, (invoking) these three names, "Baltala, Thallal, Melchal," and I heal them.[67]

Rather than addressing Lix Tetrax directly and commanding him to leave, other names are invoked, presumably those of higher powers believed to have influence over the demon.[68] Later, in chapter 18 of the *Testament of Solomon*, there is an extended list of thirty-six "heavenly bodies, the world rulers of the darkness of this age."[69] They all give their name, the damage they can inflict on humanity, and the means for forcing their departure. In this list is a veritable catalogue of the physical ailments known to the author, including, among other things, headache, sore throat, eye and ear diseases, nerve damage, fever, digestive ailments, and organ pain. Also listed are interpersonal conflicts and mental health concerns. Of these thirty-six, all but a handful are thwarted by means of calling on a higher power, and about half of these heavenly bodies

---

[66] *Sepher ha-Razim*, the first firmament, lines 28–9.

[67] *T. Sol.* 7.5–6.

[68] In this passage, the ritual for securing protection against a fever-causing demon is a spoken invocation. As in the *Sepher ha-Razim*, however, other rituals from the *Testament of Solomon* give instructions that include writing. For example, a demon named Obyzouth instructs Solomon that writing the name of the archangel Raphael on a piece of papyrus will ensure safety against her attacks on women in childbirth (*T. Sol.* 13.6).

[69] *T. Sol.* 18.2.

explain that they can be gotten rid of by the recitation of verbal formulae. The very first one can serve as an example: "I am the first decan of the zodiac (and) I am called Ruax. I cause heads of men to suffer pain and I cause their temples to throb. Should I hear only, 'Michael, imprison Ruax,' I retreat immediately."[70] As we have already seen, this speech act presupposes an understanding that words can produce change. Through the act of issuing the command to Michael, Ruax is immediately expelled.

In this section we have seen two different types of ritual speech. In some cases, demons are addressed directly and spoken words are used to expel them and the illnesses they cause. In other cases, the practitioner invokes higher powers, who effect similar results. These two forms of ritual speech are not mutually exclusive; the same text can employ both. Together, they are premised on a shared understanding between the practitioner and the person being treated that these speech acts have real power. The desired outcome can be obtained simply by speaking the correct words.

Ritual actions

Alongside the use of speech acts to combat demons and heal diseases, some rituals employed gestures or actions, such as the imposition of hands or the application of oil. The earliest evidence for such actions in Christian healing rituals is found in the epistle of James, where the sick are instructed to have community elders anoint them with oil and pray. There is a continuous Christian tradition of anointing with oil, to which we will turn in a moment, but first a few words must be said about what took place during the elder's prayer. James 5 is somewhat ambiguous on this point, saying simply that the elders were to pray "over" the sick person (*proseuxasthōsan ep' auton*).[71] By the time that Origen referred to this passage in his *Homily on Leviticus*, or at least by the time that Origen's homily was translated into Latin by Rufinus, the prayer offered by the elders was accompanied by the imposition of hands on the sick person (*imponant ei manus*) followed by anointing with oil in the name

---

[70] *T. Sol.* 18.5. A smaller number of these heavenly bodies explain that they can be expelled by writing. Sometimes the medium for this written text is specified, such as a piece of papyrus, or in one example a "piece of wood from a ship which has run aground" (*T. Sol.* 18.24, 28). The location of the writing matters in other cases. Rhyx Alath, who inflicts croup on children, instructs that the name Rarideris be written and carried as an amulet, while Mardero, a fever-causing demon, says that his name should be written somewhere in the house (*T. Sol.* 18.25, 23). In contrast, Rhyx Manthado who damages kidneys, is particularly vague, simply saying that "Iaoth, Ouriel" is to be written in some unspecified location (*T. Sol.* 18.27).

[71] For a discussion of this preposition, see Allison 2013, 758–9.

of the Lord (*unguentes eum oleo in nomine Domini*).[72] It is difficult to determine when this ritual imposition of hands came to accompany the anointing found in James 5. One possible context for its development may be stories of charismatic holy men who healed by touch, notably Jesus and the apostles. The reference in Jas 5:17 to Elijah, who belongs to a long tradition of Palestinian holy men, could reinforce this reading. Elijah's close access to the divine and his ability to accomplish great feats simply by requesting them of God are two traits of the charismatic healer, as we will see in Chapter 6. It is worth considering whether the imposition of hands in early Christian liturgical healing rites marked a way that the *presbyteroi*, as ritual specialists within early Christian communities, assumed functions otherwise performed by charismatic holy men, thereby underscoring the authority of the institutional elite. In other words, the miraculous function that had been exercised by charismatic holy men such as Elijah and Jesus was, in the eyes of at least some, transferred to the *presbyteroi* who operated within a liturgical framework.[73] Regardless of its origin, the imposition of hands during healing rituals continued. The *Sacramentary of Serapion* is a mid-fourth-century prayer book from Egypt for use by the clergy during the eucharistic liturgy and other services.[74] Its Prayer VIII (30) is titled "Laying on of hands of the sick" and contains an implicit comparison between the touch offered by the officiant and God's hand. In conjunction with the officiant laying his hands on the individual, he is to recite "Lord God of mercies, stretch out your hand and grant that all the sick be healed."[75]

The application of oil in Christian healing rituals can more easily be traced to Jas 5. The word for oil, *elaion*, is commonly found in the wider Greek-speaking world in the context of the bath or the gymnasium. It also appears in settings that could best be described as medical or palliative, such as Isaiah's desolate prophecy about the Kingdom of Judah's future (Isa 1:6), the parable of the Good Samaritan, where oil is mixed with wine and used as an ointment (Luke 10:34), or the Mishnah's prohibition of applying oil to the body as a medical treatment on the Sabbath.[76] No details are given in Jas 5 about how — if

---

[72] Rufinus *Orig. Hom. Lev.* 2.4 reads *ungentes eum oleo in nomine Domini*.

[73] Dale Allison (2013, 758) contrasts this institutionalization with the charismatic healing gifts found in 1 Cor 12:9, 30.

[74] For the date and authorship of the *Sacramentary of Serapion*, see discussion in Barrett-Lennard 1994, 277–84.

[75] Translations of the *Sacramentary of Serapion* are from Barrett-Lennard 2010. There are two systems of numbering the prayers in the *Sacramentary of Serapion*. The first follows the order found in the original manuscript (indicated by Roman numerals), and the second follows a proposed reconstruction of the prayers' original order (Arabic numerals). For more on the order of these prayers, see discussion in Barrett-Lennard 2010, 9–11.

[76] *m. Šabb.* 8:1, 14:3–4, 19:2. Rabbinic authors made an exception for "children of kings," arguing that such people would be in the habit of applying oil on a daily basis. If it was used as a medical treatment, it was prohibited, but if it was a daily habit for non-medical reasons, then it was permitted.

RITUAL PRACTITIONERS 139

at all – this oil was prepared, but the church orders that developed in the following centuries would prescribe prayers both for the preparation of the oil and the anointing. In these liturgical texts, oil was used in two different contexts: healing and exorcism, the latter particularly in connection to baptism.

Cyril of Jerusalem, a fourth-century bishop of the holy city, confirmed the importance of oil in pre-baptismal exorcisms. In his lectures to newly baptized Christians, Cyril focused on the significance of the baptismal ritual that his audience had recently experienced:

> Then, once you had removed your clothes, you were anointed with exorcised oil from the topmost hairs of your head to the lowest parts of your body, and became sharers in Jesus Christ, the true olive. You were cut from the wild olive and grafted on to the true olive, and began to share in the richness of the genuine olive. So the exorcised oil is a symbol of this share in the richness of Christ, and it wards off every trace of the enemy power. For just as the breathing of the saints and the invocation of God burns like the fiercest flame and chases away the demons, so too the invocation of God together with prayer gives this exorcised oil such power that it can burn away the traces of sin and even repel the hidden powers of the evil one.[77]

In this passage, Cyril places exorcism within the broader context of an individual's reception into the church. The pre-baptismal anointing was symbolic of one's union with Jesus, while at the same time it was a powerful apotropaic device. Oil was the central element in Cyril's understanding of what took place. The oil "wards off" demonic influence, much as we have already seen speech acts do. Cyril made clear that it was not the oil alone that had this effect; the oil was powerful only because it was accompanied by prayer and an invocation of God. Cyril focused on the renunciation of sin, on "enemy powers," and the "hidden powers of the evil one." The purpose of the exorcism was, in other words, to ward off these demonic attacks. The popular understanding of *daimones* as the cause of disease means that these exorcisms were likely thought to offer some protection against physical ailments. Indeed, John Moschos' story about an unorthodox baptism that resulted in healing hints at this belief. Even though the pre-baptismal exorcism was not mentioned in John Moschos' story, it was a well-established part of the baptismal ritual by the time he wrote.

Prayer XXII (15) of the *Sacramentary of Serapion* likewise uses oil in reference to "the attacks of the malevolent powers upon them." The prayer requests that the oil be a "healing and strengthening power." It is clear that

---

[77] Cyril Hier. *Catech.* 20.3. Translations of Cyril of Jerusalem are from Yarnold 2000.

140 CONTESTED CURES

"healing" is used not simply in the sense of physical disease, but also in a spiritual sense to "eradicate from their soul, body and spirit, every indication of sin and transgression or satanic effect." In other words, the apotropaic element is just one of several interconnected components that included the forgiveness of sin and the individual's new Christian life.[78] Prayer XXIX (17) is labeled in the manuscript as "Prayer for oil or bread or water of the sick" and is the longest and most elaborate prayer concerning oil in the *Sacramentary of Serapion*. The bread and water, referenced in the prayer's title, are not mentioned in the prayer itself, where only oil is named.[79] As was seen earlier in the *Apostolic Tradition*, the intended use of the oil in the *Sacramentary of Serapion* includes both external anointing and ingestion:

> [W]e pray that you send forth a healing power of the only-begotten upon this oil, that it may become for those who are anointed with it, or partake of these your created elements, for a throwing off of every disease and every sickness, for a remedy against every demon, for a banishment of every unclean spirit, for a casting out of every evil spirit, for a driving out of every fever and shivering fit and every illness, for good grace and forgiveness of sins, for a medicine of life and salvation, for health and wholeness of soul, body and spirit and for complete bodily health and strength. Master let every satanic energy, every demon, every plot of the adversary, every blow, every scourge, every suffering, every pain, or slap or shaking or evil phantom fear your holy name which we have now called upon and the name of your only-begotten. And let them depart from the inner and outer being of these your servants, that his name may be glorified, he who was crucified and rose again for us, who has taken up our diseases and our infirmities, even Jesus Christ who is also coming to judge the living and the dead, because through him be to you the glory and the power in holy Spirit both now and to all the ages of ages. Amen.[80]

Illness-causing demons are not addressed directly in the passage; instead, third-person imperatives accomplish the desired effect. In the first part of this prayer, the oil is blessed with the request that God send the "healing power" of his son on the oil. The elements blessed by this prayer had wide-ranging applications. This is emphasized by the repeated use of *pas* ("all" or "every") throughout

---

[78] *Sacramentary of Serapion* Prayer XXII (15). For more examples of exorcisms in liturgical settings, see discussion in Kotansky 1994, 174–5, 177–8.

[79] Blessed water as an agent of healing was mentioned in the *Apostolic Constitutions*, but this is the first appearance of bread used in this way. See discussion in Barrett-Lennard 1994, 288.

[80] *Sacramentary of Serapion* Prayer XXIX (17).

the prayer. At the beginning, the oil is identified as efficacious against "every disease and every sickness"; later, more specific concerns are further modified by *pas*, such as fevers and evil spirits. The prayer also specifies that the blessed oil was to be the "medicine of life and salvation, for health and wholeness of soul, body and spirit," introducing an interest in eschatology. The emphasis on fevers here reflects widespread concerns about the perils of fever, especially fevers associated with malaria. William Brashear's survey of the medical complaints addressed in the *PGM* reveals fever, or fever and chills, to be by far the most common issue.[81] The same is true for the *lamellae* amulets from Roman and late antique Palestine, where more than a quarter specify fever, including the silver *lamella* from Tiberius for Ina discussed in Chapter 2. In other words, despite the eschatological concern in the *Sacramentary of Serapion*'s Prayer XXIX (17), the attention to fever means that the author was attuned to common ailments of the period. Here, then, was a liturgical alternative to counter the popularity of fever amulets.

The inclusion in Prayer XXIX (17) of a second list of foes, starting with "Master let every satanic energy . . .," seems to indicate a shift. Whereas the first part of the prayer imparted a blessing upon the elements, the second turned to their administration to the sick. The reference to "your holy name which we have now called upon" alludes to the invocation found at the prayer's beginning, after which the speaker turns his attention to "these your servants" who are awaiting cures. In this way, the object of prayer in the first half is the oil, presumably together with the water and bread, and the object in the second is the individual in need of healing.[82]

The oil used for anointing in Cyril of Scythopolis' stories about the monks of Palestine was taken from Jesus' cross, as seen above, which would have underscored divine sanction for the ritual. Other Palestinian monks seem to have made use of more traditional liturgical anointings, without recourse to the cross. The earliest such reference comes from Jerome's *Life of Hilarion*. In describing the crowds that flocked to Hilarion, Jerome wrote that one reason for their visits was to "receive from him bread or oil that he had blessed."[83] Although Jerome does not link the reception of these items to healing miracles, the common use of oil in healing rites and the combination of oil and bread in Prayer XXIX (17) of the *Sacramentary of Serapion* raises the possibility that Jerome understood Hilarion to make use of liturgical rites to heal. The connection between oil and healing is more apparent later in the text, when Jerome writes that people went out to be near to Hilarion as news of his

---

[81] Brashear 1995, 3499–501. Fever is mentioned elsewhere in the *Sacramentary of Serapion* in Prayer XVII (5).

[82] See discussion in Barrett-Lennard 1994, 285–6, 295–6.

[83] Jerome *V. Hil.* 30. Translations of Jerome's *Life of Hilarion* are from Deferrari 1952.

immanent death spread. Among these pilgrims was a woman named Constantia. According to Jerome, Hilarion "had saved her daughter and son-in-law from death by anointing them with oil."[84] The healing took place earlier in Hilarion's life and is mentioned in this passage simply as a way to identify Constantia. The only detail provided is that of the oil; there is no mention of the holy man's successful prayer, which figures prominently in the cures that will be discussed in Chapter 6. In another passage, Hilarion enjoined people to apply "blessed oil" to wounds.[85] In this case, Hilarion's involvement is limited to a recommendation that people make use of a liturgical remedy.

A sixth-century monk named Barsanuphius similarly recommended the use of "holy water" in response to a letter that he received. When asked if it was acceptable to have someone "read a spell over" a sick animal, the ascetic instructed:

> Magical spells are forbidden by God, and one should not resort to them at all. For they bring destruction to the soul through transgressing God's decree. Instead, bring your horse to other forms of healing and therapy, as proposed by veterinary doctors. For this is certainly not sinful. Furthermore, sprinkle some holy water over it.[86]

Although Christian liturgical texts for healing rites involving oil, water, and bread presume that the recipients of these rites are people – members of the Christian community – this letter suggests that similar remedies could be extended to animals. Barsanuphius made no mention of any particular prayers that were to accompany this sprinkling of holy water on the animal. However, such details are also absent in Jerome's description of Hilarion. The instructions that Barsanuphius gave his correspondent suggest that the individual is able to perform this rite himself, without needing to bring the animal to a church or to summon a priest or bishop to do it for him. As in Hilarion's instruction that people apply "blessed oil" to their injuries, Barsanuphius' recommendation in this letter seems to confirm that in at least some circumstances, people were able to save blessed oil and water for use at a later time as needed.

Despite the popularity of oil in Christian liturgical rites, the use of oil can be found in other healing contexts too. The *Testament of Solomon*, whose spoken formulae were considered in the previous section, also makes use of oil. While most of chapter 18's "heavenly powers" prescribe verbal formulae, others require more detailed rituals, such as the thirtieth one in the list:

---

[84] Jerome *V. Hil.* 44. For more Jerome's *Life of Hilarion*, see Chapter 6.

[85] Jerome *V. Hil.* 32.

[86] Letter no. 753. Translations of the letters of Barsanuphius and John come from Chryssavgis 2006–7.

"I am called Rhyx Physikoreth. I bring on long-term illnesses. If anyone puts salt into (olive) oil and massages his sickly (body with it) saying, 'Cherubim, seraphim, help (me),' I retreat immediately."[87] These instructions for the use of olive oil are reminiscent both of exorcistic anointing and of olive oil's long history as a soothing or medicinal treatment. *PGM* IV.3007–86, whose ritual text directly addressing demons and recalling the creation story was also considered above, similarly requires certain preparations. Olive oil is to be boiled together with several other ingredients. Although the text does not specify what, if anything, is to be done with the resulting oil mixture, it is not difficult to imagine it being administered to the person seeking healing, either as an ointment or as a mixture to consume.

In most of the examples considered in this section, actions such as anointing with oil or the imposition of hands accompany spoken prayers or formulae. Ritual handbooks, including early church orders and those used by freelance specialists, naturally included the texts to be spoken in a given setting. In some liturgical texts, we have little but the prayers themselves. For example, the *Sacramentary of Serapion* provides some of the most detailed prayers concerning healing and anointing with oil, but it contains virtually no rubrics, or instructions for what actions should accompany these prayers. In other types of texts, the prayers themselves are not written out, and the ritual actions take center stage. Our picture of these healing rituals is thus shaped by the types of sources that survive, but it is reasonable to expect that prescribed words would have accompanied these ritual actions rather than the extemporaneous and personal healing prayers of the charismatic wonderworkers who will be considered in Chapter 6.

Ritual settings

Scholarship on the rituals discussed in this chapter often follows a putative religion–magic divide. In general, the rituals performed by officially sanctioned practitioners within their religious community – the Maskil and Christian clergy – are studied within the history of their respective traditions, while those worked by freelance practitioners are relegated to the category of "magic." To some degree, this maps onto a distinction between corporate rituals and those performed privately for an individual in need of healing. That line, however, is not clear-cut. Certainly, there were corporate rituals officiated by designated practitioners. The *Songs of the Maskil* are one such example. These texts were not intended either for the private devotions of the Maskil himself or

---

[87] *T. Sol.* 18.34.

for use by individual community members. Rather, the prayers were to be sung by the Maskil on behalf of, and in the presence of, his entire community. Evidence for the public nature of the ritual is found in fragments 63–4 of 4Q511 II.4–5, "And with all [the me]n of the covenant . . ." and in the following column, "Peace to all men of the covenant" (III.4–5). The references to the "men of the covenant" suggest that the songs were used at gatherings when the entire community would be present.[88] The corporate nature of these rituals can also be seen in final lines of the scroll, "May all your works bless always. May your name be blessed for eternal centuries. Amen. Amen."[89] The affirmation "amen" at the conclusion of the prayer indicates that a congregation was present, whose assent and participation was confirmed in their vocal response.[90] Matthias Klinghardt, in his analysis of communal prayers in ancient religion, identifies such components as a "homophonic response" prayer, varieties of which were utilized in both Jewish and Christian liturgical settings.[91]

The earliest evidence for healing rituals in the New Testament also reflects a corporate setting. The closing verses of the epistle of James describe a rite intended to cure the faithful of their diseases:

> Are any among you suffering? They should pray. Are any cheerful? They should sing songs of praise. Are any among you sick? They should call for the elders (*presbyteroi*) of the church and have them pray over them, anointing them with oil in the name of the Lord. The prayer of faith will save the sick, and the Lord will raise them up; and anyone who has committed sins will be forgiven. Therefore confess your sins to one another, and pray for one another, so that you may be healed. The prayer of the righteous is powerful and effective.[92]

In this passage, the author of James instructs readers to seek healing through prayer and anointing with oil by the elders of their community. The admonition to "confess your sins to one another, and pray for one another, so that you may be healed" suggests that this rite was a communal event, rather than one involving only the sick individual and the elders.[93] While it is possible that the author

---

[88] Eshel proposed that this handbook was used during the annual renewal of the covenant; Nitzan argued instead that the ritual took place during the four days that marked the turning of the seasons. See Nitzan 1994, 238; Eshel 2003a, 413; Cf. Angel 2012, 3.

[89] 4Q511 63 IV, 1–3.

[90] Alexander 1997, 321; Eshel 2003a, 408.

[91] Klinghardt 1999, 20.

[92] Jas 5:13–16.

[93] Jas 5:16. For the alternative interpretation that verses 14–15 and 16 represent two distinct rituals, with the first two verses constituting a private ceremony, and verse 16 indicating a separate, public one, see Allison 2013, 768–9.

RITUAL PRACTITIONERS 145

of James understood the elders' prayers to be extemporaneous, our knowledge about communal prayer in the ancient world indicates that there may have been some form of prescribed prayers or psalms even from an early date.[94] There is evidence to support this supposition. Based on the similarities between 1 *Clement* 59.4 and these verses from the end of James, Dale Allison argued that James 5 betrays the influence of a liturgical text.[95] In fact, Allison pushed this conclusion further by arguing that the juxtaposition of this healing ritual with Elijah's rain miracle in the following verses indicates that this early church order was itself related to the Jewish tradition that produced benedictions 5–9 of the *Amidah*.[96] While the liturgical text that Allison proposed cannot be reconstructed, early church orders, such as we have already seen, offer some evidence for how such prayers developed within Christian communities. Two of the healing prayers in the *Sacramentary of Serapion*, Prayers VII (22) and VIII (30), were situated just before the *anaphora*, the part of the eucharistic liturgy when the bread and wine were consecrated.[97] The placement of these prayers immediately before the high point of the eucharistic service underscores the fact that by at least the fourth century healing rituals were seen as an integral part of the community's liturgical life.

The liturgical context of other prayers for healing is more ambiguous. The *Apostolic Constitutions* give no instructions for the administration of the water and oil to someone in need of healing. While it may be that an individual was immediately anointed with the elements or invited to consume them, this is not stated. It is also possible that in at least some circumstances the blessed oil and water were returned to the person who brought them so that they could be used whenever the need arose. We saw in Jerome's *Life of Hilarion* and in Barsanuphius' letter references to the private use of previously blessed oil and water. Somewhat more information about healing in private contexts is found in the *Canons of Hippolytus*, which states:

> The sick also, it is a healing for them to go to the church to receive the water of prayer and the oil of prayer, unless the sick person is seriously ill and close to death: the clergy shall visit him, those who know him.[98]

---

[94] After reviewing the evidence for the use of formularies that contain the exact text of communal prayers, Klinghardt (1999, 14–20) argues that it is the "magic character of prayers that requires a particular, fixed wording." In the case of a ritual such as the anointing with oil found in Jas 5, it seems that a fixed wording for the associated prayers may have developed quickly.

[95] Alison draws on work done by Hermut Löhr (2003) on the liturgical sources known to the author of 1 *Clement*.

[96] See Allison 2011, 13–15.

[97] Another prayer for healing in the *Sacramentary of Serapion*, Prayer XVII (5), probably took place following the distribution of communion. For the context of each prayer, see discussion in Barrett-Lennard 1994, 303–12, 285–97 esp. 286, 97–9.

[98] This translation is from Barrett-Lennard 1994, 287. For the date of the *Canons of Hippolytus*, see discussion in Chadwick and Dix 1992.

146 CONTESTED CURES

Here, it is clear that the oil and water are not self-administered. Rather, they are given to the individual by the clergy. The only variable is whether or not the person in need of healing is physically able to travel to the church to receive them or whether they must be brought to him or her. Similarly, it seems that the long Prayer XXIX (17) from the *Sacramentary of Serapion*, considered above, was used as needed during the visitation of the sick rather than during communal worship.

Evidence for the corporate nature of these rituals is not limited to official religious texts such as the *Songs of the Maskil* or the *Apostolic Constitutions*. In *P. Berol.* 17202, a papyrus of unknown provenience held by the Staatliche Museen zu Berlin, the use and transformation of liturgical texts is apparent. The fragmentary papyrus sheet contains six sections with instructions for different rituals. The first, and longest, bears the title, "For those troubled by [evil] dem[ons]." According to the text's editors, it includes portions for the practitioner to speak and responses to be offered by others present, the latter indicated by italics:

([. . .], *Lord in your command to* [*all men* . . .])
   "The one having lo[osed] the one being punished [. . .],
   And the one having sent forth his only begot/ten child,
      and having indwelled the womb of the Vir/gin"
(*As you have willed it*).
(*The race of mankind could not find out*
the manner of your birth, Lord Jesus Christ),
   "The one having walked upon the waters,
      having not even defiled his feet.
   The one having from five loaves
      fed five-thousand men."
(*for all have obeyed your command, Lord.*
[*Come*] *according to your mercy, upon me, the sinner!*) (the usual)[99]

This text calls to mind Origen's assertion seen earlier in this chapter that Christians expelled demons through the name of Jesus and references to his deeds. The specialist conducting the ritual recites events from the life of Jesus, including his birth from Mary, walking on water, and the feeding of the five thousand, while the participants' responses are addressed directly to Jesus in the second person.[100] Building on the work of William Brashear, Roy Kotansky argued that

---

[99] This translation is from Brashear and Kotansky 2002.
[100] Brashear and Kotansky 2002, 10–11. Credal statements also appear regularly on papyri amulets from Egypt, and one might expect that the same would have been true in Palestine, had papyri amulets survived.

RITUAL PRACTITIONERS 147

this antiphonal prayer originated in a liturgical context before being transformed into the version preserved on this papyrus. Despite this liturgical influence, the other texts in *P. Berol.* 17202 indicate that this is not a fragment of a church order to be used in official liturgical rites but rather one that had been modified for the private use of a freelance specialist and his clients.

The picture of freelance ritual specialists performing cures for a price, such as described by Lucian of Samosata, could lead one to imagine that freelance specialists worked with individuals, while liturgical practitioners worked within communal settings. Certainly, this did take place. The Maskil performed his exorcistic rites during gatherings of the Qumran community, and the *Sacramentary of Serapion* specifies healing rituals that are to take place within the church's regular eucharistic gatherings. Yet *P. Berol.* 17202 indicates that a freelance specialist could perform rituals whose antiphonal responses presupposed the presence of a group, and several Christian texts describe settings where healing rituals are performed by clergy on a case-by-case basis or where individuals could retain blessed elements and administer them to themselves.

* * *

The study of ritual healing in antiquity is often plagued by a dichotomy between "religion" and "magic." The corporate rites described in the Dead Sea Scrolls and in early church orders are placed in the former category, while the rituals performed by freelance specialists, such as those who used the *Sepher ha-Razim* or texts from the *PGM* are relegated to the latter. This division obscures the similarities present across these ritual texts. The specialists who performed them were all thought to produce cures through the correct recitation of certain words. In some cases, these words were accompanied by actions such as the imposition of hands or anointing with oil. In general, the identity of the practitioner was of little importance to the outcome of the ritual, and we have seen situations where the ritual was performed by those who did not believe in what they were doing or who were not authorized to conduct it. The identity of the practitioner is, in fact, of less concern than the source of the ritual. A common trait is the invocation of an earlier expert to lend legitimacy to the ceremony and to demonstrate its efficacy. Both Jewish and Christian practitioners recalled the heroes of the Hebrew Bible in this role, from Noah and Moses to David and Solomon.

What liturgical practitioners such as the Maskil or Christian clergy did within their communities, freelance specialists performed in other contexts. Some operated at the margins of communities or in the interstices between them, but we should not imagine that these agents were restricted to liminal spaces. A variety of healing practices were known to elite Jewish and Christian authors, who railed against members of their communities who partook of them. This means that Christians who had access to the official rituals performed by priests and bishops may have also participated in unsanctioned healing rituals alongside, or instead of, the liturgical rites. Yet this need not have been strange or surprising to anyone but the elites who wanted to label the rituals of freelance practitioners as "magic." To the sick and suffering, and those who cared for them, the rituals from the *Testament of Solomon* might have seemed just as legitimate as those from the *Sacramentary of Serapion*. Both used spoken formulae to combat physical ailments. But to the leaders who saw themselves as guardians of their community, this desired outcome could not justify extra-liturgical practices. As we will see in Chapter 7, the elites, particularly Christian authors, directed harsh criticism at anyone who administered or received such cures, from amulets to incubation to the ministrations of so-called magicians.

By labeling freelance practitioners as magicians, these elites circumscribed both the people and the rituals that they considered within the bounds of acceptable practice, but the reality was less clear. It is not difficult to imagine people desperate for a cure visiting any practitioner with a reputation for success, regardless of whether they belonged to the same cultural, religious, or ethnic community. The presence of clearly delineated boundaries themselves, especially in the realm of ritual healing, was the creation of these same elites and may have had little in common with the lived experiences of the sick and injured in Roman and late antique Palestine. Even where the practitioner and the client maintained a clear self-understanding of themselves as members of a particular community, one should not assume that the two individuals belonged to the same group. Several of the amulets of Chapters 1 and 2 hinted at the possibility that they might not, as do the conversions associated with miraculous cures related by Epiphanius and John Moschos.

In the end, the distinction between "religious" cures and "magical" cures in this chapter is a reflection of the rhetoric of ancient elite authors who sought to define their religious traditions by excluding certain rituals and practitioners. When scholars accept this polemical distinction and allow it to structure our own view of the past, we lose sight of the inherent similarities among these practices.

CHAPTER 6

Working Such Wonders and Signs: Charismatic Wonderworkers Who Offered Cures

Stories about the miraculous exploits of charismatic holy men have a long history in the southern Levant, from the prophets of the Hebrew Bible to Christian ascetics of late antiquity. Wandering the region, they were credited with "wonders and signs" that revealed their special abilities.[1] In the popular imagination, the figure of Jesus of Nazareth looms large as the charismatic healer par excellence, and his legacy influenced how literary accounts portrayed the lives of later holy men. Yet both the Hebrew Bible and the New Testament indicate that the wonderworkers they describe were not unique to their own religious traditions but were also common among neighboring groups. In this way, the charismatic healers of this chapter are little different than the other forms of ritual healing that this book has explored: methods of seeking divine cures were similar across the notional lines that separated communities, even while the traditions of each community informed the associated prayers, images, and expectations. Unlike the amulets or localized healing sites discussed earlier, evidence for charismatic healers is markedly one-sided. In Chapters 1 and 2, extant amulets counterbalance the critiques offered by elite authors, and in Chapters 3 and 4, votive offerings dedicated by visitors offer non-literary evidence. Even the ritual practitioners of Chapter 5 can be elucidated by texts discovered in the Judaean desert and by Egyptian papyri, which permit avenues of inquiry separate from the rhetoric of literary texts. In contrast, our knowledge of charismatic wonderworkers is limited to those literary texts, which rarely describe these figures with indifference, instead offering either panegyric or denunciation that necessarily complicates any understanding of their healing methods.

The sectarian lens through which these charismatic healers are viewed also obscures distinctions between the healers of this chapter and those of Chapter 5.

[1] Jerome *V. Hil.* 24.

150   CONTESTED CURES

Put simply, we frequently find ancient authors who maintain that wonders performed by their coreligionists are miracles wrought by God or his agents, while
similar feats performed by individuals outside their community are magic accomplished by trickery or incantations. This dichotomy is encoded in our own use
of English to describe healing rituals. What makes one text a prayer and another
an incantation? What makes one healer a magician and another a holy man?
For many today, as in antiquity, it is all in the eyes of the beholder. Despite this
us-versus-them rhetoric, I would argue that it is possible to discern a difference
between the performative acts of Chapter 5, which could be accomplished by
anyone who knew how to do them, and the charismatic healers of this chapter.
I propose that the latter were understood by their coreligionists to have a special charisma that gave them a personal ability to perform miracles.[2] No specific
prayers or rituals were required.

This chapter seeks to center the expectations that those in need of healing would have had as they approached charismatic wonderworkers. Before
turning to this reading of miracle stories, a few words are necessary about the
differences between the ritual practitioners of Chapter 5 and the charismatic
healers of Chapter 6. Christian authors seem to be aware of the distinction
between these two categories in some situations, although they are content
to ignore it when it suits their agenda of "othering" the rituals of which they
disapprove. In non-Jewish and non-Christian texts, a different problem surfaces, since these authors were inclined to elide differences between various
types of miracle-workers.[3] For example, the Greek philosopher Celsus saw no
reason to make a distinction between charismatic healers and ritual practitioners, arguing that Jesus' acts were no different than the works of the magicians
(*goētes*), who similarly performed wondrous deeds and sold their skills in the
marketplace. Celsus considered two possible implications – both Jesus and the
magicians were sons of god, or both performed their marvels with the help of
demons (*daimones*).[4] Either way, he saw the actions of the two as belonging to
the same category. Celsus also drew attention to the preponderance of holy

---

[2] In the New Testament, *charisma* is a grace or gift from God. In 1 Cor 12:9, the *charismata
iamatōn*, the "gifts of healing," are listed among the spiritual gifts (verse 1, *pneumatikōn*) given
to members of the Christian community. Max Weber (1947, 358) considered the charismatic to
be one of three models of leadership, defining charisma as "a certain quality of an individual
personality, by virtue of which he is set apart from ordinary men and treated as endowed with
supernatural, superhuman, or at least specifically exceptional powers or qualities." A slightly
different understanding of a charismatic healer has been put forward by Gerd Theissen (2010,
51), who uses it to refer to "the personal relationship between a charismatic healer and his
adherents." For an overview of the varieties of charismatic figures in the Hebrew Bible, Second
Temple and early rabbinic Judaism, and early Christianity, see Vermes 2012, 1–86.

[3] For literature on this type of competition, see Muir 2006.

[4] Origen *C. Cels.* 1.68.

men in "Phoenicia and Palestine,"[5] questioning the exceptionality of Jesus and identifying him as just one of many prophets from the region:

> There are many, he says, who are nameless, who prophesy at the slightest excuse for some trivial cause both inside and outside temples; and there are some who wander about begging and roaming around cities and military camps; and they pretend to be moved as if giving some oracular utterance.[6]

Since ritual practitioners were often depicted anonymously or identified simply by the function that they performed, such as the Maskil or Christian officials, Celsus' observation that many of these figures are nameless may indicate that he had the ritual practitioners of Chapter 5 in mind. Yet it is also plausible that this observation simply reflects Celsus' general disdain for the figures whom he described. According to Celsus, they loitered in the public spaces around temples and in cities, where they might expect to encounter a large number of people interested in their services. A few lines after the passage quoted above, Celsus ascribed "incomprehensible, incoherent, and utterly obscure utterances" (*agnōsta kai paroistra kai pantē adlēla*) to these individuals.[7] Given Celsus' perspective, this description could apply equally to charismatic healers and ritual practitioners, underscoring again the difficulty of distinguishing the two in his text.

The same problem exists for interpreting Lucian's description of Palestinian exorcists. While Lucian seems to have in mind a ritual practitioner, who performed ceremonies for anyone who would pay him, the pejorative tone reflected in the passage means that his description could apply to both holy men and ritual specialists.[8] In fact, the dialogue between a specialist and a *daimōn* that Lucian

---

[5] Origen *C. Cels.* 7.8.

[6] Origen *C. Cels.* 7.9.

[7] Origen *C. Cels.* 7.9.

[8] Lucian *Lover of Lies* 16. I will not explore in depth the question of payment for healing, but it should be noted that money or gifts were often exchanged for the forms of healing discussed throughout this book. At local healing cults, this could take the form of required sacrifices before incubation and votive dedications to celebrate a successful cure. In the case of amulets, we can expect that people paid for the materials as well as for the services of the scribe who wrote the text. Some of the ritual specialists discussed in the previous chapter likewise would have expected a payment for their services, which seems to be the scenario described by Lucian. However, when Jesus sent out his twelve disciples in Matt 10:8 to "cure the sick, raise the dead, cleanse the lepers, cast out demons," he explicitly instructed them to accept no money in exchange for their services, but rather to rely on the hospitality of those they met to feed and house them. See also Luke 10:1–12. For more on New Testament ideas about paying those in religious authority, including leaders to whom responsibility for liturgical healing would later be assigned, see 1 Cor 9:11–14; Phil 4:15–18; 1 Tim 5:17–18.

described recalls Jesus' healings in the New Testament.[9] At the same time, applying oaths (*horkous epagōn*) and making threats (*apeilōn*) were time-honored methods to expel demons, and can be found in sources ranging from the Dead Sea Scrolls to the *PGM* and early church orders. Neither Lucian nor Celsus was interested in distinguishing between these two types of healers, and they did not paint a particularly flattering image of either one. Nevertheless, they expected their audience to have heard of the itinerant holy men of Palestine and their habits of appearing in public spaces and attracting attention through mysterious words, bizarre affectations, and fantastic conversations with demons.

Between the rhetorical boundary-policing of Jewish and Christian authors, which will be examined in Chapter 7, and the elision of charismatic wonderworkers and ritual practitioners by authors such as Celsus and Lucian, the type of healing under consideration in this chapter is in many ways the most difficult to uncover. Most of the sources are literary creations with the explicit aim of advancing the reputation of these wonderworkers or the tradition that preserved their memory. This validation was in defense not only of Christianity and Judaism writ large, but also of smaller subsets, such as monasteries, the rabbis, or competing forms of Christianity in the aftermath of the divisive Council of Chalcedon in 451.[10] Unlike the previous chapters, in which material culture can shed light on what a person might have seen, heard, or experienced when they employed ritual cures, the nature of the texts in this chapter reveal more about the ideas and expectations of ancient authors than about the experiences of the sick and injured. In his treatment of charismatic wonderworkers in rabbinic Judaism, William Scott Green made precisely this point:

> The historical situation of redacted literature, therefore, is the situation of the redactor(s), not necessarily the situation of the figures who appear in it . . . The proper subject of investigation, therefore, is not what Ḥoni actually said or where he performed his miracle, but the way Mishnaic redaction has shaped the account of his activity.[11]

Green's contention here about Ḥoni applies equally to other charismatic wonderworkers. My goal is not to uncover the historical Jesus, Ḥanina, or Apollonius, but rather to explore the expectations of ritual healing known to the authors who

[9] The reference to oaths (*horkous*) in Lucian's description does not precisely reflect the New Testament evidence, where Jesus is described as expelling demons, but not using exorcistic formulae. Although Jesus is addressed by the Gerasene demoniac in Mark 5:7 with *horkizō*, Jesus himself never uses this or related words in reference to demons. For the argument that Lucian nevertheless explicitly wrote this passage with Jesus in mind, see Ogden 2007, 131–4, esp. 133.

[10] See discussion in Binns 1994; Griffith 1999.

[11] Green 1979, 628.

wrote about them and, by extension, to the audiences that heard these stories. This does not necessarily limit the texts' usefulness for identifying a distinct form of ritual healing, but it does mean that our perspective is necessarily on the historical context in which the texts were produced, which could be at some distance from the setting of the stories themselves.

Each of the narratives considered below recognizes that charismatic wonderworkers could perform miracles without recourse to prescribed ceremonies. Authors described the miracle-worker's power in a variety of ways, all of which attest to the individual's charisma. In some cases, the wonderworker seems to have an intrinsic healing power that can be conveyed by touch or speech. Other stories point to his extraordinary knowledge, his ability to persuade God to act, or to a particularly close relationship with the divine. Underlying them all is the idea that there is something personal about the wonderworker's ability to heal. It cannot be learned and replicated by others, and its application is entirely at the wonderworker's discretion.

Jesus, the healer par excellence

The figure of Jesus is central to any discussion of healing in Roman and late antique Palestine. Stories from the New Testament shaped accounts of later Christian wonderworkers and became sources of criticism and competition for non-Christian authors. While it is rather straightforward to point to the influence that stories of Jesus had on later texts, the experiences of individuals are somewhat more obscure. Nevertheless, it is reasonable to suppose that as the gospel stories of Jesus circulated, they would have shaped the expectations of the sick and injured who approached charismatic wonderworkers in search of a cure. A variety of miracles are ascribed to Jesus in the New Testament, but those relating to healing or the expulsion of demons are the most numerous. The story of a woman healed in Luke 13 offers a good example:

> And just then there appeared a woman with a spirit that had crippled her for eighteen years. She was bent over and was quite unable to stand up straight. When Jesus saw her, he called her over and said, "Woman, you are set free from your ailment." When he laid his hands on her, immediately she stood up straight and began praising God.[12]

Someone familiar with this story about Jesus might expect two things in his or her own encounters with charismatic healers. First, this account, like others in

---

[12] Luke 13:11–13.

154 CONTESTED CURES

the New Testament, emphasizes the immediacy of Jesus' cure. The cure does not need time to take effect, and the author leaves no doubt as to who should be credited with the miracle. A second take-away is the method of Jesus' cure. People who knew New Testament miracles, such as this one, would have readily accepted that charismatic healers could use physical touch and spoken words to bring about a cure. Sometimes, as in this case, the two are used together, and in other stories only one is mentioned. A brief overview of the forms that touch and speech take in the New Testament miracles will show the range of expectations that the sick may have had as they approached later charismatic wonderworkers for a cure.

Some of Jesus' touch miracles give no specifics as to how or where Jesus made contact with the individual.[13] In others, Jesus was said to take a person by the hand[14] or to touch specific body parts.[15] The centrality of touch to convey a cure can also be seen in those stories where Jesus is portrayed as a passive agent of healing from whom miraculous power flowed. In these cases, Jesus made no deliberate motions, but the people who touched him were immediately healed.[16] A subset of these touch miracles are those involving spittle. In John 9:6, Jesus anointed the eyes of a blind man in Jerusalem with mud made from spittle and clay. This can be compared to a similar account in Mark 8:23, where Jesus spat into a blind man's eyes in Bethsaida and laid his hands on him. In addition to touch miracles, two forms of spoken cures are attributed to Jesus. In the first, he addressed a person in need of a cure. The healing of the man at the Pool of Bethesda in John 5, discussed in Chapter 4, is an example of this type. John identified Jesus' spoken command as being the exact moment of cure, much as with the stories of healing by touch: "Jesus said to him, 'Stand up, take your mat and walk.' At once the man was made well, and he took up his mat and began to walk."[17] In other miracles, Jesus directly addressed a

---

[13] A man with leprosy: Luke 5:13; Matt 8:3; cf. Mark 1:41. A crowd in Capernaum: Luke 4:40. A crowd in Nazareth: Mark 5:5. A bent woman in a synagogue: Luke 13:13.

[14] An epileptic or demon-possessed boy near Mount Tabor: Mark 9:27. The dead or near-dead daughter of Jairus: Matt 9:25; Mark 5:41; Luke 8:54. Peter's feverish mother-in-law: Matt 8:15; Mark 1:31 (cf. Luke 4:38–9, which includes this story but not the element of touch).

[15] Two blind men in Capernaum: Matt 9:29. Two blind men near Jericho: Matt 20:34. The ear of the high priest's servant: Luke 22:51. Hearing- and speaking-impaired man: Mark 7:32–5. See also Mark 8:23 and John 9:6.

[16] The hemorrhaging woman: Matt 9:20–2; Mark 5:27–9; Luke 8:43–4. The crowds that touched the fringe of Jesus' garment: Matt 14:35–6; Mark 6:54–6; see also Mark 3:9–10 and Luke 6:18–19.

[17] John 5:8–9. There are additional examples of Jesus healing through such commands. Bartimaeus in Jericho: Mark 10:46–52; cf. Luke 18:35–43. Ten people are cured of leprosy: Luke 17:11–19. A man regains the ability to walk: Matt 9:2–8; Mark 2:1–12; Luke 5:17–26. A man with a withered hand recovers: Matt 12:9–14; Mark 3:1–6; Luke 6:6–11. Lazarus is raised from the dead:

CHARISMATIC WONDERWORKERS   155

demon, in scenes reminiscent of Lucian's derisive description of the "Syrian from Palestine."[18]

An exorcism described in all three synoptic gospels highlights another expectation about how charismatic wonderworkers performed miracles: the importance of personal faith. This exorcism involved a boy whose father first approached Jesus' disciples for help, and only sought out Jesus himself when the disciples failed to work the miracle.[19] The longest version of this story is found in Mark, where Jesus rebuked his audience as a "faithless generation" (9:19). After the father described his son's symptoms, "Jesus said to him, 'If you are able! All things can be done for the one who believes.' Immediately the father of the child cried out, 'I believe; help my unbelief!'" (9:23–4). Faith was again underscored at the end of the Matthew's version of this story, when Jesus responded to the disciples' question about why they could not heal the boy, "Because of your little faith. For truly I tell you, if you have faith the size of a mustard seed, you will say to this mountain, 'Move from here to there,' and it will move; and nothing will be impossible for you."[20] On the basis of this and other stories in which Jesus emphasized faith, we might expect that those approaching a charismatic healer expected faith to be a key factor in the cure – both their own faith and that of the wonderworker. This is in stark contrast to Epiphanius' story about Josephus, discussed in Chapter 5. In that case, Josephus was able to perform a healing miracle, even though he very clearly did not believe in either the Christian God or in the ritual that he planned to use.[21] Despite this disbelief, Josephus spoke the correct words, and it was his speech act that cured, not his faith. While the story of Josephus does not mean that faith was necessarily absent among those seeking cures from ritual practitioners, it suggests that faith may have been perceived as a some-what less important factor.

Stories about Jesus also connected him to figures from the Hebrew Bible, just as accounts of later Christian holy men drew upon details from the life of

---

John 11:38–44 (cf. Luke 7:11–17). Crowds following the healing of Peter's mother-in-law: Matt 8:16; cf. Luke 4:40–1; Mark 1:32–4. In other examples, Jesus speaks not to the individual her- or himself in need of a cure, but to someone who had come to intercede with Jesus on their behalf. A centurion for his servant: Matt 8:5–13; Luke 7:1–10. A Syrophoenician woman for her daughter: Matt 15:21–8; Mark 7:24–30. Both of these stories involve non-Jews petitioning Jesus, and Jesus commends their faith.

[18] A man in the synagogue at Capernaum: Mark 1:23–6; Luke 4:33–5. The Gerasene (Gadarene) demoniac(s): Matt 8:28–34; Mark 5:1–20; Luke 8:26–39.

[19] Matt 17:14–21; Mark 9:17–29; Luke 9:37–43.

[20] Matt 17:20. Mark provides a somewhat different answer to the question: the demon could only be expelled by prayer or, in some manuscripts, by prayer and fasting (9:29). Luke omits the disciples' question about why they could not heal the boy.

[21] Epiphanius *Pan.* 30.10.

156 CONTESTED CURES

Jesus. Even non-Christians, such as Celsus and Lucian, were familiar with a tradition of wonderworkers in Palestine. We might therefore expect that late antique Christians who visited charismatic wonderworkers understood them to belong to a long line of holy men that stretched back to the biblical prophet Elijah and his protégé Elisha, who were particularly known for bending the laws of nature and performing signs to underscore the power of God.[22] Luke's account of the beginning of Jesus' ministry relates an incident in the synagogue of Nazareth that illustrated how Jesus was perceived as an heir to these earlier wonderworkers. Jesus read from the scroll of Isaiah and claimed that the passage prophesied his coming, including his miracles, and anticipated his rejection by the people from his hometown:

> And he said, "Truly I tell you, no prophet is accepted in the prophet's hometown. But the truth is, there were many widows in Israel in the time of Elijah, when the heaven was shut up three years and six months, and there was a severe famine over all the land; yet Elijah was sent to none of them except to a widow at Zarephath in Sidon. There were also many lepers in Israel in the time of the prophet Elisha, and none of them was cleansed except Naaman the Syrian."[23]

Elsewhere, Elijah famously appears with Moses during the transfiguration on Mount Tabor, and all the synoptics suggest that people questioned whether Jesus was Elijah himself.[24] This illustrates the connections that first-century Jews and later Christians made between Iron Age prophets and contemporary miracle-workers, and which would have informed their expectations when they went in search of cures from charismatic healers.

These accounts build a picture of the cultural and religious milieu in which late antique wonderworkers operated. Popular stories about Jesus conditioned believers to expect that a holy man's touch or speech could produce instantaneous cures. The role of faith, both on the part of the supplicant and the healer, offered yet another connection between biblical and late antique stories. Taken together, the sick and injured could expect that the living holy

---

[22] Walter and Moberly 2011, 62–3. For the perception of Elijah as a healer in late antique Palestine, see Nutzman 2017, 297–300 and Chapter 3. Considerable scholarly work has been done, for example, on how Elijah became a prophetic model for later figures such as Ḥoni the Circle-Maker, John the Baptist, Jesus, and Ḥanina ben Dosa. See discussion in Vermes 1973, 53–5, 62; Martyn 1976; Horsley 1985, 439–41; Evans 1987; Miller 1988; Guillaume 1999; Poirier 2009; Vermes 2012. For Elisha as another forerunner, see Blenkinsopp 1999; Gibson 2004, 143–4.

[23] Luke 4:24–7.

[24] For the transfiguration, see Matt 17:1–8; Mark 9:2–8; Luke 9:28–36. For questions about Jesus and Elijah, see Matt 16:13–20; Mark 8:27–30; Luke 9:18–20.

men whom they visited would be able to work miracles just as spectacular as those known from the Hebrew Bible and the life of Jesus.

Christian ascetics as charismatic wonderworkers

Late antique hagiography is replete with stories of charismatic wonderworkers who healed in a variety of ways. Considerable research has been done on the role of the Christian holy man in late antique society, stimulated by Peter Brown's pioneering 1971 study. In Palestine, a number of Christian ascetics between the third and seventh centuries were remembered as wonderworking holy men. The earliest of these is Hilarion, who was born near Gaza in the late third century and who was reputed to be the founder of Palestinian monasticism. Hilarion's hagiographer, Jerome, is best known for his translation of the Bible into Latin, but he also spent the last thirty years of his life in the region of Bethlehem, and it was there, at the end of the fourth century, that he wrote about Hilarion's life.[25] Several Palestinian hagiographers, along with their subjects, were ascetics in the Judaean desert. Among them was Cyril of Scythopolis (Beth She'an), a sixth-century monk who lived at different times at the monasteries of St. Euthymius and Mar Saba, both in the hills surrounding Jerusalem. He wrote accounts of seven Palestinian ascetics from the fourth through sixth centuries. By far the longest and most detailed of his hagiographies are those concerning the monks who founded the two monasteries where he lived.[26] A contemporary of the seven monks that Cyril profiled was Peter the Iberian, a Georgian prince and anti-Chalcedonian monk in the fifth century, who founded a monastery in Bethlehem. An account of Peter's life was written by one of his disciples, John Rufus. Another of the Judaean desert monks was George of Choziba, who was likely born in the decades following the death of Cyril of Scythopolis and who himself died sometime after the Muslim conquest. He lived at the monastery now named for him in Wadi Qelt, a short distance from Jerusalem. His disciple and fellow monk in Wadi Qelt, Antony of Choziba, wrote about his life. A contemporary of George of Choziba and yet another monk from the Judaean desert was John Moschos, who lived in the sixth and early seventh centuries. He traveled to Egypt and elsewhere in the eastern Mediterranean, where he met and collected stories from holy men. Unlike the other hagiographers, who wrote extended lives devoted to single individuals, John Moschos in *Spiritual Meadow* presented windows into the

---

[25] Jerome *V. Hil.* 24. Jerome reported that Hilarion and Anthony the Great carried out a correspondence, and that whenever pilgrims from Syria came to see Anthony in Egypt, he chastised them for not visiting Hilarion instead of traveling to see him.

[26] See discussion in Griffith 1999, 143–4.

158 CONTESTED CURES

experiences of many ascetics whom he encountered during his travels. His story of the unusual baptism that resulted in a miraculous cure has already been considered in Chapter 5. Finally, there are the monks Barsanuphius and John, who lived near Gaza in the first half of the sixth century. Our knowledge of this pair comes not from a hagiographer, but from their own personal correspondence.

While an exhaustive treatment of the miracles attributed to each of these ascetics is not possible here, a few episodes will serve to demonstrate how these figures were portrayed as charismatic wonderworkers and how late antique Christians might have understood them. Taken together, the stories paint a picture of holy men who have some sort of personal ability to heal, whether through their own innate power or their close connection to God. I would suggest that such stories contributed to a world view, shared by at least some who visited them, that considered the healers of the present chapter as fundamentally different than the ritual practitioners of Chapter 5. One way that hagiographers chose to differentiate their subjects from ritual practitioners was through purposeful connections to Jesus and the tradition of Palestinian prophets. For example, Jerome emphasized the similarity of biblical precedents to Hilarion's miracles when he wrote that the monk traveled around "working such wonders and signs that he was thought to be one of the ancient saints" (*tanta miracula et signa facientem ut de veteribus sanctis putaretur*).[27] This would have affirmed that Hilarion was not one of the "magicians" condemned by patristic authors, but rather someone who worked miracles as in the famous stories told about Jesus, the apostles, and the prophets of the Hebrew Bible. A couple of centuries later, Barsanuphius recognized that just as God was able to work miracles through Jesus' disciples, he continued to work them among his contemporaries: "Therefore, as [God] acted through the first (disciples) and raised the paralytic as well as Tabitha, who had died, so is he also able to act now."[28] Later in the same letter, Barsanuphius clarified that it was God who healed, not the ascetic himself:

> I know that a certain servant of God in this present generation, in this time and this place, is able even to raise the dead in the name of our Master Jesus, and to cast out demons, and to heal incurable illnesses, and to perform other works of power no less than the apostles, as the one who gave him this gift, or rather these gifts, bears witness. For what is

[27] Jerome *V. Hil.* 38; cf. 24, 42. For parallels from the book of Acts, see 2:22, 5:12, 6:8, 7:36, 15:12. Similar expressions are also found several times in John Rufus (*V. Petr. Ib.* 25, 98, 105). In section 105, John Rufus explicitly connects these "signs and wonders" to the advancement of anti-Chalcedonian communities, which he calls "congregations of orthodox." Translations from the *Life of Peter the Iberian* are taken from Horn and Phenix 2008.

[28] Letter no. 90.

this, that even such things occur in the name of Jesus? Indeed, he does not use his own authority.[29]

Barsanuphius seems to be making a distinction here between people who credit their miracles to the power of God, and those who take personal credit for them. Even the holy man who could perform that most dramatic miracle of bringing someone back to life could act only because God gave him the authority to do so. Yet even without these clear references to Jesus or allusions to the New Testament, details of late antique miracle stories would have invited contemporaries to make comparisons to Jesus and the apostles.

A common feature found in the lives of charismatic wonderworkers is their ability to cure an individual when others have failed. This theme was already present in the New Testament; the story of the boy whom Jesus healed when his disciples could not is one example.[30] Another is the woman who had suffered from a hemorrhage for twelve years and who exhausted her resources on physicians before Jesus healed her.[31] Such details advanced their authors' theological claims and highlighted Jesus' power in contrast to other healers.[32] In the same way, Jerome emphasized Hilarion's superiority over medical practitioners as part of his agenda to portray Hilarion as the pre-eminent wonderworker in Palestine. Jerome described how Aristaenete, the wife of a high-ranking official, was returning from a visit to Anthony, the great holy man of Egypt, when her three sons suffered a malarial attack. She consulted physicians, who told her that there was nothing that they could do. Learning of Hilarion, Aristaenete sought his help: "Hilarion, servant of Christ, give me back my children; Anthony watched over them in Egypt, you must save them in Syria."[33] Despite originally refusing to leave his monastic enclosure, Hilarion was persuaded to return with Aristaenete to her sons. At each one's bedside, he called on Jesus, and through this intercession the child recovered immediately. Jerome concluded by stating that Hilarion's miracle resulted in conversions to Christianity and in the growth of monasticism:

---

[29] Letter no. 90.

[30] Matt 17:14–21; Mark 9:17–29; Luke 9:37–43.

[31] Luke 8:43. The story is also found in Matt 9:20–2 and Mark 5:25–34. Matthew did not mention anything about previous medical treatments; Mark did include this detail and pointed out that her health continued to decline despite her being under the care of physicians.

[32] In contrast to this sense of competition, Bronwen Wickkiser (2008; cf. 2006) argued that the growth of the cult of Asklepios and the concurrent professionalization of medicine in the fifth century BCE took place in tandem as part of a symbiotic relationship. Wickkiser used evidence from both the *iamata* of Asklepios and the medical treatises to argue that the god specialized in chronic ailments. The same conditions that appear repeatedly in the *iamata* are identified in the contemporary medical corpus as incurable, and the treatises encourage doctors to refuse patients suffering from these diseases.

[33] Jerome *V. Hil.* 14.

Up to that time, there had been no monasteries in Palestine nor had anyone known of any monk in Syria before St. Hilarion. He was the founder, inspiration, and teacher there of monastic life and service to God. Our Lord Jesus had his senior servant Anthony in Egypt and his junior, Hilarion, in Palestine.[34]

This origin story emphasizes how the close, personal relationship that Hilarion enjoyed with God was the source of the saint's wonderworking abilities and the impetus for the growth of Christianity and Palestinian monasticism. Elsewhere, Jerome told of a blind woman from Egypt whom Hilarion healed, calling attention to the failure of doctors to cure the woman, and put in the mouth of Hilarion the admonishment "If what you lost on physicians you had given to the poor, Jesus the true Physician would have healed you."[35] While Hilarion did eventually heal the woman, using spittle in a way that deliberately called to mind New Testament stories about Jesus restoring sight, this miracle complements the message found in the healing of Aristaenete's sons.[36] In both cases, Jerome emphasized the superiority of the holy man's cures to medicine. Pious Christians were to put their trust in God, not medicine, and God would reward their faith by working miracles through the holy men whom he had chosen.

Jerome's story about Aristaenete emphasized the fact that healing was entirely up to Hilarion's discretion. There was no guarantee that he would perform the miracle when she requested it of him, and in fact he initially refused to do so. Another refusal, this time without a subsequent change of heart, can be seen in the lengthy correspondence carried out between a sick monk named Andrew and the Gazan ascetics Barsanuphius and John. Andrew requested that Barsanuphius and John heal him, but their responses redirected

---

[34] Jerome *V. Hil.* 14. The tension between local, Palestinian forms of monasticism and the appeal of Egyptian monasticism is also seen in the first chapter of John Moschos' *Spiritual Meadow*. When the Archbishop of Jerusalem tried to appoint a certain elder as head of a monastery, the elder refused on the grounds that he wanted to go to Mount Sinai in Egypt. Along the way, the elder contracted a high fever and took shelter in a cave. When a man appeared to him in a vision and told him not to continue to Mount Sinai, the elder again refused, and his fever grew worse. When the man appeared in a second vision, he identified himself as John the Baptist and said "Do not go there (Mount Sinai). For this little cave is greater than Mount Sinai. Many times did our Lord Jesus Christ come in here to visit me. Give me your word that you will stay here and I will give you back your health" (*Prat.* 1). The elder abandoned his plans to travel to Sinai and was instantaneously cured; he remained at the cave and founded a new monastery there.

[35] Jerome *V. Hil.* 15. For another example of a cure where doctors had failed, see John Moschos *Prat.* 28.

[36] Jerome *V. Hil.* 15. See John 9:6 and Mark 8:23 for New Testament miracles involving spittle. For the treatment of medicine in Sophronius' *Miracles of Cyrus and John*, see Booth 2014, 59–69.

Andrew's attention from physical complaints to spiritual matters.[37] By demurring when pressed by the monk for a cure, Barsanuphius and John underscored the personal nature of a holy man's cure.[38] One might be hard-pressed to imagine a similar reluctance to perform the cures of Chapter 5. On the one hand, those provided by freelance specialists were likely part of a transaction in which the practitioners were remunerated for their services. If someone could make the required payment, one supposes that the practitioner would have conducted the requested ritual. On the other hand, healing rituals conducted as part of a regular cycle of services, such as some of the examples from the *Sacramentary of Serapion*, may have required no special request or petition for healing; the prayers were simply offered on behalf of whoever happened to be present. This stands in stark contrast to the examples from Jerome, Barsanuphius, and John, which presuppose that the person in need of healing had to convince the wonderworker to perform a cure. In the absence of definitive criteria whereby holy men were said to choose whom they would heal, we are left to speculate about how these decisions would have been perceived by people seeking cures in late antique Palestine. Given the apparent expectation that ascetic wonderworkers would not necessarily heal everyone who implored them for help – they could and did refuse – supplicants likely felt pressure to prove themselves worthy of a cure, such as by demonstration of their personal faith or a promise to do something if they were healed.

Both of these components can be found in a story that Cyril of Scythopolis told about Euthymius. A Persian chieftain was desperate to find a cure for his son who suffered from a paralysis that his father attributed to a demon.[39] As we have already seen in Jerome's *Life of Hilarion*, Cyril emphasized the failure of others who attempted to use "medical science and magical arts" to cure the boy.[40] In time, the son, Terebōn, became convinced that there was nothing to be gained from seeking out such remedies and reflected on his prospects for a cure:

---

[37] Letter nos. 72–123. For the monks' emphasis on spiritual health rather than physical, see Hevelone-Harper 2005, 84–9.

[38] In the end, Barsanuphius wrote to John that Andrew would be healed on a given day (Letter no. 81). When this took place, another monk claimed that the miracle was the result of "the prayers of the saints" (Letter nos. 82–3).

[39] See discussion in Griffith 1999, 143–4.

[40] Cyril Scyth. *V. Euthym.* 10. Cyril also described Sabas, Euthymius' younger contemporary, as healing where medical practitioners failed. The Patriarch of Jerusalem had a sister whom doctors could not cure. Although not specified by Cyril, one might wonder whether the original audience of this story would have expected that the patriarch also administered the church's healing rites to his sister, including prayer and anointing with oil, before turning to a wonderworking ascetic. While Cyril describes the patriarch as particularly respectful of Sabas, late antique holy men were at times seen as rivals to the institutional hierarchy of the church, which would have made his consultation of a charismatic healer for his sister particularly striking. See Cyril Scyth. *V. Sab.* 68.

162   CONTESTED CURES

Terebōn, where now is the vanity of life and all medical skill? Where are the fantasies of our magicians and the power of our rites? Where are the invocations and invented myths of the astronomers and astrologers? Where are the incantations and the sophistries of sorcerers? For see, none of these have effect unless God gives his assent . . . O God, great and terrible, creator of heaven and earth with all their panoply, if you take pity on my sickness and rescue me from this dire disorder, I will become a Christian, renouncing all lawlessness and pagan worship.[41]

With this conclusion, Euthymius appeared to Terebōn and assured him of a cure if he would fulfill his promise to become a Christian. The presumed wealth of Terebōn's father, as indicated by the "huge sums" that he spent on the boy's treatment, suggests that he would have been in the position to purchase a cure from a charismatic wonderworker, if money was all that was required. Cyril, however, gave no suggestion of a monetary payment to entice Euthymius to act on the boy's behalf. Rather, Cyril claimed that it was Terebōn's faith in God and his promise to abandon his former gods that got the attention of Euthymius and persuaded him to intervene. Other details of the story underscore the personal aspects of this cure. In Terebōn's vision of Euthymius, the saint said, "If you wish to be healed, come to me without delay, and God will cure you through me." Euthymius did not simply promise that God would answer Terebōn's prayers for healing or instruct him to visit a church to participate in a ritual anointing with oil. Instead, Euthymius told Terebōn to travel to Palestine and personally seek him out, whereupon God would use the ascetic wonderworker as the agent of a cure. Cyril emphasized that the cure was worked through the strength of Euthymius' prayer: "by praying fervently and sealing Terebōn with the sign of the cross, he restored him to health." Terebōn was healed not because Euthymius said the correct words or simply because he made the sign of the cross, but because of the sincerity of his prayers. The faith of both Euthymius and Terebōn played a pivotal role in Cyril's account.

The implication of this story about Euthymius, as in the ones about Hilarion, is that it is the strength of the holy man's prayers, perhaps made more effective by his closeness to God, that brought about the cure, rather than some inherent power possessed by the wonderworker. In other words, God healed at the request of the ascetic. This dynamic is particularly clear in a story from the life of George of Choziba. A farmer left his dead son at George's monastery, hidden in a basket covered with fruit. This man is described as particularly beloved

---

[41] Cyril Scyth. *V. Euthym.* 10. Translations of Cyril's *Lives of the Monks of Palestine* are from Price and Binns 1991.

CHARISMATIC WONDERWORKERS 163

(*agapētos*) by the monks. When the boy's body was discovered, George persuaded his brother and fellow monk to join him in prayer, recognizing that if God chose to heal the boy, it would be in spite of their sins:

> And if God overlooks our sins and, when we call upon him, raises the child, our friend will depart, according to his faith, with his child alive again. If, however, God's goodness does not wish to do this, we will cry out to God and say that, because we are sinners, we have not attained such authority (*metra ouk ephthasamen*), nor do we have the liberty to do so (*oude echomen parrēsian toiautēn*).[42]

This passage emphasizes the author's perspective that it was God who healed, not the famed ascetic. I would suggest, however, that this does not diminish the perception that a holy man's cures were deeply personal, as there is no hint that God would have chosen to raise this particular boy if it were not for the monks' prayers. They were instrumental in the miracle, but as intercessors, rather than as the direct source of healing: "They stood for prayer with tears and a heart shattered with contrition (*syntetrimmenēs kardias*). And the all-merciful Lord, the lover of humankind, who creates the will of those who fear him, heard their prayers and raised the child."[43]

In contrast to these accounts that emphasize God as the healer and the holy man simply as the one who persuaded God to act, others reflect a belief that the holy man had some sort of innate power that could be transferred by his touch, as the New Testament described some of Jesus' miracles. For example, John Rufus told the story of a man with a hearing impairment who attempted to prostrate himself at Peter the Iberian's feet. Preventing this act of obeisance, Peter nevertheless touched the man's ears and kissed him on the forehead, bringing an instantaneous cure.[44] The hagiographer makes no mention of Peter offering a prayer; the touch and the kiss alone sufficed to work this miracle. John Moschos also included an example of a touch miracle in a short anecdote about a monk in Phoenicia named John. The holy man

---

[42] Antony Choz. *V. Georg. Choz.* 2.8. Antony, the text's author, further claims that he was personally healed by George: "When ... I endured numerous battles and illness and temptations and afflictions, the old man eased my pains and healed me body and soul." Although Antony provides neither the specifics of his ailments nor details about how George effected these cures in this passage, this is further evidence of his portrayal of George as a charismatic wonderworker. All translations of this text are from Vivian and Athanassakis 1994.

[43] Antony Choz. *V. Georg. Choz.* 2.8. John Rufus' account of the life of Peter the Iberian also attests to the idea that God chose to heal people on the strength of Peter's prayers for them (*V. Petr. Ib.* 60, 127).

[44] John Rufus *V. Petr. Ib.* 132.

164   CONTESTED CURES

received a "vision from God" telling him "Whatever <disorder> you lay your hand on, it shall be healed."[45] The episode concluded with an example of John performing exactly this kind of miracle, even though he at first demurred on account of his sinfulness, much as we saw with George of Choziba. A third example comes from Cyril's *Life of Sabas*; the holy man encountered a hemorrhaging woman, who guided Sabas' hand to touch the source of her hemorrhage. Before touching the woman, Sabas said "I trust in the God I worship that you will be cured."[46] As soon as he touched her, she recovered.[47] While these miracles convey the idea of powerful wonderworkers who only needed to touch individuals to cure them, hagiographers at times still emphasized that it was God who acted through the holy man, as Cyril did in this last example.

Up to this point, these miracles have involved the holy man choosing to act on behalf of a supplicant. In some cases, this action was a prayer, and in others it was a deliberate touch. Hagiographers at times portrayed a dialogue or encounter between the person who was sick and the ascetic whom they asked for healing, in which the former persuaded the latter to act. While these stories presuppose the possibility that the holy man might choose not to intervene, other accounts portrayed charismatic healers as having such an abundance of power that they radiated it, even without their conscious thought. This, then, offered the late antique Christian the possibility of an alternative path to a cure. Rather than having to convince the holy man to act, the individual only had to get close enough to tap into his power. New Testament antecedents for this idea can be found in the hemorrhaging woman who was healed when she touched Jesus' clothing, in the crowds who were healed when Peter's shadow passed over them, and in the miracles worked through articles of Paul's clothing.[48] In much the same way, Cyril described a youth freed from a demon as soon as he saw Euthymius.[49] Mere sight of Euthymius was enough to expel the demon, apparently without any specific prayers or even a physical touch. Cyril described two repercussions of this miracle. First, the youth underwent a religious transformation from a sect that Cyril considered heretical to Cyril's own form of Christianity. While the youth had not promised this conversion before the miracle, as in the account of Terebōn and Euthymius, stories such as this might reflect a popular belief that the proper response to

---

[45] John Moschos *Prat.* 56.
[46] Cyril Scyth. *V. Sab.* 62.
[47] Cyril Scyth. *V. Sab.* 62.
[48] Hemorrhaging woman: Matt 9:20–2; Mark 5:25–34; Luke 8:43–8. Peter's shadow: Acts 5:15–16. Paul's clothing: Acts 19:11–12.
[49] Cyril Scyth. *V. Euthym.* 12. See also John Moschos *Prat.* 82, which says that a certain elder named John was "feared by the demons" and could cure anyone who was possessed by a demon. The method of these cures is not stated.

a miraculous cure was a new or more pious devotion to God, the church, or a particular holy man. Second, Cyril credited this miracle as the foundation story for Euthymius' monastery, since the episode encouraged crowds to seek out the holy man, much as the growth of monasticism two centuries earlier was attributed to Hilarion's healing of Aristaenete's sons. Another example of an ascetic as a passive agent of cure can be found in Cyril's *Life of Abraamius*. A monk at Abraamius' monastery went into the church, took off his clothes, and sat down naked in the place where Abraamius typically sat. As soon as he was seated, the monk was healed of a hemorrhage.[50] Relics and the cult of the saints may have been perceived similarly to these two stories: the saint's healing power was available to anyone who came into contact with his relics. For example, Cyril told of an official from Antioch who was anointed with oil from the tomb of Euthymius and was restored to health.[51] This recalls the mechanism for collecting oil from a tomb found in the excavation of the church in Dora, discussed in Chapter 4. Hagiographers credited miracles associated with relics to the deceased saints themselves. There is also an element of place involved in the cult of the saints, as pilgrims would come to a specific location to pray at the saint's tomb. Finally, pilgrimage tokens from a saint's grave could be used as amulets, including those that contained relics or oil taken from the tomb.[52] Thus, miracles associated with relics combine several avenues of healing explored in this book: person, place, and object.

Accounts of these miracle-working ascetics give a sense for how late antique Christians may have viewed potential healing encounters with a holy man. Except for these last stories, the decision about whether or not to facilitate a miracle rested entirely with the individual holy man. Visitors in search of a cure may have come prepared to convince the wonderworker that they were worthy of being healed. Hagiographic texts gave the impression that certain factors might be offered as evidence that individuals merited a cure, including the variety of other treatments that they had pursued unsuccessfully, the length of their illnesses, or their promise to do something upon being healed.

---

[50] Cyril Scyth. *V. Abr.* 9.

[51] Cyril Scyth. *V. Euthym.* 47; cf. 49, 51–3, 56. Not all stories of miraculous relics, however, suggest that the saint was a passive agent of cure. Some report that the holy man appeared to the person whom they cured in a dream or vision or that they interceded on behalf of supplicants (e.g. John Moschos *Prat.* 40 and Antony Choz. *Miracles of the Most Holy Mother of God at Choziba* 6). The idea that the bones of a holy man could work miracles after his death did not originate in late antiquity. A story in the Hebrew Bible portrayed the remains of Elisha as miraculous. 2 Kgs 13:20 describes the death and burial of Elisha; sometime later an unnamed man died and was to be buried near Elisha. Before the man could be buried, raiders came upon the party and in haste the mourners put the dead man in the tomb of Elisha. As soon as the dead man's body came into contact with the bones of Elisha, the man came back to life.

[52] See discussion in Vikan 1995, 384–7.

166   CONTESTED CURES

Late antique hagiographers generally did not parse differences in the ways that holy men worked their miracles. The key point was rather that there was something personal about the individual's ability to heal; they did not effect cures by the correct performance of rituals or prayers. In some cases, miracles were conveyed through touch or sight, while in others it was through the holy man's prayer or a close connection to God. Regardless of these narrative details, the stories are portrayed as demonstrations of God's power, and by extension as evidence of the author's correct belief in God. Miracle stories could function as proof texts in an era of competition between Christians and non-Christians, between holy men and physicians, and between various forms of Christianity. Ultimately, these accounts perpetuated devotion to ascetics by offering hope to late antique Christians that contemporary holy men would continue to perform miracles like those attributed to Jesus, biblical prophets, and the apostles.

Charismatic wonderworkers in rabbinic texts

At the same time as sources about Christian healers multiplied, the rabbinization of late antique Judaism obscured the role of charismatic wonderworkers. Tannaitic sources downplay wonderworking as part of their efforts to reimagine a new form of Jewish life centered on the study of the Torah. Amoraic sources, in contrast, preserve stories of miracle-workers, but shape them to the support the rabbis' priorities.[53] As Michael Becker has argued,

> for the rabbis of the *talmudic era* [italics in the original], charismatic authority did not stem from the miraculous, but from the authority of the Torah. It is not the personal charisma of a rabbi, but the charisma of the Torah as the order of the whole creation that provides a rabbi with charismatic competence in these later traditions.[54]

In the later period, then, miracle stories were somewhat more likely to appear, but they were used not simply to demonstrate an individual's charisma but rather in support of halakhic positions.[55] The nature of this evidence makes

[53] A number of scholars have explored this shift in detail: Green 1979; Van Cangh 1984, 45–9; Bokser 1985; Kalmin 2003; Becker 2006.

[54] Becker 2006, 51.

[55] Géza Vermes (1972, 28–37) suggested that certain *baraitot* in later Talmudic texts, such as those about Ḥanina, preserve earlier versions of stories than those in the Mishnah. However, my intention is not to identify the historical Ḥanina, any more than it is to identify the historical Jesus or Hilarion. Rather than trying to reconstruct what the historical Ḥanina may or may not have actually done, my interest is in what types of miracles the rabbinic redactors portrayed as plausible.

CHARISMATIC WONDERWORKERS 167

it difficult to identify the sorts of expectations that those seeking cures from Jewish wonderworkers might have had. At a basic level, however, we can identify how rabbinic authors chose to portray these figures and draw some comparisons with the Christian material.

Among wonderworkers mentioned in rabbinic sources, the two most famous are Ḥoni the Circle-Maker and Ḥanina ben Dosa, who lived in the first century BCE and the first century CE respectively. No healings were attributed to Ḥoni, but stories about his rain miracle attest to a belief in charismatic wonderworkers among at least some Jews.[56] The earliest evidence for Ḥoni the Circle-Maker comes from Josephus, who wrote that Ḥoni (Onias) ended a drought through his prayers.[57] The Mishnah gives a more complete account of the miracle, opening with people asking Ḥoni to pray for rain, apparently with the expectation that his prayer would be successful.[58] The subsequent give-and-take between Ḥoni and God in the Mishnah's description illustrates the wonderworker's direct access to God and his ability to persuade God to act. This was not a simple case of a prayer for rain and a subsequent answer. After his initial prayer went unanswered, Ḥoni gave God an ultimatum, drawing a circle and promising not to leave it until God sent rain. When God relented and caused it to rain, Ḥoni objected twice – the first time because it was too little rain, and the second time because it was too much. In the end, Ḥoni got his way, and God provided the needed rain. At the end of the passage, a leading Jew compared the relationship between Ḥoni and God to that of a father and a son. Just as a father would do what a son asks, so too God would respond favorably to Ḥoni's request. Like some of the hagiographers discussed above, the rabbinic redactors portrayed Ḥoni as being able to persuade God to act through his fervent prayers.

Stories about Ḥanina ben Dosa, whom *m. Soṭah* 9:15 identified as the last of the "men of good deeds," are somewhat more plentiful.[59] Unlike Ḥoni, Ḥanina is mentioned in the context of healing:

---

[56] Elijah was also associated with the end of a drought in 1 Kgs 18:41–6, and a rain miracle was attributed to Ḥanina in *b. Taʿan.* 24b–25a. For more on Jewish rainmakers, see Lapin 1996; Kalmin 2003.

[57] Josephus *Ant.* 14.19.

[58] *m. Taʿan.* 3:8. Cf. *y. Taʿan.* 3:9–10 (66d–67a); *b. Taʿan.* 19a, 23a–b. The Tosefta also includes an account of an anonymous *ḥasid* who performed a rain miracle (*t. Taʿan* 2:13), and some scholars have identified this figure as Ḥoni. For the relationship between the two passages, see Green 1979, 631–2. For the idea that Ḥoni and Ḥanina ben Dosa were *ḥasidim*, see Berman 1979; Freyne 1980, 224–7. See also Rosenfeld 1999, 369–75, who argued that R. Simeon b. Yohai was portrayed as both a *ṣaddíq* and a *ḥasid*.

[59] Géza Vermes' two-part treatment of Ḥanina ben Dosa (1972; 1973) has served as a point of departure for more recent studies, even among scholars who disagree with his conclusions.

168 CONTESTED CURES

> They tell of R. Hanina b. Dosa that he used to pray over the sick and say, "This one will live," or "This one will die." They said to him, "How do you know?" He replied, "If my prayer is fluent in my mouth I know that he is accepted; and if it is not I know that he is rejected."[60]

This story is situated within a discussion of the correct recitation of prayers; the sentence immediately before it highlights the consequences of mistakes during prayer:

> If he that says the *Tefillah* falls into error it is a bad omen for him; and if he was the agent of the congregation it is a bad omen for them that appointed him, because a man's agent is like to himself.[61]

The rabbis used the story of Ḥanina to underscore these bad omens: they indicated to him when a prayer would not be answered and by extension when it would. Ḥanina's intimacy with the prayers was what enabled his prescient knowledge of a sick person's prognosis. An alternative interpretation was offered by Géza Vermes, who argued that Ḥanina's reference to praying fluently indicated an improvised prayer, not a set prayer to be recited correctly. Thus, Vermes saw this as "an example of the rabbinic redactors reshaping a charismatic healing" story to support their *halakha*, in this case as it related to the importance of reciting prayers correctly.[62] If Vermes was correct, it would suggest that some had originally understood that Ḥanina's prayers themselves were what persuaded God to act, much like Elijah's prayers for the widow's son or Ḥoni's prayers for rain.

While this Mishnaic anecdote about Ḥanina speaks only in generalities, both the Palestinian and the Babylonian Talmuds relate stories about the sons of leading rabbis who were healed after Ḥanina's prayers. Rabban Gamaliel sent two students to Ḥanina out of concern for his sick son. After Ḥanina met with the students, he went upstairs and then returned with news of the cure. The Yerushalmi and the Bavli offer different explanations for Ḥanina's role in the cure, attesting to a range of ideas about charismatic wonderworkers.[63] The

---

[60] *m. Ber.* 5:5.

[61] *m. Ber.* 5:5.

[62] Vermes 1972, 29–30.

[63] Ḥanina could not touch or see Gamaliel's son when he was healed, and the Yerushalmi indicates that they were not even in the same town at the time of the miracle. Similar stories of long-distance cures are told both of Jesus in the New Testament and of Sabas by Cyril of Scythopolis. For Jesus, see Matt 8:5–13 and Luke 7:1–10; Matt 15:21–8 and Mark 7:24–30. For Sabas, see Cyril Scyth. *V. Sab.* 79.

CHARISMATIC WONDERWORKERS 169

Yerushalmi does not indicate that God was influenced by Ḥanina's prayers. In fact, it does not explicitly say that Ḥanina prayed while upstairs, although this is implied since the passage is a commentary on *m. Ber.* 5:5, which connected Ḥanina's prayers to miraculous cures. Ḥanina reported that Rabban Gamaliel's son had been healed, and it was later revealed that he had recovered at the precise moment that Ḥanina announced the cure. This seems to suggest that prophetic knowledge was the primary component of Ḥanina's miracle in this story. In other words, he discovered the cure, rather than working the cure.[64] The Bavli, in contrast, assigned Ḥanina a more active role in the cure of Rabban Gamaliel's son. Ḥanina was asked to pray, presumably with the under-standing that such prayers could heal.[65] When Ḥanina announced that the fever had broken, Rabban Gamaliel's scholars inquired as to whether Ḥanina was a prophet. He denied being a prophet and instead repeated the sentiment from the Mishnah that the fluency of his prayer indicated to him whether it had been successful. Sean Freyne, discussing the differences between these two accounts, observed that the Yerushalmi "significantly omits any mention of the fluidity of Ḥanina's prayer . . . highlighting instead his personal gift of intimacy with the divine will through prayer."[66]

A few sentences after the miraculous recovery of Gamaliel's son in the Bavli, a second healing was attributed to Ḥanina when R. Yoḥanan ben Zakkai petitioned him for help:

> He [R. Yoḥanan] **said to him: Ḥanina, my son, pray for mercy on behalf of** my son **so that he will live. Rabbi Ḥanina ben Dosa placed his head between his knees** in order to meditate **and prayed for mercy upon his behalf, and** Rabbi Yoḥanan ben Zakkai's son **lived. Rabbi Yoḥanan ben Zakkai said** about himself: **Had ben Zakkai stuck his head between his knees throughout the entire day, they would have paid him no attention. His wife said to him: And is Ḥanina greater than you? He replied to her: No, but** his prayer is better received than my own because **he is like a servant before the King,** and as such he is able to enter before the King and make various requests at all times. **I,** on the other hand, **am like a minister before the King,** and I can enter only

---

[64] *y. Ber.* 5:5 (9d). A Christian example of prophetic knowledge being attributed to a charismatic wonderworker can be found in John Moschos' *Spiritual Meadow.* A monk in Jerusalem named Zachaios was asked about a plague in Caesarea. After spending two hours in silent prayer, Zachaios announced that the plague would end in two days (*Prat.* 131).

[65] *b. Ber.* 34b.

[66] Freyne 1980, 229.

when invited and can make requests only with regard to especially significant matters.[67]

As in the Bavli's account of R. Gamaliel's son, the cure in this story is attributed to Ḥanina's prayer, not his prophetic knowledge. The conversation between R. Yoḥanan and his wife portrayed a close connection between Ḥanina and God. R. Yoḥanan suggested that his own prayers would not have had the same result as Ḥanina's, even if the rabbi had spent all day praying. When R. Yoḥanan's wife interpreted this to mean that her husband was inferior, he explained that it was not a question of who is greater, but rather the relationship that each had with God. The nature of Ḥanina's relationship with God made his prayers for healing more productive.

Prophetic knowledge was also attributed to R. Pinhas ben Yair. As with Ḥoni the Circle-Maker, R. Pinhas' miracles were not associated with healing. In a discussion about tithing in the Yerushalmi, several individuals approached R. Pinhas concerning agricultural problems. He identified the source of each problem as a failure to tithe properly: a donkey refused to eat for three days because the barley it was fed had not been properly tithed, mice devoured stored grain because it had not been properly tithed, and a spring failed to produce sufficient water because the produce of the fields that it watered had not been properly tithed.[68] R. Pinhas' diagnosis of the underlying halakhic issue highlights the rabbinic lens through which traditions of wonderworkers were filtered, as all the examples reinforced the rabbinic ideology of tithing found in the tractate *Demai*. After R. Pinhas diagnosed the cause of these misfortunes and ensured that proper tithing would resume, the ill effects were immediately reversed: The donkey commenced eating, the mice stopped eating the grain, and the water level of the spring increased. R. Pinhas' role here is twofold. First, he had extraordinary knowledge that allowed him to discern the source of the problem, and second, the natural elements – donkey, mice, and spring – recognized his intervention and ceased to cause harm when the failure to tithe was rectified.[69]

Stories of both prayer and prophecy relied on God, either knowledge of what God would do or persuasive prayers that God acted upon. Lacking both

---

[67] *b. Ber.* 34b. All quotations of the Bavli are taken from the Steinsaltz edition of the Talmud, as found on the Sefaria website. In the Steinsaltz edition of the Talmud, text in bold typeface translates the words found in the Talmud, while the plain typeface indicates the translator's expansions on the text for greater clarity.

[68] *y. Demai* 1:3 (21d–22b).

[69] Another wonder ascribed to R. Pinhas is reminiscent of Moses' parting of the Red Sea during the exodus. When the Ginnai River was too high for him to cross, he addressed it: "Ginnai, Ginnai, why do you prevent me from going to the House of Assembly?" (*y. Demai* 1.3 [21d–22b]). The river parted and R. Pinhas passed to the other side.

CHARISMATIC WONDERWORKERS 171

of these components, however, is a miracle in the late antique Palestinian text *Leviticus Rabbah*. The Roman emperor Antoninus had a servant who was dying, and so the emperor asked a certain rabbi to send one of his students who were famous for raising the dead. When the student arrived and found the servant dead, he said, "How can you be lying down and your master standing on his feet?"[70] With this simple rebuke, the dead servant got up. The servant heeded the rebuke and was healed. The implication is that the cure was wrought with the spoken chastisement alone; prayer and prophecy were not mentioned. Although there are limited late antique Jewish comparanda, nevertheless, there seems little question that this student was portrayed as a charismatic healer; he had some sort of personal charisma that enabled him to perform the miracle without recourse to prescribed rituals. This invites a comparison with the New Testament stories in which Jesus commanded people to get up and to go about their business, free from what had ailed them. In both, it is the speech – whether a command or a chastisement – that brought about a cure.[71]

Elsewhere, it was the holy man's piety that enabled a miracle. In the *Pesikta de-Rab Kahana*, a midrashic text likely compiled in fifth-century Palestine, the second-century sage R. Simeon b. Yohai is described as encountering a woman in Sidon who had been unable to have children. After she subsequently conceived, the episode closes: "For, even as the Holy One remembers barren women, righteous men [such as R. Simeon] also have the power to remember barren women."[72] This observation about the ability of the righteous man – the *ṣaddiq* – to heal through prayer raises the question as to whether the author understood that such men were routinely approached for healing intercessions. The complicated redactional history of rabbinic texts and the role that miracle stories had in supporting halakhic arguments makes this difficult to determine. The extent to which these stories, either in their rabbinic formulation or in

---

[70] *Lev. R.* 10:4. The translation of this passage is from Gray 2005, 42. The identity of both the key figures in this story, the rabbi and Antoninus, is somewhat problematic. For an overview of the issues, see Naiweld 2014, 87–8.

[71] A report in *Midrash Rabbah Numbers* 20.14 may also reflect the possibility of a charismatic healer using speech to bring about a cure, but the story is met by a certain amount of skepticism by the rabbinic author. The passage describes a doctor who could cure a snakebite with his tongue. This is contrasted to the same doctor needing to use a stick to kill a dangerous lizard. The text suggests that curing a snakebite is more difficult than killing a lizard. Therefore, if he was able to work any sort of a miracle, the easier one – killing the lizard – was expected. The fact that he had to use a weapon to kill the lizard cast doubt on his ability to perform the more challenging task in a miraculous manner. Although the man is described as a doctor, the healing of the snakebite with a spoken word implies a miraculous cure rather than a medical one. See discussion in Nolland 1979, 207.

[72] *Pesikta de Rab Kahana* 22.2. The translation of this passage is from Braude and Kapstein 2002. For the date of this work, see Braude and Kapstein 2002, lxxxv–lxxxvi.

172   CONTESTED CURES

independent versions, would have circulated beyond the rabbis' immediate circles is likewise far from clear. Nevertheless, it would seem that at least some late antique Jews were open to the possibility of charismatic wonderworkers whose prayers could result in healing.

In contrast to the abundance of miracle narratives in early Christianity, details about charismatic wonderworkers in Roman and late antique Judaism are more limited. Nevertheless, stories about Honi the Circle-Maker, Hanina ben Dosa, R. Pinhas ben Yair, the rabbinic student who healed Antoninus' servant, and R. Simeon b. Yohai suggest that Jewish communities continued to recognize holy men who, like the prophets of the Hebrew Bible, could perform cures and bend the laws of nature. The strength of one's prayer or ability to convince God to act set some of these individuals apart. Others were identified by prophetic or extraordinary knowledge. Uniting them all was the wonderworker's charisma that enabled him to perform miracles at will. Yet even more than with stories of Christian wonderworkers, we must not lose sight of the fact that we have little access to the expectations of the individuals who might have approached them for help. Rather, we are constructing a picture of the types of miracles that later authors accepted as plausible.

Apollonius and imperial wonderworkers

Charismatic wonderworkers from the Greek and Roman worlds, outside Jewish and Christian communities, appear less commonly in our sources. Some explanation for this can be seen in the passage by Celsus discussed earlier in this chapter, in which Celsus was uninterested in distinguishing between ritual practitioners and charismatic wonderworkers. Scholars have also pointed to the role of miracles in advancing claims of religious exceptionalism and in inspiring conversion within monotheistic traditions.[73] Such motivations are minimalized or absent in polytheistic contexts, which may also contribute to the relative infrequence of charismatic healers within Greek, Roman, and Semitic traditions. Without Palestinian comparanda to draw on, Greek and Roman parallels must be found outside the region in stories about Apollonius, Vespasian, and Hadrian.[74]

Apollonius of Tyana was a Greek philosopher who lived in the first century CE. Philostratus' *Life of Apollonius*, written in the first half of the third century, contains several stories that identify the philosopher as a charismatic wonderworker. When Apollonius encountered a funeral procession in Rome for a young woman from

---

[73] For example, Garland 2011, 89.

[74] Much has been written on the concept of the *theios anēr* ("divine man") and its application to figures such as Apollonius. For a review of the literature and, ultimately, an argument against Apollonius as a *theios anēr*, see Koskenniemi 1998; see also Blackburn 1991; Anderson 1994.

a consular family, he stopped the mourners to inquire after the dead girl. He then touched her and "whispered something secret," after which the girl came to back life.[75] Philostratus did not provide any details about what Apollonius said, making it difficult to ascertain whether Philostratus understood this "secret" speech as a prescribed prayer from a ritual practitioner's repertoire or the spontaneous prayer of a charismatic wonderworker. However, its similarity to Jesus' raising of the widow of Nain's son in Luke 7 might suggest that Philostratus intended this episode to illustrate Apollonius' charismatic ability to work miracles. Other stories in the *Life of Apollonius* seem to support this contention.[76] For example, Apollonius expelled a demon with a spoken command, and the miracle's success was confirmed when a statue was knocked over by the demon after it left.[77] This recalls a story that appears in each of the synoptic Gospels: Jesus exorcised one or two men with a command and cast the demons into a nearby herd of pigs. Proof of the demons' expulsion was provided when the pigs stampeded down into the Sea of Galilee.[78]

Other wonders performed by Apollonius in his guise as a charismatic healer offer a comparison to the prophetic knowledge attributed to wonderworkers in rabbinic texts, such as the account of a rabid dog that bit and infected an adolescent boy.[79] When the crowd explained to Apollonius that no one had seen the animal responsible for the boy's condition, Apollonius described the rabid dog and explained where it could be found. He then instructed the dog to lick the spot where it had bitten the boy thirty days earlier, at which point the boy was immediately healed.[80] The episode concludes with a second cure.

---

[75] Philostratus *V. Apoll.* 4.45. All translations of this text are taken from Jones 2005.

[76] For comparative work on Jesus and Apollonius, see Bovon 1991, 351–2; Van Cangh 2008, 213–36.

[77] Philostratus *V. Apoll.* 4.20.

[78] Matt 8:28–34; Mark 5:1–20; Luke 8:26–39.

[79] Philostratus *V. Apoll.* 43.

[80] For examples of dogs as agents of cure at the Asklepieion in Epidauros, see *IG* IV^2 1:122, no. 26 and *IG* IV^2 1:121, no. 20 (Edelstein and Edelstein 1998, T. 423). Apollonius is also linked to Asklepios in Philostratus' story about a young Assyrian man who came as a supplicant to the healing god, but whom Asklepios refused to heal because of his intemperate lifestyle. When the sick man complained of Asklepios' failure to heal him, Asklepios appeared to him and told him to seek help from Apollonius. The man questioned Apollonius regarding the benefits of his philosophy, whereupon Apollonius explained what the young man must do to recover. The account concludes, "Apollonius restored the youth to health by expressing wise counsels in simple form" (Philostratus *V. Apoll.* 1.9). This story is somewhat different from the others under discussion, in which Apollonius' identity as a charismatic healer is more readily apparent. Here, he seems to employ his logical skills to convince a recalcitrant patient to follow common sense, as had presumably been conveyed by attendants or medical practitioners at the Asklepieion. Nevertheless, respect for Apollonius' abilities – or even deference toward Apollonius – can be inferred from Asklepios' instructions to the suppliant, "If you talk with Apollonius, you will get relief" (Philostratus *V. Apoll.* 1.9).

174   CONTESTED CURES

Not only did Apollonius cause the boy to be healed, but he also did the same for the dog. He made the dog swim across the Cydnus River and drink from its water, which healed him. A second miracle attributed to Apollonius also credited him with prophetic knowledge. The wonderworker brought an end to a plague in Ephesus when he gathered the people of the city around an old beggar and instructed them to stone him. Despite initial resistance, the crowd did as he said, and the beggar was revealed to be a demon whose demise dispelled the plague.[81] These stories about the rabid dog and the plague in Ephesus combine the idea that Apollonius possessed specialized knowledge – the location of the dog and the identity of the demon – and the power to act on that knowledge to bring about a cure. This is reminiscent of the prophetic knowledge of Ḥanina and of R. Pinhas ben Yair, the latter of which correctly diagnosed a lack of tithing as the source of certain problems and intervened in the natural order to resolve them. While I do not intend to argue for the literary dependence of the *Life of Apollonius* on Jewish or Christian texts, Philostratus' work nevertheless reflects the premise that some individuals in the wider Greco-Roman world were also understood to possess a special wonderworking ability that distinguished them from practitioners whose miracles were predicated upon the correct completion of rituals.

The persona of a charismatic wonderworker was likewise applied to two Roman emperors, Vespasian and Hadrian.[82] As in stories about Jesus, these accounts portray the emperors as conveying instantaneous cures through a simple touch. The author of the *Life of Hadrian* in the *Historia Augusta* reports somewhat skeptically that near the end of his life, Hadrian was very ill but restored sight to a blind man who touched him.[83] As with the sick people who tried to touch Jesus, the action here seems to be entirely on the part of the visually impaired man, and healing power was said to flow unconsciously from Hadrian. What sets this episode apart from the New Testament examples is that both parties involved were healed; the blind man received his sight, and Hadrian's fever abated. In fact, the role of the healer and the sick person could be open to interpretation: the blind man could be said to have healed Hadrian,

---

[81] Pythagoras, a Greek philosopher who lived in the sixth century BCE, was also credited with the ability to bring an end to plagues according to Neoplatonist biographers who lived in the third and fourth centuries CE. Neither of the authors who wrote about Pythagoras' life specified how the philosopher was understood to have accomplished this (Porphyry *V. Pyth.* 29; Iamblichus *V. Pyth.* 28.135). Diogenes Laertius, who wrote about the lives of several Greek philosophers, included in his life of Empedocles, another archaic Greek philosopher, a reference to a miracle that he performed for a woman named Pantheia, who had been deemed uncurable by the physicians whom she consulted (*Lives of Eminent Philosophers* 8.69).

[82] For a detailed analysis of the emperor's role as healer, see Luke 2010, 77–106; see also Lalleman 1997, 358–61.

[83] *V. Hadr.* 25.

CHARISMATIC WONDERWORKERS   175

instead of the other way around.[84] The episode's presence in the *HA* necessarily raises doubts about its authenticity with regard to the life of the emperor, but it nevertheless reveals that some ancient authors accepted that charismatic healers could be found outside Jewish or Christian contexts.

In contrast to the *HA* story about Hadrian, in which the author deliberately called into question the truth of the miracle, two of the three authors who recounted Vespasian's miraculous cures highlighted the large crowds who witnessed the event.[85] Tacitus added that people who were present at the miracles of Vespasian continued to maintain their veracity in his own day, even after the emperor's death. While in Alexandria following his acclamation as emperor, Vespasian was reportedly approached by two men searching for cures, one who was visually impaired and one with a diseased hand. Tacitus and Suetonius both indicated that the impetus for the men to approach Vespasian came from the god Serapis, and Suetonius specified that Serapis appeared to them in a dream.[86] The blind man asked Vespasian to use spittle to anoint his eyes, and the second man requested that Vespasian touch the heel of his foot to the injured hand.[87] Vespasian hesitated at first to grant the men's requests, but ultimately acquiesced and successfully healed them. According to Tacitus, the cure was instantaneous, as in the touch-cures seen earlier in this chapter. The use of spittle to heal the blind man is also strikingly similar to other stories in which sight was restored by Jesus and Hilarion, but the healing of the man with the injured hand offers a rare example in which a miracle was conveyed through the wonderworker's foot.

The accounts of Apollonius, Vespasian, and Hadrian do not originate in Palestine, and it is difficult to determine the degree to which they would have

[84] Immediately before this account is a story about Hadrian and a blind woman, but the nature of both the illness and the cure is more complicated. The woman's blindness was a punishment for not trying to persuade Hadrian to refrain from committing suicide, as she had been instructed in a dream. When she was told a second time to make the case to Hadrian and to kiss his knees, she complied. Her sight was returned after she washed her eyes in water from a temple. While the kiss in this story implies touch, it seems to be separated from her cure, which was instead dependent on washing in the temple water.

[85] Tacitus *Hist.* 4.81; Suetonius *Vesp.* 7. The third account, found in Cassius Dio 65.8, is much shorter and does not comment on the story's veracity.

[86] For Serapis as a healer and the therapeutic cult of Serapis-Asklepios at the Pool of Bethesda in Jerusalem, see Chapter 4. The use of Vespasian's foot may be related to the cult of Serapis, who was said to have given the two men instructions to ask the emperor to perform these miracles. Votive feet were a common dedication at shrines of Serapis and may reflect the idea that the deity's foot could convey healing. For examples of feet as votive dedications at shrines of Serapis, see Dow and Upson 1944, 58–77; Le Glay 1978, 573–89. Pyrrhus heals diseased spleens by touching his toe to the torsos of the afflicted in Plutarch *Life of Pyrrhus* 3.4; I appreciate Jane Burkowski for calling my attention to this passage.

[87] Tacitus and Cassius Dio wrote that the problem was with the man's hand, while Suetonius reported that it was with his leg.

176 CONTESTED CURES

been known in the region. The relative paucity of such stories may mean that, like Celsus, Greek and Roman authors were less interested in distinguishing between ritual practitioners and charismatic healers. Nevertheless, it must be recognized that at least some stories circulated in non-Jewish and non-Christian communities about individuals who possessed an innate ability to heal and perform other wonders.

* * *

This chapter has argued that charismatic wonderworkers were believed to have a personal trait that set them apart and enabled them to perform miracles. In some cases, this distinguishing characteristic had to do with extraordinary knowledge or prophetic abilities they possessed. In other cases, the holy man was portrayed as having an innate power that he could transfer through speech or touch. Some of these wonderworkers were even described as healing without any deliberate intention to do so, as people could be cured simply by touching or looking at them. More frequently, it was the strength of the individual's prayers and close connection with God that enabled the miracle. Despite various manifestations, these wonderworkers were all seen by their coreligionists as having some sort of personal characteristic that endowed them with special abilities. Richard Kalmin, in his study of holy men in late antique Jewish society, wrote: "It bears emphasizing at the outset that my claim is not that we are dealing with a uniform entity in late antique society and literature; that all holy men possessed the same characteristics to the same degree."[88] To the extent that this was true for the figures that Kalmin studied, his observation is all the more pertinent in present chapter. The key characteristic that unites the stories from different cultural and religious groups in this chapter is that they credited wonderworkers with miracles that were not dependent on the prescribed rituals discussed in Chapter 5. Beyond this, no uniformity is necessary.

These charismatic wonderworkers are most plentiful in Christian material, from the New Testament to hagiography. They are also present, but somewhat harder to ascertain, in rabbinic sources. In late antique Palestinian hagiographies, we can uncover some of the expectations that the sick and injured likely had as they approached holy men for cures: the necessity to convince them that they were worthy of help, the importance of faith, and the idea that contemporary ascetics were following the miracle traditions found in the New Testament and the Hebrew Bible. Among Jews and Christians, the fame and presumed power of charismatic healers became a source of tension

---

[88] Kalmin 2003, 217.

that disrupted their religious communities. The institutionalization of healing rituals, such as that seen in the liturgical ceremonies of Chapter 5, may have functioned as an alternative to charismatic holy men in an effort to mitigate this power struggle. The cures offered by these formal rituals would have been under the control of religious elites and were legitimized by the use of the prayers and performative acts that they prescribed. This power struggle between the institutional elite and charismatic holy men can be seen in some of the polemical texts that we will turn to next in Chapter 7.

PART IV

Elite Rhetoric

CHAPTER 7

It is Better to Die: Elite Rhetoric and Communal Identity

Throughout this book, we have seen how techniques employed in ritual healing were shared across the notional lines that separated the ethnic, cultural, and religious communities of ancient Palestine. People wore amulets to heal them from their illnesses and to ward off the potential for new diseases. Some of these amulets contained lengthy texts or biblical quotations, while others included only a few words or images. The sick visited sites known for producing miraculous cures, in some cases expecting to encounter a divine healer in a dream. The control of many of these places changed hands with the shifting political landscape of the region, but their association with healing was remarkably persistent. Ritual practitioners addressed speech acts to demon-causing illnesses or higher powers in order to make a demon, and the disease with it, flee, while charismatic wonderworkers drew on their innate abilities or personal connection to the divine to perform miracles for those in need.

Some of these forms of ritual healing included syncretistic elements, such as *charaktares* or *voces magicae*. Others lacked such overt characteristics, but nevertheless reflected shared techniques for seeking ritual cures. In these cases, the ritual's spoken or written components may have stayed within the parameters of a particular community's religious expression. Yet, among Christian authors in particular, it was not only the former, more explicit forms of shared practices that drew the ire of elite authors. Some of their harshest critiques were directed at the techniques themselves and at the ritual practitioners who facilitated them, even maintaining the extreme position that death would be preferable to being healed through such means. In this chapter, I argue that it is precisely the commonalties among ritual healing practices demonstrated throughout this book that prompted Jewish and Christian elites to make healing practices a litmus test for coreligionists.

My approach in this chapter mirrors that of Hagith Sivan, who used conflict theory to explain how the communities of late antique Palestine related to

182 CONTESTED CURES

each other.[1] Sivan argued that intra-communal conflicts offered the opportunity to sift through positions held by coreligionists and identify those that were acceptable, and that external conflicts focused on the shared characteristics that united a group in the face of a common enemy. While Sivan used a series of physical and rhetorical conflicts to sketch out a more comprehensive picture of group dynamics in this time period, the present chapter focuses on a relatively narrow, yet universal, aspect of daily life – health and healing – to offer insight into one way that affiliation with a given group was evaluated.

Of necessity, the focus in this final chapter will be on Jewish and Christian responses to healing rituals, such as those found in the Jerusalem Talmud and in John Chrysostom's homilies. Addressing his congregation in Antioch during the late fourth century CE, Chrysostom admonished the people to shun Jewish healing practices: "Let me go so far as to say that even if they really do cure you, it is better to die than to run to God's enemies and be cured that way."[2] Chrysostom returned to this theme a short while later: "When you stand indicted before God's tribunal, what reason will you be able to give for considering the Jews' witchcraft more worthy of your belief than what Christ has said?"[3] The Jerusalem Talmud, which was redacted in the same time period, includes a similar condemnation of Christian healers. The wonderworker Jacob of Kefar Sama offered to perform a miracle by calling upon Jesus ben Pandera, but R. Ishmael advised that it would be better to die than to accept such a cure.[4] Both Chrysostom and the redactors of the Yerushalmi forcefully rejected the use of ritual cures that originated outside their communities. Nevertheless, these passages suggest that the inevitability of sickness and injury made people willing to experiment with seemingly beneficial techniques. If they knew that these practices originated in foreign ritual contexts or that elites had forbidden these cures, it may have been of little concern, given the life-and-death situations in which they found themselves.

The non-exclusivity of other cults, in the many Greek, Roman, Semitic, and Egyptian forms that they took in ancient Palestine and throughout the Mediterranean world, means that we expect – and indeed find – no parallel critiques from authors who belong to these groups. This is not to say that "pagan" critiques are entirely absent, such those of practices labeled *superstitio*. Participants in these activities could suffer legal consequences or be perceived as having a moral failing or as being unproductive members of society, but this

---

[1] Sivan 2008.

[2] John Chrys. *Adv. Iud.* 8.5. Translations of John Chrysostom's *Adversus Iudaeos* homilies are from Harkins 1979.

[3] John Chrys. *Adv. Iud.* 8.8.

[4] *y. Šabb.* 14:4 (14c–15a). The idea that Jesus was the son of a Roman soldier Panthera is also found in Celsus (Origen *C. Cels.* 1.32).

ELITE RHETORIC AND COMMUNAL IDENTITY   183

is quite a bit different than the sorts of boundaries that were put into place around practices by Jewish and Christian authors, including those who used ritual practices as a determining factor for delineating insiders and outsiders.[5] Elite Samaritan critiques of healing rituals are likewise absent. However, the general uniformity of content and medium across the Samaritan amulets is striking and may suggest that the creation and use of amulets was policed by those who acted as guardians of Samaritan identity much as we will see in the discussion of Jewish and Christian authors to follow. Overall, the literary emphasis on circumscribing traditions reveals the preoccupation of religious elites with questions about what made someone a Jew or a Christian, or alternatively what made someone a "good" Jew or a "good" Christian in the author's eyes.[6]

Jewish criticism

There is a long tradition in ancient Palestine of repudiating foreign ritual practitioners. The most extensive list of such prohibitions in the Hebrew Bible can be found in the legal text of Deut 18.[7] This passage has traditionally been difficult for scholars to interpret, since it includes terms about which there is little or no information other than comparative Semitic philology. It identifies groups of practitioners by the rituals that they performed, but, as Gideon Bohak observed, it is not necessarily the aims, or perhaps even the methods, of these foreign specialists that the Deuteronomistic author condemned, since elsewhere the Hebrew Bible offers Israelite alternatives.[8] The biblical author's concern was that the people of Israel seek remedies within the structure of their own community, rather than turning to outsiders for help. As the present chapter demonstrates, this remains an overarching concern of Jewish and Christian authors throughout late antiquity.

The exodus story offers a narrative example of this desire to distinguish between miracles performed by insiders and outsiders. Moses, together with his brother Aaron, performed signs for the Egyptian pharaoh to convince him to release the people of Israel (Exod 7–12). Members of the Egyptian court responded by replicating several of the brothers' signs. Despite identical outcomes, the language used in Exodus stakes a rhetorical claim about the legitimacy

---

[5] For example, see discussions in Flint 1991, 13–21; Dickie 2001, 137–55.

[6] See Frankfurter 2005 for a discussion of the "discourse of ritual censure," which informs this chapter. See also Eidinow 2019.

[7] For a discussion of these biblical injunctions and their alternatives, see Bohak 2008, 11–35.

[8] Bohak 2008, 14–16. Bohak (2008, 382–5) has a similar understanding of how the label "the ways of the Amorites," applied to certain activities and practitioners in rabbinic texts.

184 CONTESTED CURES

of the Israelites' miracles and the aberration of the Egyptians'. Exod 7:11 indicates that the Egyptians' deeds were accomplished by means of enchantments or secret arts (*bĕlahăṭêhem*), while in Exod 7:9 God's command that Moses change a staff into a snake is called a wonder or divine sign (*môpēt*). When this passage was translated into Greek in the Hellenistic period, the same distinction was maintained: The Egyptians performed witchcraft (LXX: *pharmakeiais*), while Moses and Aaron performed a sign (LXX: *semeion*). In addition, the Egyptian specialists are identified in Exod 7:11 as *məkaśĕpîm*, and *ḥarṭummê miṣrayim* (LXX: *pharmakous*, and *epaoidoi tōn Aigyptiōn*), which consistently have rather negative connotations, like "magicians" and "sorcerers."[9] Exodus gives no details about how the Egyptian wonderworkers performed these miracles, and it may be that the biblical author understood their process to have been largely indistinguishable from Moses' and Aaron's. Nevertheless, the language in this passage reflects the author's belief that the Egyptians' power must be attributed to a source other than the God of Israel.

When retelling the exodus story for Roman readers, Josephus illustrated that claims of exclusivity could be made by any party. Josephus' pharaoh neatly inverted the biblical perspective by accusing Moses of "juggleries and magical arts" (*teratourgiais kai mageiais*) in contrast to the "spectacles" (*opseis*) produced by his own court officials.[10] Josephus' Moses responded with a speech that reinforced the biblical interpretation of the events:

> Indeed, O king, I too disdain not the cunning of the Egyptians, but I assert that the deeds wrought by me so far surpass their magic (*mageias*) and their art (*technēs*) as things divine are remote from what is human. And I will show that it is from no witchcraft (*goētiean*) or deception (*planēn*) of true judgement, but from God's providence (*pronoian*) and power (*dynamin*) that my miracles proceed.[11]

Josephus, like the biblical authors and translators before him, recognized that the distinction between "magic" and "miracle" was all in the eyes of the beholder. The use of such labels in Exod 7 and Josephus reflects competing claims about

---

[9] Exod 7:11 also describes these figures as *ḥăkāmîm* (LXX: *sophistas*), which has the more neutral meaning of "wise men." The Israelite and Egyptian wonderworkers were both able to transform a staff into a snake, to change water into blood, and to summon frogs. The Egyptians magicians failed to produce gnats or any of the subsequent plagues.

[10] Josephus *Ant.* 2.284–5. See discussion in Duling 1985, 9–12. Justin Martyr (*Dial.* 69) refers collectively to the performances of the Egyptian wonderworkers and the prophets of Baal in their contest with Elijah in 1 Kgs 18 as "things performed falsely by the so-called devil" (*ha parapoiēsas ho legomenos diabolos*).

[11] Josephus *Ant.* 2.286 (Thackeray 1956).

the nature of miracles but tells the reader little about what the Israelite and Egyptian wonderworkers actually would have done or how members of their audience might have interpreted their actions. It may be that in all three texts – the Hebrew Bible, the Greek translation, and Josephus' retelling – the authors and translators understood the words and actions of the Egyptians to differ significantly from those of Moses and Aaron, but it is equally possible that the two performances were understood as largely indistinguishable. The emphasis in all three texts, however, was not on the outwardly visible wonders, but rather on the power by which they were performed.

A story in 2 Macc 12 takes this denigration of foreign rituals to its inevitable conclusion: death. During a campaign against Gorgias, the Seleucid governor of Idumaea, some of Judas' soldiers died in battle. When the bodies were collected, the Jewish soldiers who died were all found wearing foreign amulets. The text explains that the amulets were not Jewish; the dead soldiers were wearing under their outer garments "sacred tokens of the idols of Jamnia (*hierōmata tōn apo Iamneias eidōlōn*), which the law forbids the Jews to wear."[12] This verse explicitly identifies the amulets as the reason that these particular Jews, and no others, died. Similar perspectives on foreign rituals, and the importance of demarcating which activities were permissible, can also be found in rabbinic texts.

One of the best-known examples of the rabbis' criticism of ritual healing is the one mentioned at the beginning of this chapter. The Yerushalmi includes the story of Eleazar b. Dama as a dire warning against Jews who accepted the cures offered by Christians or in the name of Jesus:

> It happened that Eleazar ben Dama was bitten by a snake and Jacob from Kefar-Sama came to heal him in the name of Jesus ben Pandera, but Rebbi Ismael prevented him. He told him, I shall bring a proof that he can heal me. He could not bring proof before he died. Rebbi Ismael said to him, you are blessed, ben Dama, that you left this world in peace and did not tear down the fences of the Sages . . .[13]

In its version of this story, the Tosefta included the following warning: "For whoever breaks down the hedge erected by sages eventually suffers punishment."[14] A rhetorical hedge surrounded the borders of acceptable practice

---

[12] 2 Macc 12:40.

[13] *y. Šabb.* 14:4 (14c–15a). The same story is also found in *t. Ḥul.* 2:22–3, *y. 'Abod. Zar.* 2:2 (40c–41a), and *b. 'Abod. Zar.* 27b. For more on Jesus and Christian healers in the Talmud, see Schäfer 2007, 52–62.

[14] *t. Ḥul.* 2:23; cf. *y. 'Abod. Zar.* 2:2 (40c–41a). Translations of the Tosefta are taken from Neusner 2002.

186   CONTESTED CURES

according to the rabbis, who took pains to delineate which practices were permitted within the hedge and which must be kept outside it. The rabbis placed Jacob of Kefar Sama beyond this hedge, a rejection that was clearly associated with his invocation of Jesus to effect a cure. Other rabbinic passages reveal that even rituals that draw on Jewish sacred texts and traditions could be forbidden. For example, as we saw in Chapter 2, *m. Sanh.* 10:1 identified several groups of people who would "have no share in the world to come." Among those called out are the following:

> Also he that reads the heretical books, or that utters charms over a wound and says, *I will put none of the diseases upon you which I have put upon the Egyptians: for I am the Lord that heals you.* Abba Saul says: Also he that pronounces the Name with its proper letters.

Two practices drew the rabbis' ire in this passage, both of which have parallels in the amulets discussed in Chapter 2. First, the rabbis rejected whispering a biblical quotation to bring about a cure. The passage quoted here is Exod 15:26, a verse that appears regularly on Samaritan rings and pendants. The second objection involved the recitation of the Tetragrammaton. This recalls the silver *lamella* from Tiberius which included the seventyfold repetition of *yôd-hê* (YH), the first two letters of the Tetragrammaton. Although these examples both come from amulets, it is likely that prayers were said when an amulet was originally put on, possibly including the recitation of inscribed texts, which makes these amulets useful comparanda for *m. Sanh.* 10:1. In contrast to *m. Sanh.* 10:1, a more permissive attitude was attributed to R. Yohanan in *y. Šabb.* 6:9 (8c–8d): "Anything which heals is not forbidden because of the ways of the Emorite."[15] Unlike some rabbis, who evidently cared more about the source of a ritual than its potential to heal, the opinion attributed to R. Yohanan gave more leeway if there was a possibility of a cure.

A third example of rabbis rejecting a healing practice outright concerns local healing cults, such as those seen in Chapters 3 and 4. An exchange between R. Akiba and Zunin in *b. ʿAbod. Zar.* 55a attempted to delegitimize foreign healing cults and their apparent efficacy. This passage describes a wayward Jew who experienced a cure after visiting a "temple of idol worship." R. Akiba does not deny the reality of the miracle, but rather questions the apparent *post hoc ergo propter hoc* assumption of his interlocutor. Unwilling to concede that the foreign deity of the shrine was responsible for this cure, R. Akiba concludes that the length of the illness was predetermined and that its termination was unrelated to the healing shrine. In other words, the man was healed in

---

[15] See also *b. Šabb.* 67a. Heinrich Guggenheimer's (2000) translation of the Yerushalmi uses "Emorite" instead of "Amorite."

spite of, not because of, the time spent inside the sanctuary. The redactors of this passage must have recognized the appeal of popular healing cults to Jews, who faced the same medical complaints as their non-Jewish neighbors.

An interesting contrast to this episode in the Bavli can be found in a story from the medieval *Midrash on the Ten Commandments* about a Jew who visited a therapeutic shrine. Two key details differentiate these two stories. First, *b. 'Abod. Zar.* 55a considers the idol in the shrine to be completely lifeless, while the later Midrash portrays a real demon inhabiting the shrine and using the idol to mislead the worshippers. Second, the conclusions of the two stories differ. While the Jew in the Bavli's story walked away healed, the other one was addressed by a demon: "You should know that by tomorrow your time had come to be healed, but because you have done this, you will never find a cure."[16] This reversal may highlight the greater accommodation that earlier rabbis were willing to make. Complete avoidance of images would have severely restricted Jews' ability to participate in the daily life of the cities they inhabited. A famous anecdote from the Mishnah illustrates this point. When Rabban Gamaliel was visiting the bath of Aphrodite in Akko, a man named Proclus asked how he could bathe in a complex that contained a statue of the goddess.[17] Rabban Gamaliel answered, "I came not within her limits: she came within mine!"[18] There is no miraculous cure in the story about Rabban Gamliel, but one can see in this episode an acknowledgement that Jews lived in a world whose public spaces were shaped by foreign traditions.[19] With this in mind, we return to R. Akiba's recognition in *b. 'Abod. Zar.* 55a that the miracle that took place in a non-Jewish shrine could nevertheless be attributed to God. The text provides no details about the shrine itself or the ritual activities performed within it. However, this story recalls the situation at the hot springs in Palestine. I argued in Chapter 3 that the thermal-mineral baths were patronized simultaneously by members of diverse ethnic, cultural, and religious communities. Whether under the patronage of the Roman army, the elites of Decapolis cities, or local Christian benefactors, the *thermae* would have had visual markers that set the space apart as foreign for the Jewish visitor. Nevertheless, like Rabban Gamaliel in Akko, Jewish visitors could have seen the presence of Greek gods or Christian religious symbols as intrusions into the

---

[16] See discussion in Urbach 1975, 25–6.

[17] Rosenberg 1990, 97. Although the bath of Aphrodite was not a thermal-mineral bath, such as those seen in Chapter 3, Rabban Gamaliel's attitude in this passage is nevertheless instructive for the types of accommodations that rabbinic authors were willing to make.

[18] *m. 'Abod. Zar.* 3:4.

[19] A contrasting position on statues in public places can be found in a story about R. Yohanan, who was said to have given instructions that all the statues in the public baths of Tiberias were to be destroyed (*y. 'Abod. Zar.* 4:4 [43d–44a]).

188   CONTESTED CURES

sacred space created by the hot spring. And like R. Akiba in the Bavli, Jews could have accepted the veracity of cures experienced there by attributing them to their own God, rather than to foreign gods. In this case, nothing prevented the Jewish inhabitants of Palestine from visiting the hot springs alongside their gentile neighbors. Such a situation would reflect Seth Schwartz's contention that the mechanism allowing Jews to participate in the daily life of Greco-Roman cities was "a spectacular act of misprision, of misinterpretation, whereby the rabbis defined pagan religiosity as consisting exclusively of cultic activity, but in so doing declared the non-cultic, but still religious aspects of urban culture acceptable."[20]

A ruling of R. Judah ha-Nasi invites further speculation that Jews did indeed experience miraculous cures at the hot springs. R. Judah's association with the hot springs surfaces on several occasions in rabbinic literature, as we have already seen in Chapter 3. He was said to have visited Hammat Gader multiple times, accompanied on different occasions by R. Yitzhak b. Abdimi (*b. Šabb.* 40b), R. Hanina (*y. Šabb.* 4.2 [6d–7a], 18.2 [16c]), and R. Yonathan (*y. Qidd.* 3.12 [64c–d]). The frequency of these Talmudic references suggests that later authors had no trouble envisioning R. Judah at Hammat Gader not merely once but repeatedly, and in the company of other prominent rabbis. One of the halakhic pronouncements attributed to him allowed the residents of Gadara to visit the *thermae* at Hammat Gader on the Sabbath but did not permit the people who lived at the settlement surrounding the bath complex itself to go up to the town of Gadara.[21] At issue in this ruling was the distance one was allowed to travel on the Sabbath. The Torah indicates that one is to remain in "his place" (Exod 16:29), which the sages of the Mishnah defined as two thousand cubits from one's town.[22]

R. Judah's decision was not strictly about bathing at Hammat Gader on the Sabbath, but rather about traveling to get there. This presupposes that bathing itself was in fact allowed. Indeed, the Bavli reveals that earlier rabbis had once tried to rescind permission for Jews to use the thermal-mineral baths on the Sabbath, since it had been taken as license to bathe in artificially heated water as well, a clear violation of the Sabbath. However, the prohibition could not be maintained, and the rabbis relented.[23] Thus, despite the multicultural and often promiscuous atmosphere that pervaded the *thermae*, visits were allowed, even on the Sabbath.[24] Restrictions on bathing for leisure on the Sabbath and

---

[20] Schwartz 1998, 207; cf. Schwartz 2001, 164.

[21] *t. ʿErub.* 4:16; cf. *y. ʿErub.* 5:7 (22d–23a); *b. ʿErub.* 61a.

[22] *m. ʿErub.* 4:3; 5:7.

[23] *b. Šabb.* 39b–40a.

[24] One example of this promiscuous nature is the frequency of children with mixed parentage, since Jews, both men and women, mingled freely with people of other religious traditions at the hot baths. Such children posed a halakhic problem, most importantly regarding whom they could marry. See discussion in Dvorjetski 2007, 307–8.

debate over using the hot springs for ritual immersion suggest that neither offers a likely justification for visiting *thermae* on the day of rest.[25] The thermal-mineral springs' reputation for healing offers an alternative explanation, but the fact that bathing there was permitted on the Sabbath argues against this healing being seen as medical in nature. Most medical remedies were strictly limited on the Sabbath except in life-threatening situations.[26] For example, broken bones could not be set, and cold water could not be applied to reduce swelling.[27] The issue was not simply one of avoiding work that was banned on the Sabbath, as the prohibition also applied to activities that did not belong to the thirty-nine categories of forbidden work, such as the ingestion or topical application of herbs.[28] In general, if the sole purpose of an action was to treat a minor illness or to alleviate pain, it was not permitted on the Sabbath.

In light of these sweeping prohibitions against medical treatments on the Sabbath, the rabbis' permission to visit the hot springs is exceptional. Common complaints such as digestive problems and skin conditions mentioned in connection to the hot springs were not life-threatening, and as a result, one would expect the rabbis to have forbidden their treatment on the Sabbath. Since both medical treatments and leisurely bathing were curtailed and could not be the purported justification for visiting the hot springs, I would posit that Jewish visitors came in search of miraculous cures, ones that were assigned completely to God, with no human agent subject to Sabbath restrictions. This speculation offers insight into the ruling about Hammat Gader preserved under R. Judah's name. No ritual activity would have necessitated travel from Hammat Gader to Gadara, and so it was forbidden, while travel in the opposite direction was permitted.

With this debate over bathing in the hot springs on the Sabbath, we have transitioned from rabbinic decisions that forbade certain healing rituals outright to those whose use was subject to Sabbath restrictions. As the discussion that follows will demonstrate, the rabbis were at times unconcerned with the practices

---

[25] For leisure: *b. Šabb.* 109a–b. For ritual immersion: *b. Šabb.* 109a–b; *b. Ḥul.* 106a.

[26] *t. Šabb.* 9:22, 15:11–17. Rabbinic opinions were rarely unanimous, and this ruling was no different, as some sages professed unease with medical care in even these most critical cases. In fact, several centuries before the compilation of rabbinic texts began, the Damascus Document gave a particularly strict interpretation of the Sabbath rule, authorizing life-saving measures only if they could be performed using implements that were ordinarily carried on the Sabbath (CD 11:16–17). See discussion in Doering 2008, 230–1.

[27] *m. Šabb.* 22:6.

[28] For forbidden categories of work, see *m. Šabb.* 7:2. For forbidden healing activities that did not belong to these categories of work, see *m. Šabb.* 14:3–4, 22:6; *t. Šabb.* 12:8–13. Healing by methods that did not include work prohibited on the Sabbath has been widely discussed in the context of Jesus, whom the New Testament portrays as healing by simple word or touch. For a study of this issue and review of previous scholarship, see Doering 2008.

themselves, focusing rather on ensuring that no one break the Sabbath to make use of them. A passage in the Yerushalmi takes this approach to the ritual whispering that was forbidden in *m. Sanh.* 10:1. In *y. ʿErub.* 10:11 (26c) and *y. Šabb.* 6:2 (8a–b) rabbinic authors give permission to whisper over snakes, scorpions, and body parts, and to wear certain amulets on the Sabbath. However, they differentiate between the apotropaic and exorcistic recitation of verses, permitting the former on the Sabbath but not the latter. In other words, healing through recitation of psalms was not permitted on the Sabbath but it was, presumably, at other times. Two psalms are mentioned as a "song of the afflicted." One, Ps 91 (LXX 90), we have already seen in Chapter 2, where it appeared on a Greek pendant from Caesarea with the Holy Rider image. It is also known from many other amulets outside Palestine.[29] We also encountered this passage in Chapter 5, where a version was found in the texts from the Judaean desert on 11QApocryphal Psalms. The other, Ps 3, also makes sense as a prayer for healing. It begins "O Lord, how many are my foes! Many are rising against me; many are saying to me, 'There is no help for you in God.' *Selah*. But you, O Lord, are a shield around me, my glory, and the one who lifts up my head."[30]

In the same discussion, the rabbis connected the recitation of verses for healing with *tefillin*, indicating that people would recite biblical texts while placing biblical scrolls or *tefillin* on a sick child.[31] As we will see below, *tefillin* are at times linked to amulets in rabbinic discussions, and the indication in this passage is that they, like amulets, were understood to have the potential to heal. While the rabbis here ultimately rejected this recitation and use of sacred objects on the Sabbath, a more lenient view was taken in the Tosefta, which permitted whispering on the Sabbath in certain circumstances: "They whisper (*lôḥăśîn*) over an eye, a serpent, and a scorpion."[32] The rabbis mentioned eye ailments along with snake bites and scorpion stings, or in the latter case, possibly apotropaic protection against such bites and stings. For these whispered rituals, the rabbis made no pronouncement outside the narrow scope of Sabbath observance. For whispered rituals "involving demons," in contrast, there was a difference of opinion. Rabban Simeon b. Gamaliel took the more permissive approach, apparently permitting these rituals on any day but the Sabbath, while R. Yose countered that the whispered rituals themselves must be rejected, regardless of Sabbath considerations. This calls to mind two things seen in Chapters 5 and 6. First, ritual practitioners and holy men addressed demons to expel them and the illnesses they caused. Second, Roman and

---

[29] De Bruyn and Dijkstra 2011.

[30] Ps 3:1–3. See *y. ʿErub.* 10:11 (26c).

[31] *y. Šabb.* 6:2 (8a–b).

[32] *t. Šabb.* 7:23. This passage also permits items to be held over a person's body, presumably for healing. See also *y. Šabb.* 6:2 (8a–b), 14:3 (14c).

late antique authors commonly accused foreign wonderworkers of performing miracles with the aid of demons. Such rituals "involving demons" must be shunned on any day of the week, according to R. Yose.

Amulets in rabbinic texts are also found in the context of debates over what constitutes work on the Sabbath.[33] Among the actions that were enumerated by rabbinic authors as constituting "work" was carrying items out of the home.[34] The rabbis did not understand carrying to be limited to the transportation of objects by holding them in one's hands or strapping them to one's back, but also applied this prohibition to items that in English we would typically designate as being "worn" on the body rather than "carried." Thus, rabbis debated wearing amulets on the Sabbath as part of a broader conversation about carrying items, and the Mishnah decreed that one may not wear "an amulet (*qāmêaʿ*) that has not been prepared by one that was skilled" on the Sabbath.[35] It would follow, then, that amulets *could* be worn on the Sabbath if they *were* made by a skilled practitioner.[36] The Tosefta asks and answers the obvious question: "What is an amulet made by an expert? Any one which served to bring healing and did so a second and a third time."[37] In other words, *t. Šabb.* 4:9 concludes that amulets could only be worn on the Sabbath if they were known to be effective; if it was an unproven amulet, then it could not be worn. This presupposes that any amulet, proven or unproven, could be worn on any other day of the week.

The rabbis also recognized that certain types of amulets could easily be mistaken for decoration, an issue for modern scholars as much as for ancient observers. In light of this potential for confusion, *t. Šabb.* 4:9 offered a further restriction based on the intent of the wearer, "on the condition that one not put [the amulet] into a ring or a bracelet and go out with it for appearance's sake." This underscores that it is the effectiveness of an amulet that permits an exception to rules about carrying. One may not use permission to wear amulets to get around prohibitions against wearing personal ornaments on the Sabbath. That being said, it is interesting that rings and bracelets are called

---

[33] Rabbinic texts demonstrate knowledge of numerous types of amulets, including those written on parchment or leather and those in the form of rings, bracelets, necklaces, and texts carried in tubes, the last of which likely included *lamellae* and papyri amulets. See *m. Šabb.* 8:3; *y. Šabb.* 6:2 (8a–b).

[34] An understanding of carrying as work is already present in Jer 17:19–27, and the full parameters of this principle would be worked out in subsequent centuries, for example in CD 11:7–9. See discussion in Jassen 2014. Tying as a category of work is also considered in the discussion of amulets in *t. Šabb.* 4:9.

[35] *m. Šabb.* 6:2. In *m. Šabb.* 6:10, R. Meir permitted other items used for healing, such as a nail from a crucifixion, while his colleagues forbade them on any day of the week, since they belonged to the "ways of the Amorite."

[36] No such exception for effective amulets existed for animals; no amulet was to be attached to an animal on the Sabbath. See *t. Šabb.* 4:5, 5:8; *y. Šabb.* 5:4 (7b–c); *b. Šabb.* 53a–b.

[37] *t. Šabb.* 4:9; cf. *y. Šabb.* 5:4 (7b–c), 6.2; *b. Šabb.* 61a–b.

out here, and this may suggest that the rabbis were engaged in the process of creating a border between practices that they permitted and those that they rejected. As seen in Chapters 1 and 2, both amuletic rings and bracelets have been discovered in Israel, yet none of them show any obvious Jewish influence. There are no Hebrew or Aramaic inscriptions on any of these rings or the bracelets, and while language is not the only way that Jewish influence or self-understanding can be demonstrated, it is perhaps significant. It may be that the rabbis' pronouncement in *t. Šabb.* 4:9 about rings and bracelets reflects an attempt to differentiate between Jewish practices and similar ones by outsiders, particularly, I would suggest, from amuletic rings with Samaritan inscriptions. Despite this concern about rings and bracelets, the overall opinion reflected in *m. Šabb.* and *t. Šabb.* might be described as cautious but not inherently opposed to all amulets. Furthermore, this caution is only exhibited in the context of what might be worn on the Sabbath; the text does nothing to prevent a person from wearing an amulet made by a non-expert on any other day.

Additional information about how the rabbis viewed amulets can be found in another exception to prohibitions against carrying on the Sabbath. In *m. Šabb.* 16:1, the rabbis determined that ordinary restrictions on carrying do not apply if biblical scrolls or *tefillin* are in imminent danger of being burned. The rabbis applied this principle to all biblical scrolls, even those that were not frequently read. Those not in active use, either because they were old and worn out or because they were written in a language that the community no longer used, were kept in a communal storage facility, a *genizah* (*gᵊnîzâ*), to prevent them from being discarded with other, profane rubbish.[38] The inclusion of *tefillin* in this exception likely reflects the fact that old *tefillin* were stored in *genizot* alongside the unused biblical scrolls. Of interest in the present context is *t. Šabb.* 13:4, which considers whether amulets should also be saved from fire alongside biblical scrolls and *tefillin*: "As to scrolls containing blessings [e.g., amulets],[39] even though they include the letters of the Divine Name and many citations of the Torah, they do not save them, but they are allowed to burn where they are." This passage ultimately rejects the idea that one can save amulets from fire on the Sabbath, but the fact that they are considered here is telling. The Tosefta's description of these amulets, "they include the letters of the Divine

---

[38] For further details on circumstances in which scrolls might not be read and why they might have been put in the *genizah*, see *y. Šabb.* 16:1–2 (15b–c) and *b. Šabb.* 115a.

[39] The Tosefta uses the word "blessings" in this passage, rather than the typical word for amulets. The Bavli uses both "blessings" (*bᵊrākôt*) and "amulets" (*qᵊmê'îm*) in its discussion of this ruling in *b. Šabb.* 115b. The idea that amulets were blessings is reflected in a copper *lamella* from Horvat Kanaf, which says "Blessed are you our Lord, the healer of all (people on) earth. Send healing (and) cure to Eleazar." (Translation is from Naveh and Shaked 1985, 50–5, no. 3; cf. Eshel and Leiman 2010, 191, no. 6.) For a similar blessing on a silver *lamella* from Irbid, see Naveh and Shaked 1993, 95–8, no. 28.

Name and many citations of the Torah," explains why one might be expected to save them from fire. As we saw in Chapter 2, this characterization of amulets accurately reflects many of the published examples from ancient Palestine and at the same time explains why they would have been placed in a *genizah*, thereby raising the question of rescuing them from fire. The nineteen *lamellae* amulets discovered in the apse of the Nirim synagogue, considered at the beginning of Chapters 1 and 2, offer material evidence that at least some amulets were deposited in the community's *genizah*. The best explanation for the discovery of these amulets in the synagogue apse was that they had originally been placed in a *genizah* located below its raised floor.[40] The three amulets from Nirim that have been unrolled reinforce the understanding of *t. Šabb.* 13:4 that amulets in *genizot* contained divine names and biblical quotations. One of them also engages in the common practice of manipulating verbal roots by repeating the first two consonants of the Tetragrammaton (YH) three times, while another amulet repeats the letters 'H, the first syllable of "I-am-who-I-am," six times.[41]

The link between amulets and *tefillin* in *t. Šabb.* 13:4 invites us to reconsider the relationship between these two types of objects, both of which permitted people to attach biblical texts onto their bodies. As discussed at the end of Chapter 2, Yehuda Cohn argues that the development of *tefillin* was related to the Jewish encounter with Hellenism. In light of these connections, a passage in the Bavli may be relevant:

> **A Torah scroll, phylacteries** [*tefillin*]**, or *mezuzot* that were written by a heretic** [*ṣədûqî*]**, a Samaritan** [*kûtî*]**, a gentile** [*ʿôbēd kôkābîm*]**,** a Canaanite **slave, a woman, a minor, or a Jewish apostate** [*meshummad*] **are unfit, as it is stated: "And you shall bind them** for a sign on your arm . . . **and you shall write them** on the doorposts of your house" (Deuteronomy 6:8–9). From this juxtaposition, one can derive the following: **Anyone who is** included **in** the mitzva of **binding** the phylacteries, i.e., one who is both obligated and performs the mitzva, **is** included **in** the class of people who may **write** Torah scrolls, phylacteries, and *mezuzot*; and **anyone who is not** included **in** the mitzva of **binding is not** included **in** the class of people who may **write** sacred texts.[42]

---

[40] For the publication of the synagogue, see Levy 1960; Levy 1971. For further discussion, see Bohak 2008, 315–18. For amulets found in a medieval *genizah* in Cairo, see Schäfer et al. 1994–9.

[41] For the Nirim amulets, see Naveh and Shaked 1985, 90–101, nos. 11–13.

[42] *b. Menaḥ.* 42b. A couple of notes about the translation are in order. The word translated "heretic" reads "Sadducee," and the word translated "gentile" reads "servant of the stars." These were likely substitutions of *mîn* and *gôy* respectively, to avoid Christian censorship of the Talmud. The Steinsaltz translation provides the transliteration for an apostate, while I have provided the rest. For the history of censorship of the Talmud under Christian authorities, see Steinsaltz 2006, 102–6, and especially 105.

194   CONTESTED CURES

While this is both a later text and one that originated outside the geographical scope of this book, its distinction between those who do and those who do not wear *tefillin* is interesting. I would suggest that the Bavli's rejection of certain categories of people as both wearers and writers of *tefillin* may in part be due to the similarities between *tefillin* and amulets and a desire to create boundaries between them. A Samaritan, called a Cuthean in this passage, is rejected alongside a gentile, a heretic (likely a Christian), an apostate, a slave, a woman, and a minor as wearers and writers of these texts. Yet, as we have already seen, Samaritans *did* wear biblical texts on their bodies. Inscriptions on Samaritan rings allowed a text to be worn on the hands, which could seem appropriate for anyone interpreting Deut 6:8 as a command to bind a physical sign of God's words on the hands.[43] Pendants inscribed with biblical verses could be worn around the neck and understood as a physical manifestation of the commands in Deut 6:6 and 11:18 to keep the words of God on or in one's heart. The fact that none of the Samaritan inscriptions on rings or pendants would have been obscured from view by being carried in a case like rabbinic *tefillin* also reflects the idea that wearing biblical texts would prompt people who read them to act justly, an interpretation of Deut 6:4–9 and Prov 6:20–2 expressed in the *Epistle of Aristeas* and by Philo of Alexandria, perhaps making these Samaritan amulets appear to some as attractive alternatives to rabbinic *tefillin*.[44] Ultimately, I suggested at the end of Chapter 2 that Samaritans might have seen the objects that we conventionally call "amulets" as fulfillments of the same command in the Torah from which the *tefillin* ritual developed. If so, the ruling in *b. Menaḥ*. about who is permitted to create *tefillin* could have been an attempt to distinguish between the ritual practice of rabbinic Jews and the Samaritans. *Tefillin* belonged to the world of adult, Jewish men. Other people who bound God's words on their bodies – even if they understood the practice as a physical manifestation of the command in Deut 6 – were by definition using something other than *tefillin*. Samaritans, Christians, women, and children wore amulets, but not *tefillin*.

Starting in the Hebrew Bible and continuing through late antique rabbinic texts, there was an effort to differentiate between the rituals of insiders and outsiders. Some practices were rejected outright, such as foreign amulets and the invocation of Jesus. Others were met with mixed opinions, with some rabbis accepting them while others rejected them. Still others were an issue only in so far as they related to Sabbath restrictions on work. As will be shown

---

[43] Cf. Exod 13:9, 16; Deut 11:18.

[44] *Ep. Arist.* 158–60; Philo *Spec.* 4.137–9, 141–2. It should be noted that the Samaritan scriptures only included the first five books of the Hebrew Bible, and thus excluded the passage in Prov 6. However, I would suggest that this interpretation of Deut 6:4–9 was popular for some time, based on its appearance in sources that span several centuries.

Christian criticism

At the beginning of the previous section, we saw that in the exodus story the miracles performed by Moses and Aaron were differentiated from those performed by the Egyptian wonderworkers according to the power by which they were accomplished. In the same way, early Christians used stories about Jesus and the apostles to advance their own claims: while miracles could look similar across religious traditions, what mattered was the source of a wonderworker's power. When Jesus was questioned by his followers about how they would recognize the time when persecution was at hand, he said, "False messiahs and false prophets will appear and produce signs (*sēmeia*) and omens (*terata*), to lead astray, if possible, the elect."[45] This warning recognized that while the miracles performed by Christians and non-Christians might outwardly appear identical, one must carefully distinguish them according to the group with which the miracle-workers were identified and the power on which they were said to draw. Such claims about Christians' ritual cures did not go unchallenged. As we saw in Chapter 6, Celsus insisted that all such wonders were essentially the same, arguing that Jesus and the apostles were no different than other wandering exorcists of the time. Taking advantage of Jesus' warning about false prophets, Celsus wrote of Jesus: "He explicitly confesses . . . that there will come among you others also who employ similar miracles, wicked men and sorcerers." Celsus continued: "Is it not a miserable argument to infer from the same works that he is a god while they are sorcerers?"[46] Celsus critiqued the exclusive claims in Mark 13 on the grounds that Jesus himself recognized that others could do the same miracles that he performed. In other words, if Jesus condemned the miracles worked by others, then he had to condemn himself. At issue here is the subjective difference between "magic" and "miracle," exactly as was construed in the stories told about Moses. From Celsus' perspective, a magic/miracle dichotomy simply did not exist.

Origen of Alexandria, who in the third century wrote an extensive rebuttal of Celsus' treatise, claimed that Celsus was assimilating the miracles of Jesus

---

[45] Mark 13:22. See also Matt 24:5 and Luke 21:8. The use of *sēmeia*, "signs," here for the things that will be done by false messiahs and false prophets distinguishes it from the earlier discussion of the Egyptian plagues, where *sēmeia* was restricted to the actions of Moses and Aaron, not those of the Egyptians.

[46] Origen *C. Cels.* 2.49 (*PG* 11:873).

196 CONTESTED CURES

to "human sorcery."[47] The perspectives of Celsus and Origen were diametrically opposed. Whereas Celsus prioritized the results of miracles and saw Christian authors as inventing a distinction that did not exist, Origen prioritized the power by which these acts were done and saw Celsus as creating a false equivalence. Origen went on to insist that the encounter between Moses and the Egyptians paralleled the passage in Mark 13:

> Just as the power of the Egyptian spells was not like the virtue in the miracle done by Moses, for the conclusion showed up the wonders of the Egyptians to have been produced by trickery, while those of Moses were divine; so also the wonders of the Antichrists and those who pretend to do miracles like the signs and wonders of Jesus' disciples are said to be "lying," prevailing "by all deceit of unrighteousness among them that are perishing"; whereas the wonders of Christ and his disciples bore fruit not in deceit but in the salvation of souls.[48]

The passage to which Origen was responding is not the only place where Celsus made similar claims. As we saw in Chapter 5, Celsus wrote that Christian miracles were worked by "pronouncing the names of certain *daimones* and incantations (*kataklēsesi*)."[49] Rejecting Celsus' characterization of Christian exorcisms as the product of incantations, Origen argued that Christians worked miracles by invoking the name of Jesus and reciting events from his life.[50] The implication seems to be that if a ritual was based on biblical texts, then it was a legitimate prayer; if it was not, then it was an incantation.[51] The conflicting world views of Celsus and Origen, and in particular their interpretations of Mark 13, illustrate the absence of "pagan" critiques of ritual healing as a means of demarcating communal boundaries. Unlike the rabbis' metaphorical hedge around acceptable practice, a sentiment if not an analogy shared by certain Christians, Celsus and others like him saw no reason for the hedge in the first place.

Eusebius was bishop of the provincial capital of Caesarea in the first part of the fourth century, and he also responded to critiques of Jesus that suggested

---

[47] Origen *C. Cels.* 2.49.
[48] Origen *C. Cels.* 2.50.
[49] Origen *C. Cels.* 1.6. Although Chadwick uses "incantation" to translate *kataklēsis*, "summoning" or "invocation" would be more accurate. See LSJ, s.v. *kataklēsis*.
[50] Origen *C. Cels.* 1.6; cf. *C. Cels.* 3.27.
[51] Irenaeus wrote more than half a century before Origen, and in *Adv. haeres.* 1.23.4 made a similar distinction, saying that those who performed magic used, among other things, "exorcisms and incantations" (*exorcismis et incantationibus*).

his miracles were done through "sorcery" (*goēteia*) as a "wonderworker" (*thaumatourgos*) or "druggist" (*pharmakeus*).[52] Eusebius rejected such claims first on the basis that Jesus did not heal in order to gain fame or fortune, but that he instead advocated justice, truth, philanthropy, and, ultimately, the worship of the God of all.[53] Elsewhere, Eusebius pointed out that Jesus' abilities to heal were personal, not taught by other wonderworkers or learned from books, which we might understand as a criticism of the freelance ritual practitioners discussed in Chapter 5. To Eusebius, the fact that Jesus received no ritual training and drew on no ritual manuals proved that he was divine (*theios*). Eusebius claimed that no other wonderworker could boast of either the quantity of Jesus' miracles or the multitude of his disciples.[54] Turning to the Christian wonderworkers who followed Jesus, Eusebius again made a contrast. Whereas others invoked *daimones* in order to perform miracles, Christians were the enemies (*echthros* and *polemios*) of demons and cast them out simply by calling on Jesus with the purest prayers (*euchē katharōtatai*), again apparently setting up a comparison between the freelance practitioners of Chapter 5 and the charismatic healers of Chapter 6.[55] In his *Against Hierocles*, Eusebius took direct aim at one of the wonderworkers discussed in Chapter 6: Apollonius of Tyana. Unlike Eusebius' claim that Jesus did not learn his miracles from any source, Eusebius pointed out that Apollonius did just that, beginning to work miracles upon his return from foreign lands where he had acquired the necessary skills.[56] Eusebius claimed that, unlike Jesus, Apollonius was only able to expel one *daimōn* with the help of another.[57]

A frequent foil to early Christian wonderworkers was Simon, who first appears in the Book of Acts. Simon was compared to Philip, who was said to heal many by performing divine "signs" (*sēmeia*), the same word that the Septuagint used to describe Moses' signs before the pharaoh.[58] Simon, in contrast, was said to practice "magic" (*mageuōn*).[59] While the precise nature of Simon's "magic" was not specified, the author of Acts indicated that both Philip and Simon attracted crowds and produced wonder among their audience, which suggests that Simon may also have been performing feats of

---

[52] Eusebius *Dem. ev.* 3.5.125.

[53] Eusebius *Dem. ev.* 3.6.126, 133. Irenaeus also pointed to the absence of such qualities as indicative of wonderworkers whose power comes from a source other than God (*Adv. haer.* 2.31.2).

[54] Eusebius *Dem. ev.* 3.6.130–1.

[55] Eusebius *Dem. ev.* 3.6.132–3. For a similar comparison between pure prayer and other ways of working miracles, see Irenaeus *Adv. haer.* 2.32.5.

[56] Eusebius *C. Hier.* 23.

[57] Eusebius *C. Hier.* 26, 31.

[58] Acts 8:6. See also Acts 8:13, where Philip is said to have performed "signs and great miracles" (*sēmeia kai dynameis megalas*).

[59] Acts 8:9, 11.

healing. Simon makes frequent appearances in later Christian texts. When Justin Martyr, born in modern-day Nablus around the turn of the second century CE, retold this story, he said that Simon "worked magical deeds (*magikas*) through the craft of the *daimones* who acted [on him]."[60] Justin, like the Book of Acts, emphasized that Simon belonged to that perennial "other," the Samaritans, and further indicated that the Samaritans worshipped him.[61] Elsewhere, Justin grouped together Jewish and "pagan" exorcisms. Speaking to a Jewish interlocutor, he wrote: "But some of your exorcists, as I have already noted, adjure the demons by employing the magical art (*technē*) of the Gentiles, using fumigations and amulets (*thymiamasi kai katadesmois*)."[62] To Justin, both Jewish and "pagan" wonderworkers were "others," devoid of true miracles. Writing a couple of decades after Justin Martyr, Irenaeus recognized that ritual cures could be the product of both magic (*magicam*) and the power of God (*virtute dei*).[63] Irenaeus ascribed to Simon a perspective similar to that professed by Celsus, namely that Christians worked miracles through the same techniques as everyone else: "He (Simon) thought that even the apostles themselves affected cures by magic and not by God's power." Rather than seeing the source of Christians' power as different from his own, Irenaeus' Simon simply thought that they were better at magic than he was, possessing "some greater knowledge of magic."[64] While we are dependent here on Irenaeus' imagination about how "pagans" responded to Christians' claims to a monopoly on divine cures – as, for that matter, we are for Origen's report of Celsus' argument – it nevertheless seems plausible. Christian authors separated ritual into "ours" and "theirs," while non-Christians (and non-Jews) saw little difference among them.

Discourse about figures such as Moses, Jesus, and Simon were not mere historical exercises, but rather were intimately tied to the authors' circumstances, used to convince their audience of the behavior they deemed proper. Some authors brought this articulation of communal identity into their present by condemning the practices of their contemporaries and not simply figures

---

[60] Justin Martyr 1 *Apol.* 26.

[61] Justin Martyr 1 *Apol.* 26; 56. For both Simon and Justin as Samaritans, see discussion in Kirkpatrick 2008.

[62] Justin Martyr *Dial.* 85.3. This translation is from Falls and Slusser 2003. Writing not long before Justin Martyr, Josephus was less concerned about differentiating between "prayer" and "incantation." When discussing the Israelite kings David and Solomon, Josephus applied terminology that Origen would later reject. Josephus wrote that the young David sang hymns (*tois hymnois exadein*) for Saul whenever the king was troubled by *daimones* (*Ant.* 6.214; cf. 6.168, *legōn te tous hymnous*), and that Solomon composed incantations (*epōdai*) and exorcisms (*exorkōsas*) that he passed down for posterity (*Ant.* 6.45). For more on Solomon, see Chapter 5.

[63] Irenaeus *Adv. haeres.* 1.23.1.

[64] Translations of Irenaeus are from Unger and Dillon 1992.

ELITE RHETORIC AND COMMUNAL IDENTITY   199

from the past. A telling example can be found in Justin Martyr. In discussing the exodus story, Justin took aim not only at the Egyptian wonderworkers but also the "false prophets" who lived at the time of Elijah, comparing both Moses' and Elijah's opponents to things that the devil had "forged" or "falsified" among the Greeks (*ha parapoiēsas ho legomenos diabolos en tois Hellēsi lechthēnai epoiēsen parapoiēsas*).[65] Origen also rejected contemporary practitioners and labeled them as magicians. His rhetoric in this regard should be seen as an attempt to construct borders between Christians and outsiders. In separate passages, he critiqued both Jews and devotees of Asklepios. For Jews, he admitted to the existence of miracles in earlier periods, but claimed that since the arrival of Jesus, they had been stripped of "their ancient glories."[66] Origen specified "prophets" and "miracles" as two things that were no longer present among Jews, but which did exist within the Christian community.[67] Despite this critique of contemporary Jews, Origen elsewhere championed the biblical patriarchs Abraham, Isaac, and Jacob and recognized the ritual power that came from combining their names with the name of God, producing miracles and expelling demons.[68] For him, these figures did not belong to contemporary Jews, but rather to Christians. Later, when denouncing Celsus for his disbelief in stories about Jesus while accepting cures attributed to Asklepios, Origen compared what he perceived as the Christians' simple, non-magical form of healing to cures obtained in the cult of Asklepios.[69] Origen's rejection of Asklepios is noteworthy for its similarity to his earlier discussion of Simon and the "incantations" of non-Christians. The distinction that contemporary scholarship draws, often by omission, between so-called magical and religious forms of healing is not reflected in these passages by Origen. Cures offered by ritual practitioners and the cult of Asklepios were both equally wrong because they were both located outside the boundaries of Christianity as Origen drew them.

Pseudo-Clement's *Homily* 9, an apocryphal sermon attributed to Peter, similarly highlights connections between forms of ritual healing, only to reject them.[70] Much of this text focuses on the role of demons in causing illnesses,

---

[65] Justin Martyr *Dial.* 69.1.

[66] Origen *C. Cels.* 2.8.

[67] Origen *C. Cels.* 2.8.

[68] Origen *C. Cels.* 4.33.

[69] *C. Cels.* 3.24. *Acts of Pilate* 1.1 attributes to Pilate the sentiment that only the name of Asklepios can cast out demons. Since this is not how ritual healing worked in the cult of Asklepios, this should be understood as a Christian author projecting onto a non-Christian individual the same sort of us-versus-them rhetoric commonly employed by Christian authors to disparage wonderworkers outside their community.

[70] For the structure, date, and origin of the Pseudo-Clementine literature, see discussion in Strecker 1991.

and the author repeatedly made the point that the demons deceived people into believing that they can cure illnesses, hiding the fact that they were actually the ones to inflict them. According to Pseudo-Clement, these miracles took place through the interpretation of dream oracles and prescriptions for the sick to follow.[71] This form of healing is well known from the cult of Asklepios, where the Greek healing god was portrayed as either working a medical treatment in a dream whose curative effects persisted into the waking world or as offering instructions in a dream that individuals had to follow when they woke up. Pseudo-Clement referred to these ritual cures as a "magical art" (*magikē technē*) and pointed out that in his own time people also had recourse to other forms of witchcraft (*goēteusousin*).[72] The author did not give any specifics about what these other forms of ritual healing were, but it seems reasonable that it would have encompassed amulets, as in Chapters 1 and 2, or cures performed by freelance practitioners, as in Chapter 5. As a counterpoint to these false forms of healing, Pseudo-Clement's *Homily* 9 concluded by saying that Peter healed the sick by touching them, a common form of miracle that was attributed to Jesus and other Christian holy men.[73]

Cyril of Jerusalem, whose catechetical lectures to newly baptized Christians were considered in Chapter 5, also demarcated the foreign rituals that new Christians were to avoid. In his first lecture, Cyril admonished those preparing for baptism to be on their guard:

> You are being given weapons to use against the powers ranged against you, weapons against heresies, against Jews and Samaritans and pagans. You have many enemies; take a good supply of weapons, for you have to shoot against many adversaries. You must learn how to shoot down the Greek, how to fight against the heretic, the Jew and the Samaritan. Your arms are ready, above all the sword of the Spirit. You must stretch out your right hand for the good cause to fight the Lord's fight, to conquer the powers ranged against you, and to become invincible to any heretical force.[74]

Cyril did not explicitly identify in this passage the form that the adversarial attacks would take, but it is not a stretch to read this harangue as encompassing forms of ritual healing practiced by the groups that he named. The rich evidence for Jewish and Samaritan amulets in Palestine, alongside the healing sought at the hot springs and from freelance specialists, presents but a few

---

[71] Ps.-Clement *Hom.* 9.14–18.
[72] Ps.-Clement *Hom.* 9.18.
[73] Ps.-Clement *Hom.* 9.23.
[74] Cyril Hier. *Catech.* 1.10.

examples. In fact, the section immediately before Cyril's enumeration of these various adversaries highlights the role of Christian exorcism in the baptismal ritual. Cyril wrote: "when the exorcists inspire terror by the Spirit of God, and set the soul, as it were, on fire in the crucible of the body, the hostile demon flees away, and there abide salvation and the hope of eternal life."[75] We can therefore imagine a contrast between the power of this baptismal exorcism and the false hope of outsiders' rituals that Cyril thought could tempt Christians. Later, in the post-baptismal catechetical lectures, Cyril took direct aim at the foreign rituals to which Christians were attracted, and associated them with the devil:

> The devil's worship consists of prayers in the temples of idols, honours paid to lifeless idols, the lighting of lamps or burning of incense by springs and rivers. Some people have been tricked by dreams or demons into acting in this way, thinking they will even find a cure for bodily ailments, but you must have no part in such doings.[76]

In the first part of this passage, Cyril rejected the practices of various polytheistic cults. While he did not specify healing cults per se, it is likely that they were understood within this rejection. The importance of water at healing sites in Palestine, such as at the hot springs in Chapter 3 or at Shuni/'Ein Tzur in Chapter 4, makes the injunction against springs and rivers particularly noteworthy. Following this passage, Cyril appended a list of several other ritual activities that likewise belong to the devil, including some intended to produce cures: amulets (*periammata*), amulets written on leaves (*en petalois epigraphai*), and forms of magic (*mageiai*).[77] The fact that Cyril went on to mention practices that are unquestionably related to ritual healing, especially amulets, makes it reasonable to see ritual healing as a factor in the first part of this passage as well. Cures attributed to healing shrines and those found through amulets or other forms of "magic" were simply two sides of the same coin for Cyril.

Two final authors are of note for their critiques of local healing cults. Both Jerome and John Chrysostom associated such sites with Jews. Jerome, who spent decades in Palestine at the end of his life, accused Jews of sleeping in the temples of idols (*in delubris idolorum*) in the expectation of dreams, and Chrysostom railed against the "Judaizing disease" and berated his congregation for sleeping in the synagogue of Daphne for the same purpose, taking pains to

---

[75] Cyril Hier. *Catech.* 1.10.
[76] Cyril Hier. *Catech.* 19.8.
[77] Cyril Hier. *Catech.* 19.8.

202 CONTESTED CURES

associate it with "pagan" practice.[78] This rhetorical connection between Jewish and "pagan" rituals served the authors' purpose of painting both as "others" who were to be avoided at all costs. This was also a common tactic when Christian authors took up the question of amulets.

As we have already seen in Cyril of Jerusalem, amulets drew the ire of Christian elites, who as a rule took a severe approach to them.[79] Eusebius compared amulets unfavorably to the charismatic cures attributed to Jesus and his disciples. In his defense of the disciples' cures, Eusebius pointed out the following:

> [The disciples] will not allow their sick even to do what is exceedingly common with non-Christians, to make use of charms written on leaves or amulets, or to pay attention to those promising to soothe them with songs of enchantment, or to procure ease for their pains by burning incense made of roots and herbs, or anything else of the kind. All these things at any rate are forbidden by Christian teaching, neither is it ever possible to see a Christian using an amulet, or incantations, or charms written on curious leaves, or other things which the crowd consider quite permissible.[80]

Eusebius was familiar with the popular healing practices of non-Christians, including a variety of amulets and rituals performed by the freelance practitioners considered in Chapter 5. His pronouncement was clearly proscriptive rather than descriptive. Evidence from Palestine leaves no doubt that amulets were used by Christians. Eusebius was trying in this passage to define the boundaries of acceptable practice among Christians, stating that anyone who was observed with an amulet was by definition not a Christian. Yet Eusebius' limitations on Christian identity were likely not shared by the users of amulets. While it can be difficult to determine the religious or cultural self-understanding of an amulet's user, there is no reason to doubt that there were amulet-users who identified as Christians.

John Chrysostom was particularly critical of exactly those amulets that he thought his congregation would find innocuous. For while Chrysostom was certain that a Christian mother would refuse to bring her sick child to an idol's temple, he thought that the same mother might see the use of an amulet as less

---

[78] Jerome *Comm. Isa.* 18.65. John Chrys. *Adv. Iud.* 1.1, 6. For Chrysostom and Antioch, see Wilken 1983; Sandwell 2007; Shepardson 2014.

[79] For a more complete catalogue of references to amulets in patristic writings, including those from the Latin West, which have been omitted in the following discussion, see Stander 1993.

[80] Eusebius *Dem. ev.* 3.6.127. This translation is from Ferrar 1920.

problematic.[81] This was especially true for amulets that lacked overt references to demonic powers and that only invoked the name of God, angels, or other Christian figures.[82] The *boēth(e)i* rings, such as the one from Hammat Gader, offer a good example of the sort of amulet that Chrysostom might have had in mind, as their content is thoroughly Christian. The Hammat Gader ring lacks images and contains only a simple request for help, directed to Christ using a *nomen sacrum*. Had the text, "Christ, help (so-and-so)" been spoken, rather than inscribed, it would have been an uncontroversial prayer. However, Chrysostom considered these Christian amulets to be the most destructive kind, because they were deceptive and because they insolently misused God's name.[83] In his *Third Homily on Colossians*, Chrysostom imagined congregants saying, "We call upon God, and do nothing more," or defending the person who created the amulet: "The old woman is a Christian . . . and one of the faithful." Chrysostom's response in both cases was the same: amulets are "idolatry."[84] Chrysostom repeatedly returned to the question of amulets, each time condemning their use. He even recognized that by following his advice, members of his congregation would die:

> Have you fallen into a severe sickness, and do many come, constraining you, some with charms (*epōdais*), some with amulets (*periamassin*), and others with other things, to remedy the evil? And have you borne it firmly and unflinchingly from the fear of God, and would you have chosen to suffer all things rather than submit to do any of those idolatrous practices? This brings to you the crown of martyrdom . . . For as such a one bears firmly the pains of torture, so as not to worship the image (*eidōlon*), so you also bear the sufferings of your disease, so as to want nothing of those remedies which the other offers, nor to do the things which he prescribes . . . For tell me, when fever is raging and burning within, and you reject the charm that others recommend to you, have you not bound on you the crown of martyrdom?[85]

According to Chrysostom, healing rituals could not be permitted, even if they prolonged life. It was better to die than to benefit from them. He was similarly

---

[81] John Chrys. *Hom.* 8 *in Col.* 5. For Chrysostom and Augustine on the dangers of amulets, see Sanzo 2019.

[82] John Chrys. *Catech. illum.* 2.5. For an extended treatment of Chrysostom's attitude toward demons, see Kalleres 2015, 51–112.

[83] John Chrys. *Catech. illum.* 2.5.

[84] John Chrys. *Hom.* 8 *in Col.* 5 (translations of this text are slightly modified versions of *NPNF* 1/13:298). Chrysostom again associates old women with amulets (*periapta*) and incantations (*epōdas*) in *Catech. illum.* 2.5.

[85] John Chrys. *Hom.* 3 *in* 1 *Thess.* 3 (translation is a slightly modified version of *NPNF* 1/13:336–7).

steadfast when addressing mothers of sick children. He charged women not to resort to amulets even if their children were near death, maintaining that mothers made the ultimate sacrifice when they rejected the idolatry of amulets and equating this sacrifice with martyrdom.[86] Put simply, Chrysostom considered death superior to the use of amulets and exhorted those burning with fever to be reminded of the fire of Gehenna rather than succumb to the temptation of amulets.[87] The fact that he considered this a life-or-death decision suggests that Chrysostom recognized the possibility that amulets could be efficacious. While most cures performed by non-Christians, he argued, were not done in reality but were the result of the practitioners' trickery (*magganeias*), even those that did effect true results ought to be shunned, as it was better to die than to employ such methods and risk eternal fire.[88] As models, Chrysostom offered Job and the parable of the rich man and Lazarus, who persevered in the face of illnesses and misfortunes without resorting to amulets or other forms of magic.[89] Chrysostom rejected amulets because they belonged to the rituals of non-Christians, being widespread among Jews and Greeks who did not trust in the power of the cross.[90] In fact, Chrysostom maintained that turning to "the witchcraft of these Jews" (*goēteias toutōn*) made even one who proclaimed himself to be a Christian worthy of condemnation.[91] No amulet could be rationalized by Chrysostom.[92]

---

[86] John Chrys. *Hom. 8 in Col.* 5. Gregory of Nazianzus, an older contemporary of Chrysostom, also addressed the mothers in his community and admonished them to refrain from using amulets to protect their children and to have faith that the Trinity was the only protection their children needed. The use of amulets (*periamma*) and enchantments (*epasma*), Gregory cautioned, would only invite the evil one. Instead, he argued that the Trinity was "the great and the good *phylaktērion*" (*Orationes* 40.17). *Phylaktērion* is a Greek word that was sometimes used to refer to amulets and other times used to refer to Jewish *tefillin* (e.g. Matt 23:5). Gregory's use of *phylaktērion* may hint at the New Testament use of this word for Jewish *tefillin* as a way to emphasize the "otherness" of amulets. Unlike Jews, who needed *phylaktēria*, Christians had no need for such ritual objects; all they needed was the Trinity.

[87] John Chrys. *Adv. Iud.* 8.7.

[88] John Chrys. *Adv. Iud.* 8.5.

[89] John Chrys. *Adv. Iud.* 8.6.

[90] John Chrys. *Hom.* 12 *in* 1 *Cor.* 7 and *Adv. Iud.* 8.5, 8.

[91] John Chrys. *Adv. Iud.* 8.8. Chrysostom was no stranger to the use of amulets to protect against fevers and knew of their severity if left untreated. In fact, his description of fevers treated by amulets likely reflects malaria. John Chrysostom, *Adv. Iud.* 8.7: "But if you put up with your fever for a short time, and do not honor those who want to speak an incantation or tie an amulet to your body, and after much insult you drive them out of your house, immediately you took relief as a drink from the knowledge. Even if the fever consumes you many times, your soul brings you consolation that is better and more profitable than any relief from water or moisture. For even if you regain your health after using the incantation, you will be more miserable than those who are feverish, since you are conscious of your sin."

[92] For the persistence of similar condemnations in subsequent centuries, particularly in the West, see discussion in Flint 1991, 240–53.

Epiphanius of Salamis, who was born in Palestine and would eventually found a monastery there before becoming Bishop of Salamis in Cyprus, also associated amulets with non-Christians. His compilation of heresies connected amulets with both the Sampsaeans and Manichaeans, whose practices Christians must avoid.[93] Epiphanius returned to the issue of amulets (*periapta* and *phylaktēria*) in his synopsis of Christian doctrine, rejecting amulets alongside other activities such as magic (*mageian*), incantations (*epaoidias*), murder, adultery, and attending the theater.[94] In the fifth century, Isaac of Antioch also identified amulets as something antithetical to Christian practice and lamented that they were worn even inside churches:

> The masses come to the Church,
> And they are led by Satan.
> And he is (proudly) carried upon their necks
> Like a royal necklace.
> This one (wears him) upon his neck.
> And an innocent child
> Comes wearing the names of demons.[95]

Isaac, like Chrysostom, pointed out that children were among those wearing amulets. To make matters worse, according to Isaac, it was not just the congregation that relied on amulets, but priests that actively encouraged people to visit magicians. Ultimately, he claimed that such practices belong to "pagans" and Jews but have no place among Christians.[96]

Christian elites proposed alternatives to amulets. Chrysostom said that Christians were to make the sign of the cross and say, "This I have as my only weapon, this as my remedy, and I know no other."[97] Cyril of Jerusalem made a similar recommendation, and exhorted those preparing for baptism to make the sign of the cross regularly, calling it a "protection" and a "terror to demons."[98] Another fourth-century author, Athanasius of Alexandria, also recommended an alternative to amulets: the recitation of Ps 41:4, "As for me, I said, 'O LORD, be gracious to me; heal me, for I have sinned against you.'" Athanasius went on to explain that amulets (*periapta*) are forms of magic (*goēteiai*) that are empty

---

[93] Epiphanius *Pan.* 1.5, 13.6.

[94] Epiphanius *De fide* 24.3.

[95] Isaac of Antioch *De magis*. This text was previously attributed to Ephraim the Syrian. For translation and discussion, see Kazan 1963, 93–7. For the cross as an alternative to "magic," see discussion in Flint 1991, 173–93.

[96] Kazan 1963, 96–7.

[97] John Chrys. *Hom.* 8 *in Col.* 5. He makes a similar argument in *Hom.* 12 *in* 1 *Cor.* 13–14.

[98] Cyril Hier. *Catech.* 13.36.

of any help (*mataia boēthēmata*), and making use of such things transforms one from a Christian into a foreigner, that is, a "pagan" (*ethnikon*).[99]

The rhetoric that we see in the writings of these late antique Christian elites was made more official through legal texts. The *Codex Theodosianus* preserved a number of laws that could be used to condemn wonderworkers. As a compilation of laws issued over more than a century, the *Codex Theodosianus* reflects changing opinions. The most lenient approach to ritual healing can be found in a law issued during the reign of Constantine:

> The science of those men who are equipped with magic arts (*magicis artibus*) and who are revealed to have worked against the safety of men or to have turned virtuous minds to lust shall be punished and deservedly avenged by the most severe laws. But remedies (*remedia*) sought for human bodies shall not be involved in criminal accusation, nor the assistance that is innocently employed in rural districts in order that rains may not be feared for the ripe grape harvests or that the harvests may not be shattered by the stones of ruinous hail, since by such devices no person's safety or reputation is injured, but by their action they bring it about that divine gifts and the labors of men are not destroyed.[100]

This law makes a distinction between aggressive and erotic "magic" on the one hand, and healing and protective rituals on the other. Despite this legal distinction made under Constantine, the fact that these four categories of ritual actions were grouped together here implies that they were seen as being related to each other, possibly because they could be performed by the same individual. Other laws in the *Codex Theodosianus* fail to differentiate in this manner, prosecuting anyone called a magician (*magus*)[101] and applying blanket rules to those convicted of magic (*veneficium, maleficium*) that forbade them from receiving pardons, appealing their convictions, or being spared capital punishment.[102] Laws such as these could also be turned against Christians. Jerome reported that prefects in Gaza accused Hilarion of being a magician and petitioned Julian to have him executed, and Ammianus Marcellinus, writing his history in the fourth century, stated that wearing amulets (*remedia*) was grounds for execution.[103]

---

[99] Athanasius *Fr. de amul.*

[100] *Cod. Theod.* 9.16.3. Translation of the *Codex Theodosianus* is from Pharr 1952.

[101] *Cod. Theod.* 9.16.6; see also 9.16.11.

[102] *Cod. Theod.* 9.38, 9.40, 11.38.

[103] Jerome *V. Hil.* 33; Ammianus Marcellinus 19.12.14. The one complaint that Ammianus Marcellinus associates explicitly with amulets is the quartan fever. As discussed in Chapter 2, fevers, likely associated with malaria, were the most common condition specified among *lamellae* amulets from Palestine. For a discussion of how legal proscriptions against magic could be applied, see discussion in Lotz 2019.

Church orders and synods carried similar authority to regulate acceptable practice for Christians. The *Apostolic Tradition* and *Apostolic Constitutions*, discussed in Chapter 5, specify that certain categories of people may not be admitted to the church as catechumens. Alongside charioteers, gladiators, and actors, among others, the *Apostolic Tradition* required that those who made amulets abandon such pursuits before they could be admitted to the church. No such possibility existed for one deemed a magician (*magos*), who could not be accepted at all. This latter provision is noteworthy in light of the fact that "pagan" priests could be received as catechumens provided they abandoned their idols.[104] Foreign priests could convert to Christianity but "magicians" could not. A similar list is contained in the *Apostolic Constitutions*. Unlike the earlier *Apostolic Tradition*, which forbade anyone who had once been a *magos* from becoming a catechumen, the *Apostolic Constitutions* permit a former *magos* or one who had once made amulets or used incantations to convert, provided sufficient time had elapsed to demonstrate the sincerity of his conversion.[105] The Synod of Laodicea, a local church council in Asia Minor, took official interest in the activities pursued by Christian clergy, forbidding them in canon 36 from being either a *magos* or an *epaoidos*. However, unlike the passage in the *Codex Theodosianus* that made allowances for protective or healing rites, the harshest condemnation in canon 36 was for those who made amulets (*phylaktēria*), which are called "prisons for their souls," and it instructs that anyone who wears an amulet is to be excommunicated. The canon immediately before it instructs that Christians are not to name angels (*aggelous onomazein*), equating this with idolatry and including it in a list of activities that are anathema. Such angelic invocations could be found both in amulets and in the texts used by freelance ritual specialists.

In his discussion of canon 36, Matthew Dickie wrote: "there can be no doubt of the existence of men who exploited their position within the Church to trade in amulets or phylacteries that might contain sacred material and readings from Scripture."[106] It is of course possible, and perhaps even likely, that the creation of amulets was an exploitive move by some. However, Dickie's interpretation seems to presume that amulets were uniformly acknowledged as bad, and that the only reason that the Christian clergy addressed in canon 36 of the Council of Laodicea might craft them was to exploit the gullible. This leaves no room for the possibility that some clergy created amulets because they thought that such items were genuinely beneficial for the wearer, and thus perceived their manufacture as a natural outgrowth of their ministry. Dickie seems to see amulets through the lens of exactly those elite authors

---

[104] *Trad. ap.* 16.
[105] *Const. ap.* 32.
[106] Dickie 2001, 270.

208   CONTESTED CURES

under discussion in this chapter. There is no guarantee that all clergy agreed with the authors discussed in the previous pages that any amulet, including those with uniformly Christian texts and images, was inherently evil and outside the bounds of acceptable practice for Christians. In fact, the prevalence of such amulets would perhaps suggest otherwise.

* * *

I have argued throughout this book that the people of Roman and late antique Palestine freely borrowed ritual techniques in their search for divine cures. It is likely that many people did not recognize the cosmopolitan influences that, with the benefit of hindsight, we can clearly see in their healing practices. In contrast, religious elites including rabbinic scholars and church officials were closely attuned to the similarities between various practices and were keen to articulate boundaries for members of their community. Some non-elites certainly would have been aware of this polemic, such as members of Chrysostom's congregation who heard his *Adversus Judaeos* homilies, but we remain in the dark on the degree to which such tirades would have changed the behavior of people desperate to secure a miracle for themselves or a loved one. Even if non-elites were familiar with these critiques, the rabbinic and patristic imposition of boundaries between insider and outsider practices would not necessarily have had the effect of decreasing cultural interactions. As Fredrik Barth has argued, the "cognitive fiat" of drawing the boundary does not prevent interaction, as "people . . . respond selectively and pragmatically, spinning connections in forms . . . shaped by social and material processes."[107] To use Barth's analogy, just as neighbors converse over the fences that mark the boundaries of their yards, so also the imposition of communal boundaries can do the very thing that it seeks to prevent: facilitate interactions among members of different groups. Ultimately, it would seem, this is what happened in Roman and late antique Palestine. It was the elites who contested the cures, but perhaps few others.

---

[107] Barth 2012, 30.

EPILOGUE

It Is Better to Live

This book has proposed that we can distinguish three basic categories of divine cures in ancient Palestine, and indeed in the ancient Mediterranean world more broadly: objects, places, and people. Despite differences in the identity of divine healers and the specific language and images used, the ways in which objects, places, and people served as conduits of healing transcended communal boundaries. The resulting similarities made these rituals the subject of polemical discourse among elite Jewish and Christian authors trying to police collective borders.

Chapters 1 and 2 surveyed the evidence from ancient Palestine for amulets. A variety of visual imagery was combined with Hebrew, Aramaic, Samaritan, and Greek inscriptions. By examining biblical quotations, *charaktares*, *voces magicae*, and images, one can see how some details on amulets were used by members of different ethnic, cultural, and religious groups. The prohibitions against amulets among both rabbinic and Christian authors reflect knowledge of a variety of amulets used by both their coreligionists and by outsiders. Christian authors, such as John Chrysostom and Eusebius, rejected all amulets. They took pains to associate amulets with Jews or with "pagans," but they even condemned amulets whose contents were wholly Christian, suggesting that these were the most insidious type. In other words, some Christian authors rejected not just the contents of amulets, but the form itself. However, they did not necessarily deny the efficacy of amulets and recognized that by eschewing them some people could die from their illnesses. Rabbinic authors, in contrast, were somewhat less rigid in their treatment of amulets. While the rabbis rejected certain amulets and placed limits on the use of others, they were in general more accommodating than Christian authors and seemed to accept the fact that Jews used amulets to ward off diseases. When rabbinic texts did restrict the use of amulets, it often was in order to prevent people from wearing or carrying amulets outside the home on the Sabbath. I suggest that in some rulings it is possible to infer knowledge of Samaritan amulets and their similarities to *tefillin*, and the rabbis attempted to create boundaries between these Jewish and Samaritan practices. It is perhaps telling that rings and pendants, the principal forms of Samaritan amulets, and that certain biblical texts common on Samaritan amulets are largely not found among those that can with some confidence be attributed to a Jewish user, a Jewish specialist, or both.

Local healing cults in Roman and late antique Palestine are noteworthy in at least two ways. First, water was a key feature in the sites considered in Chapters 3 and 4. While it is true that water was an integral part of healing cults across the ancient Mediterranean world, the evidence from Palestine seems to suggest that it was a defining feature, rather than simply one of several necessary components. If, as I suggested in Chapter 3, the evidence for ritual healing at Hammat Gader and Hammat Tiberias can be extended to other thermal-mineral springs, then Roman and late antique Palestine was dotted with sites where visitors might expect a healing theophany. This divine experience should not be understood as the motivation for all visitors to the hot springs, and it is clear that many people saw the baths as a leisure space and that others may have attributed healing experienced there to the natural properties of the water, but these activities need not have been mutually exclusive. Water also featured prominently in the healing sites of Chapter 4, where the Pool of Bethesda, a Jewish *miqveh*, became the site of a healing cult dedicated to Serapis-Asklepios and later to the miracle of Jesus, and where the water of ʿEin Tzur, channeled to Shuni, ultimately allowed a Christianized healing cult at the spring itself to replace non-Christian activities at Shuni. A second key characteristic of local healing cults in Palestine is that they welcomed members of different cultural and religious communities to the same site, either simultaneously or sequentially. The hot springs of Chapter 3 seem to fall into the former category, and the sites of Chapter 4 into the latter. Patristic authors associated local healing cults with "pagans" and Jews and argued that they were to be avoided at all times, defining these rituals as clearly outside acceptable forms of Christianity, yet the thermal-mineral springs were not explicitly named among these rejected sites. While Christian authors were critical of mixed bathing and the promiscuous atmosphere of baths, visits to the hot springs were not forbidden. Furthermore, excavations at these sites revealed Christian patronage, such as is demonstrated by Empress Eudokia's inscription at Hammat Gader. Unlike in their critiques of amulets, even those that outwardly appeared Christian, patristic authors do not take up the issue of local healing cults that were clearly Christian in nature, such as the Pool of Bethesda and Emmaus where Christian pilgrims sought cures apparently without censure. Rabbinic attitudes toward local healing cults varied. Visits to the hot springs were permitted, albeit after earlier rejections, even on the Sabbath.

Rabbinic stories reflected the popularity of local healing cults and raised the possibility that they could attract Jewish visitors. Some rabbis held that such a visit would prevent an individual from ever being healed of his or her disease, while others claimed that the sites were inhabited by demons who tried to deceive people with the promise of cures, and still others thought that God would heal the sick despite their visit to a foreign healing shrine.

In the first four chapters, archaeological evidence of amulets and local healing sites formed the basis for our understanding of these rituals. For the most part, no such evidence from Palestine exists for the rituals of Chapters 5 and 6, which makes our interpretation of them inextricably connected to the elite criticisms explored in Chapter 7. Miracles, whether cures or other wonders that defied the laws of nature, invited questions about the power by which those acts were done. This was already seen in the Hebrew Bible's account of Moses' and Aaron's demonstration before the pharaoh in Egypt, as well as in later disagreements over the source of Jesus' ability to work miracles. One of the inherent problems in studying these forms of healing is the tendency of Jewish and Christian authors to differentiate this last group of ritual cures according to the individuals who performed them. If it was performed by someone within one's own community, it was a miracle; if performed by someone outside one's community, it was magic. With this in mind, Chapter 5 considered cures that anyone could perform through the use of prescribed words and actions, while Chapter 6 looked at cures by charismatic healers believed by their coreligionists to have some sort of special power, unique to that individual. Yet some are no doubt wondering: Were these indeed two separate categories of healing? Or is the distinction simply one invented by an elite rhetorical strategy intended to restrict people to the cures offered by their community? I maintain that the evidence examined in Chapters 5 and 6 argues for these being two separate categories of healing in the minds of at least some ancient observers, but there is no doubt that our understanding of them is influenced by sweeping renunciations of certain practitioners and rituals as "magic." One of the strongest arguments in favor of these being two separate categories of healing comes from my approach in Chapter 5 of treating freelance and liturgical practitioners alongside each other, since both used designated words and actions to effect cures. The individuals performing the ritual were immaterial; what mattered was their knowledge of the correct form of the ritual, whether by dint of using specialized handbooks or by the knowledge they gained through official roles within their religious community. Christian authors, as we saw in Chapter 7, would say that non-Christians performing cures did so by means of "magic" or "incantations," based simply on the fact that they were non-Christians. Yet when authors such as Origen described what actually took place in some Christian miracles – calling on the name of Jesus and reciting stories about him – the form is strikingly similar to other cures in Chapter 5. In the same way, Chapter 6 offered evidence that multiple communities recognized miracles that could be worked with no special words or actions, but simply by means of the charismatic wonderworker's innate power or close connection to the divine. Nevertheless, as these chapters demonstrated, a fine line separated magic from miracle in the eyes of many late antique authors.

In closing, let us return to the hypothetical situation with which the book began. A mother, the wife of a skilled artisan in Caesarea, has a young son with malaria. The child's body is racked with an endless cycle of fever and chills. He seems to recover, only to become deathly ill again after some time. She has already consulted physicians, but nothing they did made any difference. Her child continues to get sick. The mother believes that divine intervention is her only hope. What can she do? Our modern scholarly conventions for studying ritual healing, divided into categories of "religion" and "magic," fail to capture the full range of ritual options that this mother had available to her. While ideological concerns, such as those outlined in Chapter 7, may have informed her decisions, I would suggest that other considerations such as cost, proximity, and reputation would have had as much, if not more, influence. Encountering other women at a well or fountain, she might hear of the ritual words that a neighbor spoke daily over a sick child who later recovered. With nothing to lose, our mother might have given this a try, regardless of whether these prayers, hymns, or psalms originated within her own community, or even if she understood the words she was saying. Another option would be to bring her son to a church and ask someone to pray for him and anoint him with oil. While we would typically think of this as an option restricted to Christians, evidence from Chapter 5 indicates that a successful cure of this sort might motivate a person to convert to Christianity. If the family still has a bit of money, she could pay a ritual practitioner to exorcise the demon that is causing the illness or purchase an amulet to protect him from future attacks. The practitioner might have a supply of ready-made, generic amulets for sale, or the mother might commission one that named both her son and herself and that specified the fevers and chills from which he suffered. Alternatively, she could try to buy an amulet previously owned by someone else. If its original owner had been healed, its proven efficacy might make the amulet all the more attractive. With the ability to travel, other options would have presented themselves. She could seek out a holy man, perhaps a monk in the desert with a reputation for cures, or she could travel to a sacred site such as Hammat Gader in expectation of a healing theophany. The cheaper options, and those nearer to home, would have likely been the ones she tried first. Only when those failed would she venture further afield. Throughout all of this, her underlying concern would be to find a cure for her son. Faced with the thought of losing him, she would do whatever it took to keep him from getting sick again. Even if she was aware that religious elites forbade her from pursuing certain cures, her desperation would have led her to try anything. In her mind, it was better that her son live through these rituals, than that he die without them. The availability and attractiveness of cures to women such as this is precisely why religious elites felt compelled to police the ideological border that separated permissible cures from the forbidden ones of neighboring groups.

Bibliography

Abed Rabbo, Omar. 2011. "New Arabic Inscriptions from the South Pool Excavations in Jerusalem." *PrOrChr* Special issue: *La Piscine Probatique de Jésus à Saladin: Le projet Béthesda*: 190–8.

Alexander, Philip S. 1997. "'Wrestling against Wickedness in High Places': Magic in the Worldview of the Qumran Community." In *The Scrolls and the Scriptures: Qumran Fifty Years After*, edited by Stanley E. Porter and Craig A. Evans, 319–30. *Journal for the Study of the Pseudepigrapha* Supplement Series 26. Sheffield: Sheffield Academic Press.

Allison, Dale C. 2011. "A Liturgical Tradition behind the Ending of James." *JSNT* 34, no. 1: 3–18.

Allison, Dale C. 2013. *A Critical and Exegetical Commentary on the Epistle of James*. The International Critical Commentary on the Holy Scriptures of the Old and New Testaments. London: Bloomsbury.

Amitai-Preiss, Nitzan. 1997. "The Arabic Inscriptions, Graffiti, and Games." In *The Roman Baths of Hammat Gader: Final Report*, edited by Yizhar Hirschfeld and Nitzan Amitai-Preiss, 267–78. Jerusalem: Israel Exploration Society.

Amitai-Preiss, Nitzan. 2004. "Glass and Metal Finds." In *Excavations at Tiberias, 1989–1994*, edited by Yizhar Hirschfeld and Roni Amir, 177–90. Jerusalem: Israel Antiquities Authority.

Amorai-Stark, Shua. 2016. *Ancient Gems, Finger Rings and Seal Boxes from Caesarea Maritima: The Hendler Collection*. Tel Aviv: Shay Hendler.

Anderson, Graham. 1994. *Sage, Saint, and Sophist: Holy Men and Their Associates in the Early Roman Empire*. London: Routledge.

Angel, Joseph L. 2012. "Maskil, Community, and Religious Experience in the 'Songs of the Sage' (4Q510–511)." *DSD* 19, no. 1: 1–27.

Applbaum, Nachum and Amihai Mazar. 2006. "Area L: Stratigraphy and Architecture." In *Excavations at Tel Beth-Shean, 1989–1996*, edited by Amihay Mazar, 292–301. Vol. 1. Jerusalem: Israel Exploration Society.

Arnould-Béhar, Caroline. 2011. "La stèle 'Au blé et au serpent' de Béthesda: Étude iconographique." *PrOrChr* Special issue: *La Piscine Probatique de Jésus à Saladin: Le projet Béthesda*: 45–56.

Ashkenazi, Dana. 2015. "The Khirbet al-'Aura/Tel Barukh Cemetery: Magical Objects." In *Samaritan Cemeteries and Tombs in the Central Coastal Plain: Archaeology and History of the Samaritan Settlement outside Samaria (ca. 300–700 ce)*, edited by Oren Tal and Itamar Taxel, 119–21.

Ägypten und Altes Testament: Studien zu Geschichte, Kultur und Religion Ägyptens und des Alten Testaments 82. Münster: Ugarit Verlag.

Aune, David Edward. 1980. "Magic in Early Christianity." *ANRW* 2.23.2: 1507–57.

Aupert, Pierre. 1991. "Les thermes comme lieux de culte." In *Les thermes romains: Actes de la table ronde*, edited by M. Lenoir, 185–92. Collection de l'École française de Rome 142. Rome: L'École française de Rome.

Austin, J. L. 1962. *How To Do Things with Words*. William James Lectures. Oxford: Clarendon Press.

Avi-Yonah, Michael. 1942. "Greek Inscriptions from Ascalon, Jerusalem, Beisan, and Hebron." *QDAP* 10: 160–9.

Avi-Yonah, Michael. 1976. *Gazetteer of Roman Palestine*. Qedem 5. Jerusalem: Institute of Archaeology, Hebrew University of Jerusalem.

Aviam, Mordechai. 2004. *Jews, Pagans, and Christians in the Galilee. 25 Years of Archaeological Excavations and Surveys: Hellenistic to Byzantine Periods*. Land of Galilee 1. Rochester, NY: University of Rochester Press.

Baert, Barbara. 2005. "The Pool of Bethsaïda: The Cultural History of a Holy Place in Jerusalem." *Viator* 36: 1–22.

Baldi, Donato. 1982. *Enchiridion locorum sanctorum: Documenta S. Evangelii loca respicientia*. 2nd ed. Jerusalem: Franciscan Printing Press.

Bar, Doron. 2003. "The Christianisation of Rural Palestine during Late Antiquity." *JEH* 54, no. 3: 401–21.

Baramki, D. C. 1932. "Note on a Cemetery at Karm Al-Shaich, Jerusalem." *QDAP* 1: 3–9.

Barkay, Gabriel. 1989. "The Priestly Benediction on the Ketef Hinnom Plaques." *Cathedra: For the History of Eretz Israel and Its Yishuv* 52: 37–76 (Heb.).

Barkay, Gabriel. 1992. "The Priestly Benediction on Silver Plaques from Ketef Hinnom in Jerusalem." *TA* 19, no. 2: 139–92.

Barkay, Gabriel, Marilyn J. Lundberg, Andrew G. Vaughn, and Bruce Zuckerman. 2004. "The Amulets from Ketef Hinnom: A New Edition and Evaluation." *BASOR* 334: 41–71.

Barkay, Rachel. 1997. "Roman and Byzantine Coins." In *The Roman Baths of Hammat Gader: Final Report*, edited by Yizhar Hirschfeld, 279–300. Jerusalem: Israel Exploration Society.

Barkay, Rachel. 2000a. "The Byzantine Period Wishing Spring of Ein Tzur in the Holy Land." In *XII. Internationaler Numismatischer Kongress Berlin 1997: Akten*, edited by Bernd Kuge and Bernhard Weisser. Vol. 2. Berlin: Staatliche Museen zu Berlin.

Barkay, Rachel. 2000b. "The Coins of Ḥorvat ʿEleq." In *Ramat Hanadiv Excavations: Final Report of the 1984–1998 Seasons*, edited by Yizhar Hirschfeld, 377–419. Jerusalem: Israel Exploration Society.

Barrett-Lennard, R. J. S. 1994. *Christian Healing after the New Testament: Some Approaches to Illness in the Second, Third, and Fourth Centuries*. Lanham, MD: University Press of America.

Barrett-Lennard, R. J. S. 2010. *The Sacramentary of Sarapion of Thmuis*. Piscataway, NJ: Gorgias Press.

Barth, Fredrick. 2012. "Boundaries and Connections." In *Signifying Identities: Anthropological Perspectives on Boundaries and Contested Identities*, edited by Anthony Cohen, 17–36. Hoboken, NJ: Taylor and Francis.

Becker, Adam H. and Annette Yoshiko Reed, eds. 2003. *The Ways That Never Parted: Jews and Christians in Late Antiquity and the Early Middle Ages*. Texts and Studies in Ancient Judaism 95. Tübingen: Mohr Siebeck.

Becker, Michael. 2006. "Miracle Traditions in Early Rabbinic Literature: Some Questions on Their Pragmatics." In *Wonders Never Cease: The Purpose of Narrating Miracle Stories in the New Testament and Its Religious Environment*, edited by Michael Labahn and L. J. Lietaert Peerbolte, 48–69. Library of New Testament Studies 288. London: T & T Clark.

216 CONTESTED CURES

Belayche, Nicole. 2001. *Iudaea-Palaestina: The Pagan Cults in Roman Palestine (Second to Fourth Century)*. Religion der römischen Provinzen 1. Tübingen: Mohr Siebeck.

Belayche, Nicole. 2017. "Épigraphie et expériences religieuses: Le cas des 'bains' de Gadara (*Palaestina IIa*)." In *Gnose et manichéisme entre les oasis d'Égypte et la route de la soie: Hommage à Jean-Daniel Dubois*, edited by Anna van den Kerchove and Gabriela Soares Santoprete, 669–82. Bibliothèque de l'École des hautes études, sciences religieuses 176. Turnhout: Brepols.

Ben Abed, Aïcha and John Scheid. 2003. "Sanctuaire des eaux, sanctuaire de sources, une catégorie ambiguë: L'exemple de Jebel Oust (Tunisie)." In *Sanctuaires et sources dans l'antiquité: Les sources documentaires et leurs limites dans la description des lieux de culte*, edited by Olivier de Cazanove and John Scheid, 7–14. Collection du Centre Jean Bérard 22. Naples: Centre Jean Bérard.

Ben-Zvi, Itzhak. 1961. "A Lamp with a Samaritan Inscription: 'There is none like unto the God of Jeshurun'." *IEJ* 11, no. 3: 139–42.

Benoit, P. 1967. "Découvertes archéologiques autour de la piscine de Bethesda." In *Jerusalem through the Ages*, edited by Charles F. Pfeiffer, 48–57. Baker Studies in Biblical Archaeology 6. Grand Rapids, MI: Baker Book House.

Berman, Ariel. 2011. "Catalogue of Coins from the Excavation of the Fossil-Hump in the South Bethesda Pool." *PrOrChr* Special issue: *La Piscine Probatique de Jésus à Saladin: Le projet Béthesda*: 187–9.

Berman, Dennis. 1979. "Hasidim in Rabbinic Tradition." In *Society of Biblical Literature 1979 Seminar Papers*, edited by Paul J. Achtemeier, 15–33. Missoula, MT: Scholars Press.

Betz, Hans Dieter. 1992. *The Greek Magical Papyri in Translation, Including the Demotic Spells*. 2nd ed. Chicago: University of Chicago Press.

Binns, John. 1994. *Ascetics and Ambassadors of Christ: The Monasteries of Palestine, 314–631*. Oxford: Clarendon Press.

Blackburn, Barry. 1991. *Theios Anēr and the Markan Miracle Traditions: A Critique of the Theios Anēr Concept as an Interpretative Background of the Miracle Traditions Used by Mark*. Wissenschaftliche Untersuchungen zum Neuen Testament 2, no. 40. Tübingen: Mohr Siebeck.

Blenkinsopp, Joseph. 1999. "Miracles: Elisha and Hanina ben Dosa." In *Miracles in Jewish and Christian Antiquity: Imagining Truth*, edited by John C. Cavadini, 57–81. Notre Dame Studies in Theology 3. Notre Dame, IN: University of Notre Dame Press.

Bliss, Frederick Jones and Archibald Campbell Dickie. 1898. *Excavations at Jerusalem, 1894–1897*. London: Committee of the Palestine Exploration Fund.

Bohak, Gideon. 1996. *Traditions of Magic in Late Antiquity*. Ann Arbor: University of Michigan Library.

Bohak, Gideon. 1999. "Greek, Coptic, and Jewish Magic in the Cairo Genizah." *BASP* 36, no. 1/4: 27–44.

Bohak, Gideon. 2003. "Hebrew, Hebrew Everywhere? Notes on the Interpretation of *Voces Magicae*." In *Prayer, Magic, and the Stars in the Ancient and Late Antique World*, edited by Scott B. Noegel, Joel Thomas Walker, and Brannon M. Wheeler, 69–82. University Park: Pennsylvania State University Press.

Bohak, Gideon. 2008. *Ancient Jewish Magic: A History*. Cambridge: Cambridge University Press.

Bohak, Gideon. 2012. "From Qumran to Cairo: The Lives and Times of a Jewish Exorcistic Formula." In *Ritual Healing: Magic, Ritual and Medical Therapy from Antiquity until the Early Modern Period*, edited by Ildikó Csepregi and Charles Burnett, 31–46. Florence: SISMEL edizioni del Galluzzo.

Bohak, Gideon. 2014. "Greek–Hebrew Linguistic Contacts in Late Antique and Medieval Magical Texts." In *The Jewish–Greek Tradition in Antiquity and the Byzantine Empire*, edited by James K. Aitken and James Carleton Paget, 247–60. New York: Cambridge University Press.

Bohak, Gideon. 2017. "Magic in the Cemeteries of Late Antique Palestine." In *Expressions of Cult in the Southern Levant in the Greco-Roman Period: Manifestations in Text and Material Culture*, edited by Oren Tal and Zeev Weiss, 163–80. Contextualizing the Sacred 6. Turnhout: Brepols.

Bokser, Baruch M. 1985. "Wonder-Working and the Rabbinic Tradition: The Case of Ḥanina ben Dosa." *JSJ* 16, no. 1: 42–92.

Bonner, Campbell. 1950. *Studies in Magical Amulets: Chiefly Graeco-Egyptian*. University of Michigan Humanistic Series 49. Ann Arbor: University of Michigan Press.

Booth, Phil. 2014. *Crisis of Empire: Doctrine and Dissent at the End of Late Antiquity*. Transformation of the Classical Heritage 52. Berkeley: University of California Press.

Boustan, Raʿanan and Michael Beshay. 2015. "Sealing the Demons, Once and for All: The Ring of Solomon, the Cross of Christ, and the Power of Biblical Kingship." *ARG* 16, no. 1: 99–130.

Boustan, Raʿanan and Joseph E. Sanzo. 2017. "Christian Magicians, Jewish Magical Idioms, and the Shared Magical Culture of Late Antiquity." *HTR* 110, no. 2: 217–40.

Bovon, François. 1991. "The Suspension of Time in Chapter 18 of *Protevangelium Jacobi*." In *The Future of Early Christianity: Essays in Honor of Helmut Koester*, edited by Birger A. Pearson, A. Thomas Kraabel, George W. E. Nickelsburg, and Norman R. Petersen, 393–405. Minneapolis: Fortress Press.

Boyarin, Daniel. 1999. *Dying for God: Martyrdom and the Making of Christianity and Judaism*. Figurae: Reading Medieval Culture. Stanford: Stanford University Press.

Boyarin, Daniel. 2004. *Border Lines: The Partition of Judaeo-Christianity*. Divinations: Rereading Late Ancient Religion. Philadelphia: University of Pennsylvania Press.

Braarvig, Jens. 1999. "Magic: Reconsidering the Grand Dichotomy." In *The World of Ancient Magic: Papers from the First International Samson Eitrem Seminar at the Norwegian Institute at Athens, 4–8 May 1997*, edited by David R. Jordan, Hugo Montgomery, and Einar Thomassen, 21–54. Bergen: Norwegian Institute at Athens.

Brashear, William M. 1995. "The Greek Magical Papyri: An Introduction and Survey; Annotated Bibliography (1928–1994)." *ANRW* 2.18.5: 3380–684.

Brashear, William M. and Roy David Kotansky. 2002. "A New Magical Formulary." In *Magic and Ritual in the Ancient World*, edited by Paul Allan Mirecki and Marvin W. Meyer, 3–24. Leiden: Brill.

Braude, William G. and Israel J. Kapstein, eds. 2002. *Pĕsiḵta dĕ-Raḇ Kahăna*. 2nd ed. Philadephia: Jewish Publication Society.

Bremmer, Jan N. 2002. "Magic and Religion." In *The Metamorphosis of Magic from Late Antiquity to the Early Modern Period*, edited by Jan N. Bremmer and Jan R. Veenstra, 267–71. Groningen Studies in Cultural Change 1. Leuven: Peeters.

Brock, S. P. 1977. "A Letter Attributed to Cyril of Jerusalem on the Rebuilding of the Temple." *Bulletin of the School of Oriental and African Studies, University of London* 40, no. 2: 267–86.

Brown, Peter. 1971. "The Rise and Function of the Holy Man in Late Antiquity." *JRS* 61: 80–101.

Brown, Raymond E. 1966. *The Gospel According to John (i–xii)*. Anchor Bible 29. Garden City, NY: Doubleday.

Brubaker, Rogers and Frederick Cooper. 2000. "Beyond 'Identity.'" *Theory and Society* 29, no. 1: 1–47.

218 CONTESTED CURES

Bruyn, Theodore S. de. 2010. "Papyri, Parchments, Ostraca, and Tablets Written with Biblical Texts in Greek and Used as Amulets: A Preliminary List." In *Early Christian Manuscripts: Examples of Applied Method and Approach*, edited by Thomas J. Kraus and Tobias Nicklas, 145–89. Texts and Editions for New Testament Study. Leiden: Brill.

Bruyn, Theodore S. de. 2017. *Making Amulets Christian: Artefacts, Scribes, and Contexts*. Oxford Early Christian Studies. Oxford: Oxford University Press.

Bruyn, Theodore S. de and Jitse H. F. Dijkstra. 2011. "Greek Amulets and Formularies from Egypt Containing Christian Elements: A Checklist of Papyri, Parchments, Ostraka, and Tablets." *BASP* 48: 163–216.

Burke, Paul F., Jr. 1995. "Malaria in the Greco-Roman World: A Historical and Epidemiological Survey." *ANRW* 2.37.3: 2252–81.

Chadwick, Henry. 1953. *Contra Celsum*. Cambridge: Cambridge University Press.

Chadwick, Henry and Gregory Dix, eds. 1992. *The Treatise on the Apostolic Tradition of St Hippolytus of Rome Bishop and Martyr: Apostolike Paradosis*. London: Alban Press; Ridgefield, CT: Morehouse Publishing.

Charlesworth, James H. 2011. "Tale of Two Pools: Archaeology and the Book of John." *NEASB* 56: 1–14.

Chryssavgis, John, ed. 2006–7. *Barsanuphius and John: Letters*. 2 vols. Fathers of the Church: A New Translation 113–14. Washington, DC: Catholic University of America Press.

Clark, Elizabeth A. 1986. "Claims on the Bones of Saint Stephen: The Partisans of Melania and Eudocia." In *Ascetic Piety and Women's Faith: Essays on Late Ancient Christianity*, edited by Elizabeth A. Clark, 95–123. Studies in Women and Religion 20. Lewiston, NY: E. Mellen.

Cline, Rangar. 2011. *Ancient Angels: Conceptualizing Angeloi in the Roman Empire*. Religions in the Graeco-Roman World 172. Leiden: Brill.

Cline, Rangar. 2019. "Amulets and the Ritual Efficacy of Christian Symbols." In *The Oxford Handbook of Early Christian Archaeology*, edited by William R. Caraher, Thomas W. Davis, and David K. Pettegrew, 351–68. Oxford: Oxford University Press.

Cohn, Yehudah. 2008a. *Tangled Up in Text: Tefillin and the Ancient World*. Brown Judaic Studies 351. Providence, RI: Brown University.

Cohn, Yehudah. 2008b. "Were *Tefillin* Phylacteries?" *JJS* 59, no. 1: 39–61.

Cotton, Hannah M. and Joseph Geiger. 1995. "A Greek Inscribed Ring from Masada." *IEJ* 45, no. 1: 52–4.

Croon, J. H. 1967. "Hot Springs and Healing Gods." *Mnemosyne* 20, no. 3: 225–46.

Csepregi, Ildikó. 2012. "Changes in Dream Patterns between Antiquity and Byantium: The Impact of Medical Learning on Dream Healing." In *Ritual Healing: Magic, Ritual and Medical Therapy from Antiquity until the Early Modern Period*, edited by Ildikó Csepregi and Charles Burnett, 131–45. Micrologus Library. Florence: SISMEL edizioni del Galluzzo.

Csepregi, Ildikó. 2015. "Christian Transformation of Pagan Cult Places: The Case of Aegae, Cilicia." In *Continuity and Destruction in the Greek East: The Transformation of Monumental Space from the Hellenistic Period to Late Antiquity*, edited by Sujatha Chandrasekaran and Anna Kouremenos, 49–57. British Archaeological Reports International Series 2765. Oxford: BAR Publishing.

Csepregi, Ildikó and Charles Burnett. 2012. *Ritual Healing: Magic, Ritual and Medical Therapy from Antiquity until the Early Modern Period*. Micrologus Library 48. Florence: SISMEL edizioni del Galluzzo.

Dalton, O. M. 1901. *Catalogue of Early Christian Antiquities and Objects from the Christian East in the Department of British and Mediaeval Antiquities and Ethnography of the British Museum*. London: British Museum.

Dan, Joseph. 1982. "The Seventy Names of Metatron." In *Proceedings of the Eighth World Congress of Jewish Studies*, 19–23. Division C: *Talmud and Midrash, Philosophy and Mysticism, Hebrew and Yiddish Literature*. Jerusalem: World Union of Jewish Studies.

Danby, Herbert, ed. 1933. *The Mishnah*. Oxford: Clarendon Press.

Daniel, Robert W. and Franco Maltomini. 1990. *Supplementum Magicum*. Abhandlungen der Rheinisch-Westfälischen Akademie der Wissenschaften Sonderreihe Papyrologica Coloniensia 16. Opladen: Westdeutscher Verlag.

Dasan, Véronique and Árpád M. Nagy. 2019. "Gems." In *Guide to the Study of Ancient Magic*, edited by David Frankfurter, 416–55. Religions in the Graeco-Roman World 189. Leiden: Brill.

Dauphin, Claudine. 1979. "Dor, Byzantine Church." *IEJ* 29, no. 3/4: 235–6.

Dauphin, Claudine. 1986. "Temple grec, église byzantine et cimetière musulman: La basilique de Dor en Israel." *PrOrChr* 36: 14–22.

Dauphin, Claudine. 1993. "Dora-Dor: A Station for Pilgrims in the Byzantine Period on Their Way to Jerusalem." In *Ancient Churches Revealed*, edited by Yoram Tsafrir, 90–7. Jerusalem: Israel Exploration Society; Washington, DC: Biblical Archaeology Society.

Dauphin, Claudine. 1996–7. "Lust, Leprosy, and Lice: Health and Hygiene in Byzantine Palestine." *BAIAS* 15: 55–80.

Dauphin, Claudine. 1997. "On the Pilgrim's Way to the Holy City of Jerusalem: The Basilica of Dor in Israel." In *Archaeology and Biblical Interpretation*, edited by John R. Bartlett, 145–65. London: Routledge.

Dauphin, Claudine. 1998. *La Palestine byzantine: Peuplement et populations*. 3 vols. British Archaeological Reports International Series 726. Oxford: BAR Publishing.

Dauphin, Claudine. 1999. "From Apollo and Asclepius to Christ: Pilgrimage and Healing at the Temple and Episcopal Basilica of Dor." *LASBF* 49: 397–430.

Dauphin, Claudine. 2000. "The Roman Baths of Hammat Gader Review Article." *PEQ* 132: 71–5.

Dauphin, Claudine. 2005. "Bethesda Project at St. Anne's in the Old City of Jerusalem." *PrOrChr* 55, no. 3/4: 263–9.

Dauphin, Claudine. 2011a. "Au service de la foi et de la France: L'archéologie au domaine national français de Sainte-Anne de Jérusalem." *PrOrChr* Special issue: *La Piscine Probatique de Jésus à Saladin: Le projet Béthesda*: 5–16.

Dauphin, Claudine. 2011b. "Destruction – Reconstruction: La probatique de l'invasion perse au califat abbasside." *PrOrChr* Special issue: *La Piscine Probatique de Jésus à Saladin: Le projet Béthesda*: 135–80.

Dauphin, Claudine. 2011c. "Un *kontakion* de pierres pour la *Théotokos*: La mosaïque du martyrion." *PrOrChr* Special issue: *La Piscine Probatique de Jésus à Saladin: Le projet Béthesda*: 57–134.

Dauphin, Claudine and Shimon Gibson. 1994–5. "The Byzantine City of Dor/Dora Discovered." *BAIAS* 14: 9–38.

Dauphin, Claudine, Sebastian P. Brock, Robert C. Gregg, and Alfred F. L. Beeston. 1996. "Païens, juifs, judéo-chrétiens, chrétiens et musulmans: Les inscriptions de Na'aran, Kafr Naffakh, Farj et Er-Ramthaniyye." *PrOrChr* 46: 305–40.

Davies, Stevan L. 1995. *Jesus the Healer: Possession, Trance, and the Origins of Christianity*. New York: Continuum.

de Cazanove, Olivier. 2015. "Water." In *A Companion to the Archaeology of Religion in the Ancient World*, edited by Rubina Raja and Jörg Rüpke, 181–93. Chichester: Wiley-Blackwell.

Deferrari, Roy J., ed. 1952. *Early Christian Biographies*. Fathers of the Church: A New Translation 15. Washington, DC: Catholic University of America.

Delatte, Armand and Philippe Derchain. 1964. *Les intailles magiques gréco-égyptiennes*. Paris: Bibliothèque nationale.

Deubner, Ludovicus. 1900. *De incubatione capita quattuor*. Leipzig: Teubner.

Devillers, Luc. 1999. "Une Piscine peut en cachet une autre: À propos de Jean 5, 1–9a." *RB* 106: 175–205.

Di Segni, Leah. 1994. "Εἷς θεός in Palestinian Inscriptions." *SCI* 13: 94–115.

Di Segni, Leah. 1997. "The Greek Inscriptions of Hammat Gader." In *The Roman Baths of Hammat Gader: Final Report*, edited by Yizhar Hirschfeld, 185–266. Jerusalem: Israel Exploration Society.

Di Segni, Leah. 1998. "The Samaritans in Roman-Byzantine Palestine: Some Misapprehensions." In *Religious and Ethnic Communities in Later Roman Palestine*, edited by Hayim Lapin, 51–66. Studies and Texts in Jewish History and Culture 5. Bethesda: University Press of Maryland.

Di Segni, Leah and Yoram Tsafrir. 2012. "The Ethnic Composition of Jerusalem's Population in the Byzantine Period (312–638 CE)." *LASBF* 62: 405–54.

Dickie, Matthew. 2001. *Magic and Magicians in the Greco-Roman World*. London: Routledge.

Dieleman, Jacco. 2019. "The Greco-Egyptian Magical Papyri." In *Guide to the Study of Ancient Magic*, edited by David Frankfurter, 283–321. Religions in the Graeco-Roman World 189. Leiden: Brill.

Doering, Lutz. 2008. "Much Ado about Nothing? Jesus' Sabbath Healings and Their Halakhic Implications Revisited." In *Judaistik und neutestamentliche Wissenschaft*, edited by Lutz Doering, Hans-Günther Waubke, and Florian Wilk, 217–41. Göttingen: Vandenhoeck & Ruprecht.

Donaldson, Terence L. 2000. *Religious Rivalries and the Struggle for Success in Caesarea Maritima*. Studies in Christianity and Judaism 8. Waterloo, ON: Wilfrid Laurier University Press.

Dothan, Moshe. 1983. *Hammath Tiberias*. Vol. 1: *Early Synagogues and the Hellenistic and Roman Remains*. Jerusalem: Israel Exploration Society.

Douglass, Laurie. 1996. "A New Look at the *Itinerarium Burdigalense*." *JECS* 4, no. 3: 313–33.

Dow, Sterling and Frieda S. Upson. 1944. "The Foot of Sarapis." *Hesperia* 13, no. 1: 58–77.

Drbal, Vlastimil. 2017. "Pilgrimage and Multi-Religious Worship: Palestinian Mamre in Late Antiquity." In *Excavating Pilgrimage: Archaeological Approaches to Sacred Travel and Movement in the Ancient World*, edited by Wiebke Friese and Troels Myrup Kristensen, 245–62. New York: Routledge.

Duling, Dennis C. 1983. "*Testament of Solomon*: A New Translation and Introduction." In *The Old Testament Pseudepigrapha*, edited by James H. Charlesworth, 935–87. Vol. 1. Garden City, NY: Doubleday.

Duling, Dennis C. 1985. "The Eleazar Miracle and Solomon's Magical Wisdom in Flavius Josephus's "Antiquitates Judaicae" 8.42–49." *HTR* 78, no. 1/2: 1–25.

Duprez, Antoine. 1970. *Jésus et les dieux guérisseurs; à propos de Jean, V*. Cahiers de la revue biblique 12. Paris: J. Gabalda.

Durkheim, Émile. 1912. *Les formes élémentaire de la vie religieuse, le système totémique en Australie*. Travaux de l'année sociologique. Paris: F. Alcan.

Dvorjetski, Esti. 1997. "Roman Emperors at the Thermo-Mineral Baths in Eretz-Israel." *Latomus* 56, no. 3: 567–81.

Dvorjetski, Esti. 2000. "The Diseases of Rabbi Judah the Patriarch in Light of Modern Medicine." *Harefuah* 139, no. 5–6: 232–6.

Dvorjetski, Esti. 2001. "'What Was Perpetrated by the Coastal Cities Was Not Perpetrated by the Generation of the Flood': The Maioumas Festivals at Ascalon during the Roman-Byzantine

Period." In *Ashkelon: A City on the Seashore*, edited by Avi Sasson, Ze'ev Safrai, and Nahum Sagiv, 99–118. Ashkelon: Ashkelon Academic College (Heb.).

Dvorjetski, Esti. 2002. "The Medical History of Rabbi Judah the Patriarch: A Linguistic Analysis." *HS* 43: 39–55.

Dvorjetski, Esti. 2007. *Leisure, Pleasure and Healing: Spa Culture and Medicine in Ancient Eastern Mediterranean*. Supplements to the Journal for the Study of Judaism 116. Leiden: Brill.

Dvorjetski, Esti. 2012. "Maioumas Festivities in the Eastern Mediterranean Basin: Maioumas-Shuni as a Case Study." *Strata* 30: 89–125.

Eade, John and Michael J. Sallnow. 2013 [1991]. *Contesting the Sacred: The Anthropology of Pilgrimage*. Eugene, OR: Wipf and Stock Publishers.

Eck, Werner. 2014. "The Armed Forces and the Infrastructure of Cities during the Roman Imperial Period:The Example of Judaea/Syria Palaestina." In *Cura Aquarum in Israel II: Water in Antiquity*, edited by Christoph Ohlig and Tsvika Tsuk, 207–14. Schriften der Deutschen Wasserhistorischen Gesellschaft e.V. 21. Clausthal-Zellerfeld: Papierflieger Verlag.

Edelstein, Emma J. and Ludwig Edelstein. 1998. *Asclepius: Collection and Interpretation of the Testimonies*. 2 vols. Baltimore: Johns Hopkins University Press.

Ehrenheim, Hedvig von. 2009. "Identifying Incubation Areas in Pagan and Early Christian Times." *Proceedings of the Danish Institute at Athens* 6: 237–76.

Ehrenheim, Hedvig von. 2016. "Pilgrimage for Dreams in Late Antiquity and Early Byzantium: Continuity of the Pagan Ritual or Development within Christian Miracle Tradition?" *Scandinavian Journal of Byzantine and Modern Greek Studies* 2: 53–95.

Eidinow, Esther. 2019. "Magic and Social Tension." In *Guide to the Study of Ancient Magic*, edited by David Frankfurter, 746–74. Religions in the Graeco-Roman World 189. Leiden: Brill.

Elgavish, Yosef. 1994. *Shiqmona: On the Coast of Mount Carmel*. Tel Aviv: Hakibbutz Hameuchad (Heb.).

Eliav, Yaron Z. 2005. *God's Mountain: The Temple Mount in Time, Place, and Memory*. Baltimore: Johns Hopkins University Press.

Elitzur, Yoel. 2008. "The Siloam Pool – 'Solomon's Pool' – was a Swimming Pool." *PEQ* 140, no. 1: 17–25.

Elsner, Jaś. 2000. "The *Itinerarium Burdigalense*: Politics and Salvation in the Geography of Constantine's Empire." *JRS* 90: 181–95.

Elsner, Jaś. 2018. "Place, Shrine, Miracle." In *Agents of Faith: Votive Objects in Time and Place*, edited by Ittai Weinryb and Fatima Bercht, 3–25. New York: Bard Graduate Center Gallery.

Eshel, Esther. 2003a. "Genres of Magical Texts in the Dead Sea Scrolls." In *Die Dämonen: Die Dämonologie der israelitisch-jüdischen und frühchristlichen Literatur im Kontext ihrer Umwelt*, edited by Armin Lange, Hermann Lichtenberger, and Diethard Römheld, 395–415. Tübingen: Mohr Siebeck.

Eshel, Esther. 2003b. "Apotropaic Prayers in the Second Temple Period." In *Liturgical Perspectives: Prayer and Poetry in Light of the Dead Sea Scrolls. Proceedings of the Fifth International Symposium of the Orion Center for the Study of the Dead Sea Scrolls and Associated Literature, 19–23 January, 2000*, edited by Esther G. Chazon, Ruth Clements, and Avital Pinnick, 69–88. Studies on the Texts of the Desert of Judah. Leiden: Brill.

Eshel, Hanan and Rivka Leiman. 2010. "Jewish Amulets Written on Metal Scrolls." *JAJ* 1: 189–99.

Eshel, Esther, Hanan Eshel, and Armin Lange. 2010. "'Hear, O Israel' in Gold: An Ancient Amulet from Halbturn in Austria." *JAJ* 1, no. 1: 43–64.

Evans, Craig A. 1987. "Luke's Use of the Elijah/Elisha Narratives and the Ethic of Election." *JBL* 106, no. 1: 75–83.

Evans-Pritchard, E. E. 1937. *Witchcraft, Oracles and Magic among the Azande*. Oxford: Clarendon Press.

Eve, Eric. 2009. *The Healer from Nazareth: Jesus' Miracles in Historical Context*. London: SPCK.

Falls, Thomas B. and Michael Slusser, eds. 2003. *Dialogue with Trypho*. Selections from the Fathers of the Church 3. Washington, DC: Catholic University of America Press.

Faraone, Christopher A. 2009. "Stopping Evil, Pain, Anger and Blood: The Ancient Greek Tradition of Protective Iambic Incantations." *GRBS* 49: 73–102.

Faraone, Christopher A. 2011. "Magical and Medical Approaches to the Wandering Womb in the Ancient Greek World." *ClAnt* 30, no. 1: 1–32.

Faraone, Christopher A. 2018. *Transformation of Greek Amulets in Roman Imperial Times*. Empire and After. Philadelphia: University of Pennsylvania Press.

Farhi, Yoav. 2010. "Note on a New Type of Samaritan Amulet." *LASBF* 60: 395–6.

Ferrar, William John. 1920. *The Proof of the Gospel, Being the Demonstratio evangelica of Eusebius of Caesarea*. 2 vols. Translations of Christian Literature. Series I: Greek Texts London: SPCK. New York: Macmillan.

Fine, Steven. 1997. *This Holy Place: On the Sanctity of the Synagogue during the Greco-Roman Period*. Christianity and Judaism in Antiquity 11. Notre Dame: University of Notre Dame Press.

Finkielsztejn, Gérald. 1986. "Asklepios Leontoukhos et le mythe de la coupe de Césarée Maritime." *RB* 93: 419–28.

Fischer, Moshe L. 2008. "Sculpture in Roman Palestine and Its Architectural and Social Milieu: Adaptability, Imitation, Originality? The Ascalon Basilica as an Example." In *The Sculptural Environment of the Roman Near East: Reflections on Culture, Ideology, and Power*, edited by Yaron Z. Eliav, Elise A. Friedland, and Sharon Herbert, 483–508. Interdisciplinary Studies in Ancient Culture and Religion 9. Leuven: Peeters.

Flannery-Dailey, Frances. 2004. *Dreamers, Scribes, and Priests: Jewish Dreams in the Hellenistic and Roman Eras*. Supplements to the *Journal for the Study of Judaism*. Leiden: Brill.

Flannery, Frances. 2017. "Talitha Qum! An Exploration of the Image of Jesus as Healer-Physician-Savior in the Synoptic Gospels in Relation to the Asclepius Cult." In *Coming Back to Life: The Permeability of Past and Present, Mortality and Immortality, Death and Life in the Ancient Mediterranean*, edited by Frederick S. Tappenden and Carly Daniel-Hughes, 407–34. Montreal: McGill University Library.

Flint, Valerie I. J. 1991. *The Rise of Magic in Early Medieval Europe*. Princeton, NJ: Princeton University Press.

Frankfurter, David. 1994. "The Magic of Writing and the Writing of Magic: The Power of the Word in Egyptian and Greek Traditions." *Helios* 21, no. 2: 189–221.

Frankfurter, David. 1995. "Narrating Power: The Theory and Practice of the Magical *Historiolae* in Ritual Spells." In *Ancient Magic and Ritual Power*, edited by Marvin W. Meyer and Paul Allan Mirecki, 243–77. Religions in the Graeco-Roman World 129. New York: Brill.

Frankfurter, David. 1997. "Ritual Expertise in Roman Egypt and the Problem of the Category 'Magician.'" In *Envisioning Magic: A Princeton Seminar and Symposium*, edited by Peter Schäfer and Hans G. Kippenberg, 115–35. Leiden: Brill.

Frankfurter, David. 2005. "Beyond Magic and Superstition." In *Late Ancient Christianity*, edited by Virginia Burrus, 255–84, 309–12. A People's History of Christianity 2. Minneapolis: Fortress Press.

Frankfurter, David. 2019a. "Ancient Magic in a New Key: Refining an Exotic Discipline in the History of Religions." In *Guide to the Study of Ancient Magic*, edited by David Frankfurter, 3–20. Religions in the Graeco-Roman World 189. Leiden: Brill.

BIBLIOGRAPHY 223

Frankfurter, David. 2019b. "Spell and Speech Act: The Magic of the Spoken Word." In *Guide to the Study of Ancient Magic*, edited by David Frankfurter, 608–25. Religions in the Graeco-Roman World 189. Leiden: Brill.

Frazer, James George. 1911–15. *The Golden Bough: A Study in Magic and Religion*. 12 vols. 3rd ed. London: Macmillan.

Fredriksen, Paula. 2018. *When Christians Were Jews: The First Generation*. New Haven, CT: Yale University Press.

Frey, Jean Baptiste. 1952. *Corpus inscriptionum iudaicarum: Recueil des inscriptions juives qui vont du IIIe siècle avant Jésus-Christ au VIIe siècle de notre ère*. Vol. 2: *Asie–Afrique*. Sussidi allo studio delle antichità cristiane 1.3. Rome: Pontificio istituto di archeologia cristiana.

Freyne, Sean. 1980. "The Charismatic." In *Ideal Figures in Ancient Judaism: Profiles and Paradigms*, edited by John J. Collins and George W. E. Nickelsburg, 223–58. Missoula, MT: Scholars Press.

Friedheim, Emmanuel. 2006. *Rabbinisme et paganisme en Palestine romaine: Étude historique des Realia talmudiques (Ier–IVème siècles)*. Religions in the Graeco-Roman World 157. Leiden: Brill.

Friedheim, Emmanuel and Shimon Dar. 2010. "Some Historical and Archaeological Notes about Paganism in Byzantine Palestine." *RB* 117, no. 3: 397–409.

Friedland, Elise Anne. 1997. "Roman Marble Sculpture from the Levant: The Group from the Sanctuary of Pan at Caesarea Philippi (Panias)." Ph.D., University of Michigan.

Frova, Antonio. 1966. "Il Tesoretto Aureo e il Reliquiario." In *Scavi di Caesarea Maritima*, edited by Giordano dell'Amore, Dinu Adamesteanu, Virginio Borroni, and Antonio Frova, 235–44. Rome: L'Erma di Bretschneider.

Ganneau, M. Clermont. 1882. "Expedition to Amwās." *PEFQS*: 22–37.

García Martínez, Florentino and Eibert J. C. Tigchelaar. 1997. *The Dead Sea Scrolls Study Edition*. 2 vols. Leiden: Brill.

Garland, Robert. 2011. "Miracles in the Greek and Roman World." In *The Cambridge Companion to Miracles*, edited by Graham H. Twelftree, 75–94. Cambridge Companions to Religion. Cambridge: Cambridge University Press.

Geiger, Joseph. 1998. "Aspects of Palestinian Paganism in Late Antiquity." In *Sharing the Sacred: Religious Contacts and Conflicts in the Holy Land: First–Fifteenth centures ce*, edited by Arieh Kofsky and Guy G. Stroumsa, 3–16. Jerusalem: Yad Izhak Ben Zvi.

Geiger, Joseph. 2012. "Asclepius Λεοντοῦχος." *Mnemosyne* 65, no. 2: 315–18.

Germer-Durand, J. 1895. "Exploration épigraphique de Gerasa." *RB* 4, no. 3: 374–400.

Germer-Durand, J. 1899. "Nouvelle exploration épigraphique de Gérasa." *RB* 8, no. 1: 5–39.

Gersht, Rivka. 1996. "Roman Copies Discovered in the Land of Israel." In *Classical Studies in Honor of David Sohlberg*, edited by Ranon Katzoff, Yaakov Petroff, and David M. Schaps, 433–50. Ramat Gan: Bar-Ilan University Press.

Giannobile, Sergio. 2002. "Medaglioni magico-devozionali della Sicilia tardoantica." *JAC* 45: 170–201.

Gibson, Shimon. 2004. *The Cave of John the Baptist: The First Archaeological Evidence of the Truth of the Gospel Story*. London: Century.

Gibson, Shimon. 2005. "The Pool of Bethesda in Jerusalem and Jewish Purification Practices of the Second Temple Period." *PrOrChr* 55, no. 3/4: 270–93.

Gibson, Shimon. 2009. *The Final Days of Jesus: The Archaeological Evidence*. New York: HarperOne.

Gibson, Shimon. 2011. "The Excavations at the Bethesda Pool in Jerusalem: Preliminary Report on a Project of Stratigraphic and Structural Analysis (1999–2009)." *PrOrChr* Special issue: *La Piscine Probatique de Jésus à Saladin: Le projet Béthesda*: 17–44.

Gichon, Mordechai. 1979. "The Roman Bath at Emmaus: Excavations in 1977." *IEJ* 29, no. 2: 101–10.

Glazier-McDonald, Beth and C. Thomas McCollough. 2009. "A Silver Amulet from Sepphoris." In *Studies on Patristic Texts and Archaeology*, 201–18. Lewiston, NY: Edwin Mellen Press.

Gnuse, Robert. 1993. "The Temple Experience of Jaddus in the Antiquities of Josephus: A Report of Jewish Dream Incubation." *JQR* 83, no. 3/4: 349–68.

Goodenough, Erwin Ramsdell. 1953. *Jewish Symbols in the Greco-Roman Period*. 13 vols. New York: Pantheon Books.

Gordon, Richard. 2011. "*Signa nova et inaudita*: The Theory and Practice of Invented Signs (*charaktêres*) in Graeco-Egyptian Magical Texts." *Revista internacional de investigación sobre magia y astrología antiguas* 11: 15–44.

Gordon, Richard. 2014. "*Charaktêres* between Antiquity and Renaissance: Transmission and Reinvention." In *Les savoirs magiques et leur transmission de l'Antiquité à la Renaissance*, edited by Véronique Dasen and Jean-Michel Spieser, 253–300. Micrologus Library 60. Florence: SISMEL Edizioni del Galluzzo.

Graf, Fritz. 1991. "Prayer in Magical and Religious Ritual." In *Magika Hiera*, edited by Christopher A. Faraone and Dirk Obbink, 188–213. New York: Oxford University Press.

Graf, Fritz. 1997. *Magic in the Ancient World*. Translated by Franklin Philip. Revealing Antiquity 10. Cambridge, MA: Harvard University Press.

Graf, Fritz. 2014. "Dangerous Dreaming: The Christian Transformation of Dream Incubation." *ARG* 15, no. 1: 117–42.

Graf, Fritz. 2015. *Roman Festivals in the Greek East: From the Early Empire to the Middle Byzantine Era*. Greek Culture in the Roman World. Cambridge: Cambridge University Press.

Gray, Alyssa M. 2005. "The Power Conferred by Distance from Power: Redaction and Meaning in b. A.Z. 10a–11a." In *Creation and Composition: The Contribution of the Bavli Redactors (Stammaim) to the Aggada*, edited by Jeffrey L. Rubenstein, 23–69. Texte und Studien zum antiken Judentum 114. Tübingen: Mohr Siebeck.

Green, Judith and Yoram Tsafrir. 1982. "Greek Inscriptions from Hammat Gader: A Poem by the Empress Eudocia and Two Building Inscriptions." *IEJ* 32: 77–96.

Green, William Scott. 1979. "Palestinian Holy Men: Charismatic Leadership and the Rabbinic Tradition." *ANRW* 2.19.2: 619–47.

Gregg, Robert C. 2000. "Marking Religious and Ethnic Boundaries: Cases from the Ancient Golan Heights." *CH* 69, no. 3: 519–57.

Gregg, Robert C. and Dan Urman. 1996. *Jews, Pagans, and Christians in the Golan Heights: Greek and Other Inscriptions of the Roman and Byzantine Eras*. South Florida Studies in the History of Judaism 140. Atlanta: Scholars Press.

Griffith, Sidney H. 1999. "The Signs and Wonders of Orthodoxy: Miracles and Monks' Lives in Sixth-Century Palestine." In *Miracles in Jewish and Christian Antiquity: Imagining Truth*, edited by John C. Cavadini, 139–68. Notre Dame Studies in Theology 3. Notre Dame: University of Notre Dame Press.

Grmek, Mirko D. 1989. *Diseases in the Ancient Greek World*. Baltimore: Johns Hopkins University Press.

Gruen, Erich S. 1998. *Heritage and Hellenism: The Reinvention of Jewish Tradition*. Hellenistic Culture and Society 30. Berkeley: University of California Press.

Gudovitch, Shlomo. 1996. "A Late Roman Burial Cave at Moza ʿIllit." *ʿAtiqot* 29: 63*–70* (Heb.).

Guggenheimer, Heinrich W., ed. 2000. *The Jerusalem Talmud*. 17 vols. Studia Judaica 18–21, 23, 29, 31, 34, 39, 43, 45, 51, 61, 68. Berlin: De Gruyter.

Guillaume, Philippe. 1999. "Miracles Miraculously Repeated: Gospel Miracles as Duplication of Elijah-Elisha's." *BN* 98: 21–3.

Gurevich, David. 2017. "The Water Pools and the Pilgrimage to Jerusalem in the Late Second Temple Period." *PEQ* 149, no. 2: 103–34.

Guttmann, Alexander. 1954. "The Patriarch Judah I: His Birth and His Death." *HUCA* 25: 256–60.

Hamburger, Anit. 1959. "A Greco-Samaritan Amulet from Caesarea." *IEJ* 9, no. 1: 43–5.

Hamburger, Anit. 1968. "Gems from Caesarea Maritima." *'Atiqot* 8: 1–38.

Hamilton, Gordon J. 1996. "A New Hebrew–Aramaic Incantation Text from Galilee: 'Rebuking the Sea.'" *JSS* 41, no. 2: 215–49.

Harari, Yuval. 2017. *Jewish Magic before the Rise of Kabbalah*. Detroit: Wayne State University Press.

Harkins, Paul W., ed. 1979. *John Chrysostom: Discourses against Judaizing Christians*. Fathers of the Church: A New Translation 68. Washington, DC: Catholic University of America Press.

Harnack, Adolf von. 1962. *The Mission and Expansion of Christianity in the First Three Centuries*. Translated by James Moffatt. New York: Harper.

Harrisson, Juliette. 2014. "The Development of the Practice of Incubation in the Ancient World." In *Medicine and Healing in the Ancient Mediterranean World*, edited by Demetrios Michaelides, 284–90. Oxford: Oxbow Books.

Hauck, Albert. 1880. "Die Entstehung des Christustypus in der abendländischen Kunst." *Sammlung von Vorträgen für das deutsche Volk* 3, no. 2: 39–62.

Henderson, W. J. 1992. "Excavations at Shuni, Israel." *Akroterion* 37, no. 1: 23–30.

Henig, Martin, Mary Whiting, and Robert Wilkins. 1987. *Engraved Gems from Gadara in Jordan: The Sa'd Collection of Intaglios and Cameos*. Oxford University Committee for Archaeology Monographs 6. Oxford: Oxford University Committee for Archaeology.

Hevelone-Harper, Jennifer L. 2005. *Disciples of the Desert: Monks, Laity, and Spiritual Authority in Sixth-Century Gaza*. Baltimore: Johns Hopkins University Press.

Hirschfeld, Yizhar. 1987. "The History and Town-Plan of Ancient Hammat-Gader." *ZDPV* 103: 101–16.

Hirschfeld, Yizhar. 1995. "The Early Roman Bath and Fortress at Ramat Hanadiv near Caesarea." In *The Roman and Byzantine Near East: Some Recent Archaeological Research*, edited by John H. Humphrey, 28–55. Journal of Roman Archaeology Supplementary Series 14. Ann Arbor, MI: Journal of Roman Archaeology.

Hirschfeld, Yizhar, ed. 1997. *The Roman Baths of Hammat Gader: Final Report*. Jerusalem: Israel Exploration Society.

Hirschfeld, Yizhar. 1998. "The Fountain of Fertility at Ramat Hanadiv." *Qad* 31: 109–16 (Heb.).

Hirschfeld, Yizhar. 2000a. *Ramat Hanadiv Excavations: Final Report of the 1984–1998 Seasons*. Jerusalem: Israel Exploration Society.

Hirschfeld, Yizhar. 2000b. "General Discussion: Ramat Hanadiv in Context." In *Ramat Hanadiv Excavations: Final Report of the 1984–1998 Seasons*, edited by Yizhar Hirschfeld, 679–735. Jerusalem: Israel Exploration Society.

Hirschfeld, Yizhar. 2000c. "Architecture and Stratigraphy." In *Ramat Hanadiv Excavations: Final Report of the 1984–1998 Seasons*, edited by Yizhar Hirschfeld, 235–370. Jerusalem: Israel Exploration Society.

Hirschfeld, Yizhar. 2004a. "Architecture and Stratigraphy." In *Excavations at Tiberias, 1989–1994*, edited by Yizhar Hirschfeld and Roni Amir, 75–134. IAA Reports 22. Jerusalem: Israel Antiquities Authority.

Hirschfeld, Yizhar. 2004b. "Conclusions." In *Excavations at Tiberias, 1989–1994*, edited by Yizhar Hirschfeld and Roni Amir, 219–22. IAA Reports 22. Jerusalem: Israel Antiquities Authority.

Hirschfeld, Yizhar and Roni Amir. 2004. *Excavations at Tiberias, 1989–1994*. IAA Reports 22. Jerusalem: Israel Antiquities Authority.

Hirschfeld, Yizhar and Giora Solar. 1981. "The Roman Thermae at Hammat-Gader: Preliminary Report of Three Seasons of Excavations." *IEJ* 31: 197–219.

Hirschfeld, Yizhar and Giora Solar. 1984. "Sumptuous Roman Baths Uncovered Near Sea of Galilee." *BAR* 10, no. 6: 22–40.

Hoftijzer, J., G. van der Kooij, and H. J. Franken. 1976. *Aramaic Texts from Deir Alla*. Documenta et monumenta Orientis antiqui 19. Leiden: Brill.

Holum, Kenneth G. 1998. "Identity and the Late Antique City: The Case of Caesarea." In *Religious and Ethnic Communities in Later Roman Palestine*, edited by Hayim Lapin, 157–77. Studies and Texts in Jewish History and Culture 5. Bethesda: University Press of Maryland.

Horn, Cornelia B. and Robert R. Phenix, eds. 2008. *John Rufus: The Lives of Peter the Iberian, Theodosius of Jerusalem, and the Monk Romanus*. Writings from the Greco-Roman World 24. Atlanta: Society of Biblical Literature.

Horsley, Richard A. 1985. "'Like One of the Prophets of Old': Two Types of Popular Prophets at the Time of Jesus." *CBQ* 47, no. 3: 435–63.

Horsley, Richard A. 1995. "Archaeology and the Villages of Upper Galilee: A Dialogue with Archaeologists." *BASOR* 297: 5–16.

Horsley, Richard A. 2014. *Jesus and the Politics of Roman Palestine*. Columbia: University of South Carolina Press.

Hulse, E. V. 1975. "The Nature of Biblical 'Leprosy' and the Use of Alternative Medical Terms in Modern Translations of the Bible." *PEQ* 107: 87–105.

Hunt, E. D. 1982. *Holy Land Pilgrimage in the Later Roman Empire, AD 312–460*. Oxford: Clarendon Press.

Ilan, Zvi. 1982. "A Ring with a Samaritan Inscription Found at Caesarea: Another Testimony to the Large Samaritan Settlement There." *A. B. – The Samaritan News* 305 (1/3/1982): 1, 4 (Heb.).

Irshai, Oded. 2009. "The Christian Appropriation of Jerusalem in the Fourth Century: The Case of the Bordeaux Pilgrim." *JQR* 99, no. 4: 465–86.

Israeli, Yael and David Mevorah. 2000. *Cradle of Christianity*. Jerusalem: Israel Museum.

Jackson-Tal, Ruth E. 2015a. "The Khirbet al-Hadra Burial Cave: Magical Objects." In *Samaritan Cemeteries and Tombs in the Central Coastal Plain: Archaeology and History of the Samaritan Settlement Outside Samaria (ca. 300–700 CE)*, edited by Oren Tal and Itamar Taxel, 170–2. Ägypten und Altes Testament: Studien zu Geschichte, Kultur und Religion Ägyptens und des Alten Testaments 82. Münster: Ugarit Verlag.

Jackson-Tal, Ruth E. 2015b. "The Tell Qasile Burial Cave: Magical Objects." In *Samaritan Cemeteries and Tombs in the Central Coastal Plain: Archaeology and History of the Samaritan Settlement Outside Samaria (ca. 300–700 CE)*, edited by Oren Tal and Itamar Taxel, 190. Ägypten und Altes Testament: Studien zu Geschichte, Kultur und Religion Ägyptens und des Alten Testaments 82. Münster: Ugarit Verlag.

Jacobs, Andrew S. 2004. *Remains of the Jews: The Holy Land and Christian Empire in Late Antiquity*. Divinations: Rereading Late Ancient Religion. Stanford: Stanford University Press.

Jacobs, Andrew S. 2012. "Matters (Un-)Becoming: Conversions in Epiphanius of Salamis." *CH* 81, no. 1 (March): 27–47.

Jakoel, Eriola. 2013. "Tombs and Burials in Jaffa (Joppa) during the Roman Period (1st Century BCE–4th Century CE)." M.A., Tel Aviv University (Heb.).

Jassen, Alex P. 2014. *Scripture and Law in the Dead Sea Scrolls*. New York: Cambridge University Press.

Jaubert, A. 1953. "Le calendrier des Jubilés et de la secte de Qumrân: Ses origines bibliques." *VT* 3, no. 3: 250–64.

Jaubert, A. 1957. "Le calendrier des Jubilés et les jours liturgiques de la semaine." *VT* 7, no. 1: 35–61.

Jefferson, Lee M. 2014. *Christ the Miracle Worker in Early Christian Art*. Minneapolis: Fortress.

Jeffreys, Elizabeth, Michael Jeffreys, and Roger Scott, eds. 1986. *The Chronicle of John Malalas*. Byzantina Australiensia 4. Melbourne: Brill.

Jeremias, Joachim. 1966. *The Rediscovery of Bethesda: John 5:2*. New Testament Archaeology Monographs 1. Louisville, KY: Southern Baptist Theological Seminary.

Johnson, Barbara L. 2008. "The Pottery." In *Archaeological Excavations at Caesarea Maritima: Areas CC, KK and NN, Final Reports*, edited by Joseph Patrich, 13–206. Vol. 1: *The Objects*. Jerusalem: Israel Exploration Society.

Jones, C. P., ed. 2005. *Philostratus: The Life of Apollonius of Tyana*. 2 vols. Loeb Classical Library 16–17. Cambridge, MA: Harvard University Press.

Jones, W. H. S. and E. T. Withington. 1977. *Malaria and Greek History*. New York: AMS Press.

Kaizer, Ted. 2008. "Introduction." In *The Variety of Local Religious life in the Near East in the Hellenistic and Roman Periods*, edited by Ted Kaizer, 1–36. Religions in the Graeco-Roman World 164. Leiden: Brill.

Kalleres, Dayna S. 2015. *City of Demons: Violence, Ritual, and Christian Power in Late Antiquity*. Berkeley: University of California.

Kalmin, Richard. 2003. "Holy Men, Rabbis, and Demonic Sages in Late Antiquity." In *Jewish Culture and Society under the Christian Roman Empire*, edited by Richard Lee Kalmin and Seth Schwartz, 211–53. Interdisciplinary Studies in Ancient Culture and Religion 3. Leuven: Peeters.

Kaplan, Jacob. 1949–50. "Ancient Jewish Tomb-Caves near Tel-Aviv." *BJPES* 15: 71–4 (Heb.).

Kaplan, Jacob. 1967. "Two Samaritan Amulets." *IEJ* 17, no. 3: 158–62.

Kaplan, Jacob. 1968. "Ancient Jewish Cemetery at Tel Baruch." *Museum Haaretz Bulletin* 10: 70–1.

Kaplan, Jacob. 1971. "A Second Samaritan Amulet from Tel Aviv." *ErIsr* 10: 255–7 (Heb.).

Kaplan, Jacob. 1975. "A Second Samaritan Amulet from Tel Aviv." *IEJ* 25, no. 2/3: 157–9.

Kartveit, Magnar. 2009. *The Origin of the Samaritans*. Leiden: Brill.

Kazan, Stanley. 1963. "Isaac of Antioch's Homily against the Jews (III)." *OrChr* 47: 89–97.

Kee, Howard Clark. 1983. *Miracle in the Early Christian World: A Study in Sociohistorical Method*. New Haven, CT: Yale University Press.

Keel, Othmar and Christoph Uehlinger. 1998. *Gods, Goddesses, and Images of God in Ancient Israel*. Minneapolis: Fortress.

Khamis, Elias. 2006. "A Byzantine Magical Amulet." In *Excavations at Tel Beth-Shean, 1989–1996*, edited by Amihai Mazar, 675–76. Beth-Shean Valley Archaeological Project Publication 1. Jerusalem: Israel Exploration Society.

Kimelman, Reuven. 1999. "Identifying Jews and Christians in Roman Syria-Palestine." In *Galilee through the Centuries: Confluence of Cultures*, edited by Eric M. Meyers, 301–33. Duke Judaic Studies 1. Winona Lake, IN: Eisenbrauns.

Kingsley, Sean A. 2011. "Bethesda 1999 – A Preliminary Pottery Report." *PrOrChr* Special issue: *La Piscine Probatique de Jésus à Saladin: Le projet Béthesda*: 181–6.

Kippenberg, Hans G. 1971. *Garizim und Synagoge: Traditionsgeschichtliche Untersuchungen zur samaritanischen Religion der aramäischen Periode*. Berlin: De Gruyter.

Kirkpatrick, Jonathan. 2008. "How to Be a Bad Samaritan: The Local Cult of Mt Gerizim." In *The Variety of Local Religious Life in the Near East in the Hellenistic and Roman Periods*, edited by Ted Kaizer, 155–78. Religions in the Graeco-Roman World 164. Leiden: Brill.

Klinghardt, Matthias. 1999. "Prayer Formularies for Public Recitation: Their Use and Function in Ancient Religion." *Numen* 46, no. 1: 1–52.

Knoppers, Gary N. 2013. *Jews and Samaritans the Origins and History of Their Early Relations*. New York: Oxford University Press.

Kofsky, Arieh. 1998. "Mamre: A Case of Regional Cult?" In *Sharing the Sacred: Religious Contacts and Conflicts in the Holy Land, First–Fifteenth Centures ce*, edited by Arieh Kofsky and Guy G. Stroumsa, 19–30. Jerusalem: Yad Izhak Ben Zvi.

Kogan-Zehavi, Elena. 2006. "A Burial Cave of the Byzantine Period in the Naḥalat Aḥim Quarter, Jerusalem." *'Atiqot* 54: 61*–86* (Heb.).

Koskenniemi, Erkki. 1998. "Apollonius of Tyana: A Typical θεῖος ἀνήρ?" *JBL* 117, no. 3: 455–67.

Kotansky, Roy. 1991. "An Inscribed Copper Amulet from 'Evron." *'Atiqot* 20: 81–7.

Kotansky, Roy. 1994. *Greek Magical Amulets: The Inscribed Gold, Silver, Copper, and Bronze Lamellae: Text and Commentary*. Abhandlungen der Nordrhein-Westfälischen Akademie der Wissenschaften Sonderreihe Papyrologica Coloniensia 22. Opladen: Westdeutscher Verlag.

Kraus, Thomas J. 2005. "Septuaginta-Psalm 90 in apotropäischer Verwendung: Vorüberlegungen für eine kritische Edition und (bisheriges) Datenmaterial." *BN* 125: 39–73.

Kraus, Thomas J. 2007. "Psalm 90 der Septuaginta in apotropäischer Verwendung – erste Anmerkungen und Datenmaterial." In *Proceedings of the 24th International Congress of Papyrology*, edited by J. Frösén, T. Purola, and E. Salmenkivi, 497–514. Vol 1. Helsinki: Societas Scientarum Fennica.

Kropp, Amina. 2010. "How Does Magical Language Work? The Spells and *Formulae* of the Latin *defixionum tabellae*." In *Magical Practice in the Latin West: Papers from the International Conference Held at the University of Zaragoza, 30 Sept.–1 Oct. 2005*, edited by R. L. Gordon and Francisco Marco Simón, 357–80. Religions in the Graeco-Roman World 168. Leiden: Brill.

Küchler, Max. 1994. "Die 'Probatische' und Betesda mit den fünf στοαί." In *Peregrina curiositas. Eine Reise durch den orbis antiquus: Zu Ehren von Dirk van Damme*, edited by Andreas Kessler, Thomas Ricklin, and Gregor Wurst, 127–54. Novum Testamentum et orbis antiquus 27. Fribourg: Universitätsverlag; Göttingen: Vandenhoeck & Ruprecht.

Laird, Lance D. 2013. "Boundaries and *Baraka*: Christians, Muslims, and a Palestinian Saint." In *Muslims and Others in Sacred Space*, edited by Margaret Cormack, 40–73. Religion, Culture, and History. Oxford: Oxford University Press.

Lalleman, Pieter J. 1997. "Healing by a Mere Touch as a Christian Concept." *TynBul* 48, no. 2: 355–61.

Lapin, Hayim. 1996. "Rabbis and Public Prayers for Rain in Later Roman Palestine." In *Religion and Politics in the Ancient Near East*, edited by Adele Berlin, 105–29. Studies and Texts in Jewish History and Culture. Potomac: University Press of Maryland.

Lapin, Hayim. 1998. "Locating Ethnicity and Religious Community in Later Roman Palestine." In *Religious and Ethnic Communities in Later Roman Palestine*, edited by Hayim Lapin, 1–28. Studies and Texts in Jewish History and Culture 5. Bethesda: University Press of Maryland.

Lapin, Hayim. 2012. *Rabbis as Romans: The Rabbinic Movement in Palestine, 100–400 CE*. Oxford: Oxford University Press.

BIBLIOGRAPHY 229

Le Blant, Edmond. 1898. "750 inscriptions de pierres gravées inédites ou peu connues." *Mémoires de l'Institut national de France* 36, no. 1: 1–210.

Le Glay, M. 1978. "Un pied de Sarapis à Timgad, en Numidie." In *Hommages à Maarten J. Vermaseren*, edited by Margreet de Boer and T. A. Edridge, 573–89. Études préliminaires aux religions orientales dans l'Empire romain 68. Leiden: Brill.

Lévi-Strauss, Claude. 1962. *La pensée sauvage*. Paris: Plon.

Levine, Lee I. 1989. *The Rabbinic Class of Roman Palestine in Late Antiquity*. Jerusalem: Yad Izhak Ben-Zvi; New York: Jewish Theological Seminary of America.

Levine, Lee I. 1998. *Judaism and Hellenism in Antiquity: Conflict or Confluence*. Seattle: University of Washington Press.

Levine, Lee I. 2000. *The Ancient Synagogue: The First Thousand Years*. New Haven, CT: Yale University Press.

Levy, Shalom. 1960. "The Ancient Synagogue of Ma'on (Nirim). A: Excavation Report." *Bulletin of the Louis M. Rabinowitz Fund for the Exploration of Ancient Synagogues* 3: 6–13.

Levy, Shalom. 1971. "The Ancient Synagogue of Ma'on (Nirim)." In *Roman Frontier Studies, 1967: The Proceedings of the Seventh International Congress held at Tel Aviv*, edited by Shimon Applebaum, 206–10. Tel Aviv: Students' Organization of Tel Aviv University.

Levy, Yosef. 1991. "Gelilot." *ESI* 10: 120–1.

LiDonnici, Lynn R. 1995. *The Epidaurian Miracle Inscriptions*. Texts and Translations 36. Atlanta: Scholars Press.

Lifshitz, Baruch. 1964. "Einige Amulette aus Caesarea Palaestinae." *ZDPV* 80, no. 1: 80–4.

Lindbeck, Kristen H. 2010. *Elijah and the Rabbis: Story and Theology*. New York: Columbia University Press.

Lindblom, Johannes. 1961. "Theophanies in Holy Places in Hebrew Religion." *HUCA* 32: 91–106.

Löhr, Hermut. 2003. *Studien zum frühchristlichen und frühjüdischen Gebet: Untersuchungen zu 1 Clem 59 bis 61 in seinem literarischen, historischen und theologischen Kontext*. Wissenschaftliche Untersuchungen zum Neuen Testament 160. Tübingen: Mohr Siebeck.

Lotz, Almuth. 2019. "Libanius and Theodoret of Cyrrhus on Accusations of Magic: Between Legal Norm and Legal Practice in Late Antiquity." *Magic, Ritual & Witchcraft* 14, no. 2: 211–29.

Louth, Andrew, ed. 1989. *Eusebius: History of the Church from Christ to Constantine*. Translated by G. A. Williamson. Penguin Classics. London: Penguin Books.

Luke, Trevor S. 2010. "A Healing Touch for Empire: Vespasian's Wonders in Domitianic Rome." *GR* 57, no. 1: 77–106.

Ma'oz, Zvi. 1996. "Banias, Temple of Pan – 1993." *ESI* 15: 1–5.

Ma'oz, Zvi. 1998. "The Sanctuary of Pan at Baniyas." *Qad* 54: 18–25 (Heb.).

Macalister, R. A. Stewart. 1912. *The Excavation of Gezer: 1902–1903 and 1907–1909*. 3 vols. London: Palestine Exploration Fund.

McCasland, S. Vernon. 1939a. "Religious Healing in First-Century Palestine." In *Environmental Factors in Christian History*, edited by J. T. McNeill, M. Spinka and H. R. Willoughby, 18–34. Chicago: University of Chicago Press.

McCasland, S. Vernon. 1939b. "The Asklepios Cult in Palestine." *JBL* 58: 221–7.

Mackowski, Richard M. and Garo Nalbandian. 1980. *Jerusalem, City of Jesus: An Exploration of the Traditions, Writings, and Remains of the Holy City from the Time of Christ*. Grand Rapids, MI: Eerdmans.

McLean, Bradley H. 1999. "The Inscriptions of Caesarea and Their Relation to the Physical Remains of the City, Part II." *AncW* 30: 3–28.

Mader, Evaristus. 1957. *Mambre: Die Ergebnisse der Ausgrabungen im heiligen Bezirk Râmet el-Halîl in Südpalästina, 1926–1938*. Freiburg: Erich Wewel.

Magen, Yitzhak. 1991. "Elonei Mamre – Herodian Cult Site." *Qad* 24: 46–55 (Heb.).

Magen, Yitzhak. 2008. "Jewelry Bearing Samaritan Inscriptions (Amulets?)." In *The Samaritans and the Good Samaritan*, edited by Izchak Magen, 249–56. Judea and Samaria Publications 7. Jerusalem: Israel Antiquities Authority.

Magness, Jodi. 2005. "Heaven on Earth: Helios and the Zodiac Cycle in Ancient Palestinian Synagogues." *DOP* 59: 1–52.

Makhouly, N. 1939. "Rock-Cut Tombs at El-Jish." *QDAP* 8: 45–50.

Manns, Frédéric. 1977. "Nouvelles traces des cultes de Neotera, Serapis et Poseidon en Palestine." *LASBF* 27: 229–38.

Margain, Jean. 1984. "Un anneau samaritain provenant de Naplouse." *Syria* 61, no. 1/2: 45–7.

Margalioth, Mordechai. 1966. *Sepher Ha-Razim: A Newly Recovered Book of Magic from the Talmudic Period*. Tel Aviv: Yediot Acharonot (Heb.).

Markschies, Christoph. 2006. "Gesund werden im Schlaf: Einige Rezepte aus der Antike." *Berichte und Abhandlungen* 12: 187–216.

Markschies, Christoph. 2007. "Gesund werden im Schlaf: Einige Rezepte aus der Antike." In *Salute e guarigione nella tarda antichità: Atti della giornata tematica dei Seminari di archeologia cristiana, Roma, 20 maggio 2004*, edited by Hugo Brandenburg, Stefan Heid, and Christoph Markschies, 165–98. Sussidi allo studio delle antichità cristiane 19. Vatican City: Pontificio istituto di archeologia cristiana.

Markus, R. A. 1994. "How on Earth Could Places Become Holy? Origins of the Christian Idea of Holy Places." *JECS* 2, no. 3: 257–71.

Martyn, J. Louis. 1976. "We Have Found Elijah." In *Jews, Greeks and Christians: Religious Cultures in Late Antiquity. Essays in Honor of William David Davies*, edited by Robert Hamerton-Kelly and Robin Scroggs, 161–219. Studies in Judaism in Late Antiquity 21. Leiden: Brill.

Maspero, Jean. 1908. "Bracelets-amulettes d'époque byzantine." *Annales du service des antiquités de l'Égypte* 9: 246–58.

Masterman, E. W. G. 1905. "The Pool of Bethesda." *Biblical World* 25, no. 2: 88–102.

Mastrocinque, Attilio. 2004. "Le gemme gnostiche." In *Sylloge gemmarum gnosticarum*, edited by Attilio Mastrocinque, 49–112. Bollettino di numismatica monografia 8.2.1. Rome: Istituto poligrafico e Zecca dello Stato.

Mastrocinque, Attilio. 2011. "Magical Gems as a Documentary Source for Ancient Religion." *TAPhS* 101, no. 5: 3–8.

Mauss, Charles. 1888. *La piscine de Béthesda à Jérusalem*. Paris: Ernest Leroux.

Mauss, Marcel and Henri Hubert. 1902. "Esquisse d'une théorie générale de la magie." *AnSoc* 7: 1–146.

Mazar, Amihai. 2006. "Beth-Shean from the Late Bronze Age IIB to the Medeival Period: A Summary." In *Excavations at Tel Beth-Shean, 1989–1996*, edited by Amihay Mazar, 26–47. Beth-Shean Valley Archaeological Project Publication 1. Jerusalem: Israel Exploration Society.

Melfi, Milena. 2007. *I santuari di Asclepio in Grecia*. Vol. 1. Rome: L'Erma di Bretschneider.

Meri, Josef W. 1999. "Re-Appropriating Sacred Space: Medieval Jews and Muslims Seeking Elijah and Al-Khadir." *Medieval Encounters* 5, no. 3: 237.

Meshel, Ze'ev. 1978. *Kuntillet 'Ajrud: A Religious Centre from the Time of the Judaean Monarchy on the Border of Sinai*. Jerusalem: Israel Museum.

Meshel, Ze'ev, A. Ahituv, and Liora Freud. 2012. *Kuntillet 'Ajrud (Horvat Teman): An Iron Age II Religious Site on the Judah–Sinai Border*. Jerusalem: Israel Exploration Society.

Meshorer, Ya'akov. 1982. "Hygieia in Aelia Capitolina." *Israel Museum Journal* 1: 17–18.

Meshorer, Ya'akov. 1985. *City-Coins of Eretz-Israel and the Decapolis in the Roman Period*. Jerusalem: Israel Museum.

Meshorer, Ya'akov. 1989. *The Coinage of Aelia Capitolina*. Jerusalem: Israel Museum.

Meyer, Marvin W. and Richard Smith. 1999. *Ancient Christian Magic: Coptic Texts of Ritual Power*. Princeton, NJ: Princeton University Press.

Meyers, Eric M. 1985. "Galilean Regionalism: A Reappraisal." In *Approaches to Ancient Judaism*, edited by W. S. Green, 115–31. Vol. 5. Atlanta: Scholars Press.

Michel, Simone. 2004. *Die Magischen Gemmen: Zu Bildern und Zauberformeln auf geschnittenen Steinen der Antike und Neuzeit*. Studien aus dem Warburg-Haus 7. Berlin: Akademie Verlag.

Millar, Fergus. 1993. *The Roman Near East, 31 BC–AD 337*. Cambridge, MA: Harvard University Press.

Miller, Robert J. 1988. "Elijah, John, and Jesus in the Gospel of Luke." *NTS* 34, no. 4: 611–22.

Mitchell, Hinckley G. 1919. "The Modern Wall of Jerusalem." *Annual of the American School of Oriental Research in Jerusalem* 1: 28–50.

Montgomery, James A. 1911. "Some Early Amulets from Palestine." *JAOS* 31, no. 3: 272–81.

Morgan, Michael A. 1983. *Sepher ha-Razim: The Book of the Mysteries*. Texts and Translations 25. Chico, CA: Scholars Press.

Mouterde, R. 1942–3. "Objets magiques, Recueil S. Ayvaz." *MUSJ* 25: 105–28.

Muir, Steven C. 2006. "Mending yet Fracturing: Healing as an Arena of Conflict." In *The Changing Face of Judaism, Christianity and Other Greco-Roman Religions in Antiquity*, edited by Ian H. Henderson and Gerbern S. Oegema, 57–71. Gütersloh: Gütersloher Verlagshaus.

Müller-Kessler, Christa, T. C. Mitchell, and Marilyn I. Hockey. 2007. "An Inscribed Silver Amulet from Samaria." *PEQ* 139, no. 1: 5–19.

Murphy-O'Connor, J. 2012. "Review of Sainte-Anne de Jérusalem. La Piscine Probatique de Jésus à Saladin: Le projet Béthesda (1994–2010), Numéro spécial de "Proche-Orient Chrétien" 2011." *RB* 119, no. 3: 429–33.

Nagy, Árpád. 2012. "*Daktylios Pharmakites*: Magical Healing Gems and Rings in the Graeco-Roman World." In *Ritual Healing: Magic, Ritual and Medical Therapy from Antiquity until the Early Modern Period*, edited by Ildikó Csepregi and Charles Burnett, 71–106. Micrologus Library. Florence: SISMEL Edizioni del Galluzzo.

Naiweld, R. O. N. 2014. "There Is Only One Other: The Fabrication of Antoninus in a Multilayered Talmudic Dialogue." *JQR* 104, no. 1: 81–104.

Naveh, Joseph. 1998. "Fragments of an Aramaic Magic Book from Qumran." *IEJ* 48, no. 3–4: 252–61.

Naveh, Joseph and Shaul Shaked. 1985. *Amulets and Magic Bowls: Aramaic Incantations of Late Antiquity*. Jerusalem: Magnes Press.

Naveh, Joseph and Shaul Shaked. 1993. *Magic Spells and Formulae: Aramaic Incantations of Late Antiquity*. Jerusalem: Magnes Press.

Negev, Avraham. 1977. "The Inscriptions of Wadi Haggag, Sinai." *Qedem*, no. 6: 1–100.

Neusner, Jacob, ed. 2002. *The Tosefta: Translated from the Hebrew, with a New Introduction*. Peabody, MA: Hendrickson.

Newsom, Carol A. 1990. "The Sage in the Literature of Qumran: The Functions of the Maskil." In *The Sage in Israel and the Ancient Near East*, edited by John G. Gammie and Leo G. Perdue, 373–82. Winona Lake, IN: Eisenbrauns.

Nitzan, Bilha. 1992. "Hymns from Qumran: 4Q510–4Q511." In *The Dead Sea Scrolls: Forty Years of Research*, edited by Devorah Dimant and Uriel Rappaport, 53–63. Studies on the Texts of the Desert of Judah 10. Leiden: Brill.

Nitzan, Bilha. 1994. *Qumran Prayer and Religious Poetry*. Studies on the Texts of the Desert of Judah 12. Leiden: Brill.

Nolland, John. 1979. "Classical and Rabbinic Parallels to 'Physician, Heal Yourself' (Lk. IV 23)." *NovT* 21, no. 3: 193–209.

Nongbri, Brent. 2013. *Before Religion: A History of a Modern Concept.* New Haven, CT: Yale University Press.

Nutton, Vivian. 2004. *Ancient Medicine.* London: Routledge.

Nutzman, Megan. 2017. "'In This Holy Place': Incubation at Hot Springs in Roman and Late Antique Palestine." In *Gods, Objects, and Ritual Practice*, edited by Sandra Blakely, 281–304. Studies in Ancient Mediterranean Religions 1. Atlanta: Lockwood Press.

Ogden, Daniel. 2007. *In Search of the Sorcerer's Apprentice: The Traditional Tales of Lucian's Lover of Lies.* Swansea: Classical Press of Wales.

Oppenheim, A. Leo. 1956. "The Interpretation of Dreams in the Ancient Near East, with a Translation of an Assyrian Dream-Book." *TAPhS* 46, no. 3: 179–373.

Ovadiah, Asher and Yehudit Turnheim. 2011. *Roman Temples, Shrines and Temene in Israel.* Supplementi alla *Rivista di archeologia* 30. Rome: Giorgio Bretschneider.

Patrich, Joseph. 1996. "Warehouses and Granaries in Caesarea Maritima." In *Caesarea Maritima: A Retrospective after Two Millennia*, edited by Avner Raban and Kenneth G. Holum, 146–76. Documenta et monumenta Orientis antiqui 21. Leiden: Brill.

Patrich, Joseph. 2002a. "Caesarea: The Palace of the Roman Procurator and the Byzantine Governor, a Storage Complex and the Starting Stalls at the Herodian Stadium." *Kadmoniyot* 35: 68–86 (Heb.).

Patrich, Joseph. 2002b. "Four Christian Objects from Caesarea Maritima." *Israel Museum Studies in Archaeology* 1: 21–32.

Patrich, Joseph. 2008. "The Excavations 1993–1998, 2000–2001." In *Archaeological Excavations at Caesarea Maritima: Areas CC, KK and NN, Final Reports*, edited by Joseph Patrich, 1–11. Vol. 1: *The Objects*. Jerusalem: Israel Exploration Society.

Patrich, Joseph and Kate Rafael. 2008. "The Jewelry." In *Archaeological Excavations at Caesarea Maritima: Areas CC, KK and NN, Final Reports*, edited by Joseph Patrich, 419–31. Vol. 1: *The Objects*. Jerusalem: Israel Exploration Society.

Patrich, Joseph, D. Reshef, D. Ben-Yosef, S. Rotgaizer, S. Pinkas, Z. Bar-Or, H. Van-Dam, and A. Moscu. 1999. "The Warehouse Complex and Governor's Palace (areas KK, CC, and NN, May 1993–December 1995)." In *Caesarea Papers 2: Herod's Temple, the Provincial Governor's Praetorium and Granaries, the Later Harbor, a Gold Coin Hoard, and Other Studies*, edited by Kenneth G. Holum, Avner Raban, and Joseph Patrich, 70–107. *Journal of Roman Archaeology* Supplementary Series 35. Portsmouth, RI: Journal of Roman Archaeology.

Patton, Kimberley C. 2004. "'A Great and Strange Correction': Intentionality, Locality, and Epiphany in the Category of Dream Incubation." *HR* 43, no. 3: 194–223.

Pearcy, Lee T. 1988. "Theme, Dream, and Narrative: Reading the Sacred Tales of Aelius Aristides." *Transactions of the American Philological Association* 118: 377–91.

Penney, Douglas L. and Michael O. Wise. 1994. "By the Power of Beelzebub: An Aramaic Incantation Formula from Qumran (4Q560)." *JBL* 113, no. 4: 627–50.

Perdrizet, Paul. 1914. "ΥΓΙΑ ΖΩΗ ΧΑΡΑ." *REG* 27: 266–80.

Peterson, Erik. 1926. *Eis Theos: Epigraphische, formgeschichtliche und religionsgeschichtliche untersuchungen.* Forschungen zur religion und literatur des Alten und Neuen Testaments 24. Göttingen: Vandenhoeck & Ruprecht.

Pharr, Clyde, ed. 1952. *The Theodosian Code and Novels, and the Sirmondian Constitutions.* The Corpus of Roman Law (*Corpus Juris Romani*) 1. Princeton, NJ: Princeton University Press.

Philipp, Hanna and Margarete Büsing. 1986. *Mira et magica: Gemmen im Äyptischen Museum der Staatlichen Museen Preussischer Kulturbesitz, Berlin-Charlottenburg.* Mainz: Philipp von Zabern.

Pierre, Marie-Joseph and Jourdain-Marie Rousée. 1981. "Sainte-Marie de la probatique, état et orientation des recherches." *PrOrChr* 31: 23–42.

BIBLIOGRAPHY 233

Pietersma, Albert and Benjamin G. Wright, eds. 2007. *A New English Translation of the Septuagint and the Other Greek Translations Traditionally Included under That Title*. New York: Oxford University Press.

Pilcher, E. J. 1920. "A Samaritan Periapt." *Journal of the Royal Asiatic Society of Great Britain and Ireland* 3: 343–6.

Ploeg, Ghislaine E. van der. 2018. *The Impact of the Roman Empire on the Cult of Asclepius*. Impact of Empire 30. Leiden: Brill.

Poirier, John C. 2009. "Jesus as an Elijianic Figure in Luke 4:16–30." *CBQ* 71, no. 2: 349–63.

Preisendanz, Karl and Albert Henrichs. 1973. *Papyri graecae magicae*. 2 vols. Sammlung wissenschaftlicher Commentare. Stuttgart: Teubner.

Prentice, William K. 1908. *Greek and Latin Inscriptions*. Publications of an American Archaeological Expedition to Syria, 1899–1900 3. New York: Century.

Preuschen, Erwin. 1903. *Origenes Werke*. Johanneskommentar 4. Leipzig: J. C. Hinrichs.

Price, Richard and John Binns, eds. 1991. *Cyril of Scythopolis: Lives of the Monks of Palestine*. Cistercian Studies Series 114. Kalamazoo, MI: Cistercian Publications.

Puech, Emile. 1992. "Les deux derniers Psaumes davidiques du rituel d'exorcisme: 11QPsAp^a IV4–V14." In *The Dead Sea Scrolls: Forty Years of Research*, edited by Devorah Dimant and Uriel Rappaport, 64–89. Studies on the Texts of the Desert of Judah 10. Leiden: Brill.

Pummer, Reinhard. 1987. "Samaritan Amulets from the Roman-Byzantine Period and Their Wearers." *RB* 94: 251–63.

Pummer, Reinhard. 1989. "Samaritan Rituals and Customs." In *Samaritans*, edited by Alan D. Crown, 650–90. Tübingen: Mohr Siebeck.

Pummer, Reinhard. 2016. *The Samaritans: A Profile*. Grand Rapids, MI: Eerdmans.

Pummer, Reinhard. 2020. "What Was the Meaning and Purpose of Amulets with Samaritan Writing in the Byzantine Period?" *RB* 127, no. 1: 82–104.

Purvis, James D. 1968. *The Samaritan Pentateuch and the Origin of the Samaritan Sect*. Harvard Semitic Monographs 2. Cambridge, MA: Harvard University Press.

Raffaeli, Samuel. 1920–1. "A Recently Dicovered Samaritan Charm." *JPOS* 1: 143–4.

Rahmani, L. Y. 1985. "On Some Byzantine Brass Rings in the State Collections." '*Atiqot* 17: 168–81.

Rajak, Tessa. 2001. *The Jewish Dialogue with Greece and Rome: Studies in Cultural and Social Interaction*. Arbeiten zur Geschichte des antiken Judentums und des Urchristentums 48. Leiden: Brill.

Ravid, Liora. 2003. "The Book of Jubilees and Its Calendar: A Reexamination." *DSD* 10, no. 3: 371–94.

Reed, Annette Yoshiko. 2020. *Demons, Angels, and Writing in Ancient Judaism*. New York: Cambridge University Press.

Reed, Jonathan L. 2000. *Archaeology and the Galilean Jesus: A Re-Examination of the Evidence*. Harrisburg: Trinity Press International.

Reich, Ronny. 1985. "A Samaritan Amulet form Nahariya." *RB* 92: 383–8.

Reich, Ronny. 1989. "A Samaritan Ring from Apollonia." In *Apollonia and Southern Sharon*, edited by Israel Roll and Etan Ayalon, 269–71. Tel Aviv: Hakibutz Hameuhad (Heb.).

Reich, Ronny. 1994. "Two Samartian Rings from Gelilot (El Galil) near Herzliyya." '*Atiqot* 25: 135–8.

Reich, Ronny. 2002. "Samaritan Amulets from the Late Roman and Byzantine Periods." In *Sefer ha-Shomronim*, edited by Ephraim Stern and Hanan Eshel, 289–309. Jerusalem: Yad Yitshak Ben Tsevi (Heb.).

Reich, Ronny and Eli Shukron. 2005. "The Shiloaḥ Pool during the Second Temple Period." *Qad* 38, no. 130: 91–6.

Reich, Ronny and Eli Shukron. 2011. "The Pool of Siloam in Jerusalem of the Late Second Temple Period and Its Surroundings." In *Unearthing Jerusalem: 150 Years of Archaeological Research in the Holy City*, edited by Katharina Galor and Gideon Avni, 241–55. Winona Lake, IN: Eisenbrauns.

Reich, Ronny, Eli Shukron, and Omri Lernau. 2007. "Recent Discoveries in the City of David, Jerusalem." *IEJ* 57, no. 2: 153–69.

Remus, Harold. 2004. "The End of 'Paganism'?" *SR* 33, no. 2: 191–208.

Renberg, Gil H. 2016. *Where Dreams May Come: Incubation Sanctuaries in the Greco-Roman World*. 2 vols. Religions in the Graeco-Roman World 184. Leiden: Brill.

Riethmüller, Jügen W. 2005. *Asklepios: Heiligtümer und Kulte*. 2 vols. Studien zu Antiken Heiligtümern. Heidelberg: Verlag Archäologie und Geschichte.

Ringel, Joseph. 1975. *Césarée de Palestine: Étude historique et archéologique*. Paris: Éditions Ophrys.

Robinson, Thomas A. 2009. *Ignatius of Antioch and the Parting of the Ways: Early Jewish–Christian Relations*. Peabody, MA: Hendrickson.

Roll, Israel and Oren Tal. 2008. "A New Greek Inscription from Byzantine Apollonia-Arsuf/Sozousa: A Reassessment of the Εἷς θεὸς μόνος Inscriptions of Palestine." *SCI* 28: 139–47.

Rosenberg, Joel. 1990. "Midrash on the Ten Commandments." In *Rabbinic Fantasies: Imaginative Narratives from Classical Hebrew Literature*, edited by David Stern and Mark Mirsky, 91–119. Philadelphia: Jewish Publication Society.

Rosenberger, Mayer. 1977. *City Coins of Palestine (The Rosenberger Israel Coin Collection)*. Vol. 3: *Hippos-Sussita, Neapolis, Nicopolis, Nysa-Scytopolis, Caesarea-Panias, Pelusium, Raphia, Sebaste, Sepphoris-Diocaesarea, Tiberias*. Jerusalem: Rosenberger.

Rosenfeld, Ben-Zion. 1999. "R. Simeon b. Yohai: Wonder Worker and Magician, Scholar, *Saddiq* and *Hassid*." *REJ* 158, no. 3–4: 349–84.

Safrai, Ze'ev. 1998a. *The Missing Century: Palestine in the Fifth Century: Growth and Decline*. Leuven: Peeters.

Safrai, Ze'ev. 1998b. "The Institutionalization of the Cult of Saints in Christian Society." In *Sanctity of Time and Space in Tradition and Modernity*, edited by Alberdina Houtman, Marcel Poorthuis, and Joshua Schwartz, 193–214. Leiden: Brill.

Sallares, Robert. 2002. *Malaria and Rome: A History of Malaria in Ancient Italy*. Oxford: Oxford University Press.

Sanders, E. P. 1992. *Judaism: Practice and Belief, 63 bce–66 ce*. London: SCM Press.

Sandwell, Isabella. 2007. *Religious Identity in Late Antiquity: Greeks, Jews, and Christians in Antioch*. Greek Culture in the Roman World. Cambridge: Cambridge University Press.

Sanzo, Joseph E. 2017. "Magic and Communal Boundaries: The Problems with Amulets in Chrysostom, *Adv. Iud.* 8, and Augustine, *In Io. tra.* 7." *Henoch: studi storico-testuali su giudaismo e cristianesimo in età antica e medievale* 39, no. 2: 227–46.

Sanzo, Joseph E. 2019. "At the Crossroads of Ritual Practice and Anti-Magical Discourse in Late Antiquity: Taxonomies of Licit and Illicit Rituals in Leiden, Ms. AMS 9 and Related Sources." *Magic, Ritual & Witchcraft* 14, no. 2: 230–54.

Sanzo, Joseph E. 2020. "Deconstructing the Deconstructionists: A Response to Recent Criticisms of the Rubric 'Ancient Magic.'" In *Ancient Magic: Then and Now*, edited by Attilio Mastrocinque, Joseph E. Sanzo, and Marianna Scapini, 25–48. Stuttgart: Steiner.

Sauer, Eberhard W. 2005. *Coins, Cult and Cultural Identity: Augustan Coins, Hot Springs and the Early Roman Baths at Bourbonne-les-Bains*. Leicester Archaeology Monographs 10. Leicester: School of Archaeology and Ancient History, University of Leicester.

Schäfer, Peter. 2007. *Jesus in the Talmud*. Princeton, NJ: Princeton University Press.

BIBLIOGRAPHY 235

Schäfer, Peter, Shaul Shaked, Martin Jacobs, Claudia Rohrbacher-Sticker, and Giuseppe Veltri. 1994–9. *Magische Texte aus der Kairoer Geniza*. Texte und Studien zum antiken Judentum 42, 64, 72. Tübingen: Mohr Siebeck.

Scheid, John. 1991. "Sanctuaires et thermes sous l'Empire." In *Les thermes romains: Actes de la table ronde*, edited by M. Lenoir, 205–14. Collection de l'École française de Rome 142. Rome: L'École française de Rome.

Scheidel, Walter. 2001. *Death on the Nile: Disease and the Demography of Roman Egypt*. *Mnemosyne*, bibliotheca classica Batava Supplementum 228. Leiden: Brill.

Schnackenburg, Rudolf. 1990. *The Gospel According to St. John*. Translated by Cecily Hastings, Francis McDonagh, David Smith, and Richard Foley. Vol. 2: *Commentary on Chapters 5–12*. New York: Crossroad.

Schremer, Adiel. 2010. *Brothers Estranged: Heresy, Christianity, and Jewish Identity in Late Antiquity*. Oxford: Oxford University Press.

Schwab, Moïse. 1906. "Une amulette judéo-araméenne." *JA* 2e série, vol 7: 5-17.

Schwab, Moïse. 1917. "Amulets and Bowls with Magic Inscriptions." *JQR* 7, no. 4: 619-28.

Schwabe, Moshe. 1936. "Three Rings." *Tarbits* 7: 345-51 (Heb.).

Schwartz, Seth. 1998. "Rabban Gamaliel in Aphrodite's Bath." In *The Talmud Yerushalmi and Graeco-Roman Culture*, edited by Peter Schäfer, 203–17. Texte und Studien zum antiken Judentum 93. Tübingen: Mohr Siebeck.

Schwartz, Seth. 2001. *Imperialism and Jewish Society, 200 B.C.E. to 640 C.E.* Jews, Christians, and Muslims from the Ancient to the Modern World. Princeton, NJ: Princeton University Press.

Segal, Arthur. 1994. *Theatres in Roman Palestine and Provincia Arabia*. *Mnemosyne*, bibliotheca classica Batava Supplementum 140. Leiden: Brill.

Seyrig, Henri. 1935. "Invidiae medici." *Ber* 2: 50.

Shanks, Hershel, ed. 2013. *Partings: How Judaism and Christianity Became Two*. Washington, DC: Biblical Archaeology Society.

Shaw, Frank. 2014. *The Earliest Non-Mystical Jewish Use of Iαω*. Contributions to Biblical Exegesis and Theology 70. Leuven: Peeters.

Shenhav, Eli. 1990a. "Shuni/Miamas." *Qad* 89–90: 58–62.

Shenhav, Eli. 1990b. "Le théâtre romain de Shuni, rival de celui de Césarée." *MdB* 67: 58–60.

Shenhav, Eli. 1993. "Shuni." In *The New Encyclopedia of Archaeological Excavations in the Holy Land*, edited by Ephraim Stern, Ayelet Lewison-Gilboa, and J. Aviram, 1382–4. Jerusalem: Israel Exploration Society & Carta; New York: Simon & Schuster.

Shenhav, Eli. 1997. "The Maiumas Cult in Light of the Excavations at Shuni." In *New Studies on the Coastal Plain: Proceedings of the Seventeenth Annual Conference of the Department of Land of Israel Studies. In Honor of Prof. Yehuda Feliks, May 20th 1997*, edited by Eyal Regev, 56–70. Ramat Gan: Bar Ilan University (Heb.).

Shenhav, Eli. 1999. "Speakers in Shuni According to the Epigraphic Finds and Choricus of Gaza's Testimony." In *Judea and Samaria Research Studies: Proceedings of the Eighth Annual Meeting 1998*, edited by Ya'acov Eshel, 127–33. Kedumim-Ariel: Research Institute, College of Judea and Samaria (Heb.).

Shepardson, Christine. 2014. *Controlling Contested Places: Late Antique Antioch and the Spatial Politics of Religious Controversy*. Berkeley: University of California Press.

Shoshan, A. 1977. "The Illness of Rabbi Judah the Patriarch." *Korot* 7: 522–3 (Heb.).

Sivan, Hagith. 2008. *Palestine in Late Antiquity*. Oxford: Oxford University Press.

Smith, Jonathan Z. 1982. *Imagining Religion: From Babylon to Jonestown*. Chicago Studies in the History of Judaism. Chicago: University of Chicago Press.

Smith, Jonathan Z. 1987. *To Take Place: Toward Theory in Ritual*. Chicago Studies in the History of Judaism. Chicago: University of Chicago Press.

Smith, Jonathan Z. 1995. "Trading Places." In *Ancient Magic and Ritual Power*, edited by Marvin W. Meyer and Paul Allan Mirecki, 13–27. Religions in the Graeco-Roman World 129. New York: Brill.

Smith, Jonathan Z. 2002. "Great Scott! Thought and Action One More Time." In *Magic and Ritual in the Ancient World*, edited by Paul Allan Mirecki and Marvin W. Meyer, 73–91. Leiden: Brill.

Smith, Morton. 1978. *Jesus the Magician*. San Francisco: Harper & Row.

Smoak, Jeremy Daniel. 2016. *The Priestly Blessing in Inscription and Scripture: The Early History of Numbers 6:24–26*. New York: Oxford University Press.

Sowers, Brian P. 2008. "Eudocia: The Making of a Homeric Christian." Ph.D., University of Cincinnati.

Spier, Jeffrey. 2007. *Late Antique and Early Christian Gems*. Spätantike-frühes Christentum-Byzanz: Reihe B, Studien und Perspektiven 20. Wiesbaden: Reichert.

Stander, H. F. 1993. "Amulets and the Church Fathers." *Ekklesiastikos Pharos* 75: 55–66.

Steger, Florian. 2004. *Asklepiosmedizin: Medizinischer Alltag in der römischen Kaiserzeit*. Stuttgart: Steiner.

Steger, Florian. 2016. *Asklepios: Medizin und Kult*. Stuttgart: Steiner.

Steinsaltz, Adin. 2006. *The Essential Talmud*. 30th anniversary ed. New York: Basic Books.

Strack, Hermann Leberecht, Günter Stemberger, and Markus N. A. Bockmuehl. 1996. *Introduction to the Talmud and Midrash*. 2nd ed. Minneapolis: Fortress.

Strecker, Georg. 1991. "The Pseudo-Clementines: Introduction." In *New Testament Apocrypha*, edited by Wilhelm Schneemelcher, 2:483–93. Louisville, KY: Westminster/John Knox Press.

Sukenik, Eleazar. 1935. *The Ancient Synagogue of El-Ḥammeh (Ḥammath-by-Gadara): An Account of the Excavations Conducted on Behalf of the Hebrew University, Jerusalem*. Jerusalem: Rubin Mass.

Swartz, Michael D. 1990. "Scribal Magic and Its Rhetoric: Formal Patterns in Medieval Hebrew and Aramaic Incantation Texts from the Cairo Genizah." *HTR* 83, no. 2: 163–80.

Tal, Oren. 1995. "Roman-Byzantine Cemeteries and Tombs around Apollonia." *TA* 22, no. 1: 107–20.

Tal, Oren. 2009. "A Winepress at Apollonia-Arsuf: More Evidence on the Samaritan Presence in Roman-Byzantine Southern Sharon." *LASBF* 59: 319–42.

Tal, Oren. 2015. "A Bilingual Greek–Samaritan Inscription from Apollonia-Arsuf/Sozousa: Yet More Evidence of the Use of εἷς θεὸς μόνος Formula Inscriptions among the Samaritans." *ZPE* 194: 169–75.

Tal, Oren and Itamar Taxel. 2014. "Samaritan Burial Customs outside Samaria: Evidence from Late Roman and Byzantine Cemeteries in the Southern Sharon Plain." *ZDPV* 130, no. 2: 155–77, pl. 19–29.

Tal, Oren and Itamar Taxel. 2015. *Samaritan Cemeteries and Tombs in the Central Coastal Plain: Archaeology and History of the Samaritan Settlement Outside Samaria (ca. 300–700 CE)*. Ägypten und Altes Testament: Studien zu Geschichte, Kultur und Religion Ägyptens und des Alten Testaments 82. Münster: Ugarit Verlag.

Talbot, Alice-Mary. 2002. "Pilgrimage to Healing Shrines: The Evidence of Miracle Accounts." *DOP* 56: 153–73.

Tambiah, Stanley J. 1973. "Form and Meaning of Magical Acts: A Point of View." In *Modes of Thought: Essays on Thinking in Western and Non-Western Societies*, edited by Robin Horton and Ruth Finnegan, 199–229. London: Faber & Faber.

Taylor, Joan E. 1993. *Christians and the Holy Places: The Myth of Jewish–Christian Origins*. Oxford: Clarendon Press; New York: Oxford University Press.

Testa, Emmanuele. 1962. *Il simbolismo dei giudeo-cristiani.* Studium biblicum franciscanum, collectio maior 14. Jerusalem: Franciscan Printing Press.

Thackeray, Henry St John. 1956. *Josephus: With an English Translation.* 9 vols. Loeb Classical Library. Cambridge, MA: Harvard University Press.

Theissen, Gerd. 2010. "Jesus and His Followers as Healers: Symbolic Healing in Early Christianity." In *The Problem of Ritual Efficacy,* edited by William Sturman Sax, Johannes Quack, and Jan Weinhold, 45–65. Oxford Ritual Studies. Oxford: Oxford University Press.

Thomassen, Einar. 1999. "Is Magic a Subclass of Ritual?" In *The World of Ancient Magic: Papers from the First International Samson Eitrem Seminar at the Norwegian Institute at Athens, 4–8 May 1997,* edited by David R. Jordan, Hugo Montgomery, and Einar Thomassen, 55–66. Bergen: Norwegian Institute at Athens.

Thomsen, Peter. 1921. "Die lateinischen und griechischen Inschriften der Stadt Jerusalem und ihrer nächsten Umgebung (Fortsetzung)." *Zeitschrift des Deutschen Palästina-Vereins* 44, no. 1/2: 1–61.

Trebilco, Paul R. 1991. *Jewish Communities in Asia Minor.* Society for New Testament Studies Monograph Series 69. Cambridge: Cambridge University Press.

Trombley, Frank R. 2001. *Hellenic Religion and Christianization c. 370–529.* 2 vols. 2nd ed. Boston: Brill.

Tsafrir, Yoram. 1998. "The Fate of Pagan Cult Places in Palestine: The Archaeological Evidence with Emphasis on Bet Shean." In *Religious and Ethnic Communities in Later Roman Palestine,* edited by Hayim Lapin, 197–218. Studies and Texts in Jewish History and Culture 5. Bethesda: University Press of Maryland.

Tsafrir, Yoram. 1999. "The Holy City of Jerusalem in the Madaba Map." In *The Madaba Map Centenary, 1897–1997: Travelling through the Byzantine Umayyad Period. Proceedings of the International Conference Held in Amman, 7–9 April 1997,* edited by Michele Piccirillo and Eugenio Alliata, 155–63. Jerusalem: Studium biblicum franciscanum.

Tsafrir, Yoram, Leah Di Segni, and Judith Green. 1994. *Tabula Imperii Romani Iudaea-Palaestina: Eretz Israel in the Hellenistic, Roman and Byzantine Periods, Maps and Gazetteer.* Publications of the Israel Academy of Sciences and Humanities Section of Humanities. Jerusalem: Israel Academy of Sciences and Humanities.

Turner, Victor. 1973. "The Center out There: Pilgrim's Goal." *HR* 12, no. 3: 191–230.

Turner, Victor W. and Edith L. B. Turner. 2011 [1978]. *Image and Pilgrimage in Christian Culture.* Columbia Classics in Religion. New York: Columbia University Press.

Tzaferis, Vassilios and Shoshana Israeli. 1996. "Banias – 1993." *ESI* 15: 5–6.

Tzaferis, Vassilios and Shoshana Israeli. 1997. "Banias – 1994." *ESI* 16: 11–14.

Unger, Dominic J. and John J. Dillon, eds. 1992. *St. Irenaeus of Lyons: Against the Heresies.* Ancient Christian Writers 55. New York: Newman Press.

Urbach, Efraim E. 1975. *The Sages, Their Concepts and Beliefs.* Jerusalem: Magnes Press.

Uzzielli, Tania Coen. 1997. "The Oil Lamps." In *The Roman Baths of Hammat Gader: Final Report,* edited by Yizhar Hirschfeld, 319–46. Jerusalem: Israel Exploration Society.

Vakaloudi, Anastasia D. 2000. "Δεισιδαιμονία and the Role of the Apotropaic Magic Amulets in the Early Byzantine Empire." *Byzantion* 70: 182–210.

Van Cangh, Jean-Marie. 1984. "Miracles de rabbins et miracles de Jésus: La tradition sur Honi et Hanina." *RTL* 15, no. 1: 28–53.

Van Cangh, Jean-Marie. 2008. "Miracles grecs, rabbiniques et évangéliques." In *Miracles and Imagery in Luke and John: Festschrift Ulrich Busse,* edited by Jozef Verheyden, Gilbert van Belle, and J. G. van der Watt, 213–36. Bibliotheca Ephemeridum theologicarum Lovaniensium 218. Leuven: Peeters.

238 CONTESTED CURES

Van Dam, Raymond. 1985. "From Paganism to Christianity at Late Antique Gaza." *Viator* 16: 1–20.

Vermes, Géza. 1972. "Hanina ben Dosa: A Controversial Galilean Saint from the First Century of the Christian Era, Part 1." *JJS* 23, no. 1: 28–50.

Vermes, Géza. 1973. "Hanina ben Dosa: A Controversial Galilean Saint from the First Century of the Christian Era, Part 2." *JJS* 24, no. 1: 51–64.

Vermes, Géza. 2012. *Christian Beginnings from Nazareth to Nicaea.* New Haven, CT: Yale University Press.

Versnel, H. S. 1990. *Inconsistencies in Greek and Roman Religion.* Vol. 1: *Ter Unus. Isis, Dionysos, Hermes. Three Studies in Henotheism.* Studies in Greek and Roman Religion 6/1. Leiden: Brill.

Versnel, H. S. 1991. "Some Reflections on the Relationship Magic–Religion." *Numen* 38, no. 2: 177–97.

Versnel, H. S. 2011. *Coping with the Gods: Wayward Readings in Greek Theology.* Religions in the Graeco-Roman World 173. Leiden: Brill.

Vikan, Gary. 1995. "Early Byzantine Pilgrimage *Devotionalia* as Evidence of the Appearance of Pilgrimage Shrines." In *Akten des XII. Internationalen Kongresses für christliche Archäologie, Bonn, 22.–28. September 1991,* edited by Ernst Dassmann and Josef Engemann, 377–88. Münster: Aschendorffsche Verlagsbuchhandlung.

Vikan, Gary. 2010. *Early Byzantine Pilgrimage Art.* Rev. ed. Dumbarton Oaks Byzantine Collection Publications 5. Washington, DC: Dumbarton Oaks Research Library and Collection.

Vincent, H. 1908. "Amulette Judeo-Araméenne." *RB* 17: 382–94.

Vincent, H. 1926. "Le sanctuaire de Sainte-Anne et la piscine probatique a Jérusalem." In *Jerusalem nouvelle,* 669–742. Jerusalem: Recherches de topographie, d'archéologie et d'histoire 2. Paris: J. Gabalda.

Vitto, Fanny. 2008. "A Jewish Mausoleum of the Roman Period at Qiryat Shemu'el, Tiberias." *'Atiqot* 58: 7*–29*.

Vivian, Tim and Apostolos N. Athanassakis, eds. 1994. *Antony of Choziba: The Life of Saint George of Choziba and The Miracles of the Most Holy Mother of God at Choziba.* San Francisco: International Scholars Publications.

Vliet, N. van der. 1938. *"Saint Marie où elle est née" et la piscine probatique.* Jerusalem: Franciscan Printing Press.

Wacholder, Ben Zion and Martin G. Abegg. 1995. *A Preliminary Edition of the Unpublished Dead Dea Scrolls: The Hebrew and Aramaic Texts from Cave Four. Fascicle Three.* Washington, DC: Biblical Archaeology Society.

Wahlde, Urban C. von. 2006a. "The 'Upper Pool,' Its 'Conduit,' and 'the Road of the Fuller's Field' in Eighth Century BC Jerusalem and Their Significance for the Pools of Bethesda and Siloam." *RB* 113, no. 2: 242–62.

Wahlde, Urban C. von. 2006b. "Archaeology and John's Gospel." In *Jesus and Archaeology,* edited by James H. Charlesworth, 523–86. Grand Rapids, MI: Eerdmans.

Wahlde, Urban C. von. 2009. "The Pool(s) of Bethesda and the Healing in John 5: A Reappraisal of Research and of the Johannine Text." *RB* 116, no. 1: 111–36.

Wahlde, Urban C. von. 2013. "The Great Public Miqvaot at Bethesda and Siloam, the Development of Jewish Attitudes toward Ritual Purity in Late Second Temple Judaism, and Their Implications for the Gospel of John." In *Rediscovering John: Essays on the Fourth Gospel in Honour of Frédéric Manns,* edited by L. Daniel Chrupcala, 267–81. Milan: Edizioni Terra Santa.

Walter, R. and L. Moberly. 2011. "Miracles in the Hebrew Bible." In *The Cambridge Companion to Miracles,* edited by Graham H. Twelftree, 55–74. Cambridge Companions to Religion. Cambridge: Cambridge University Press.

BIBLIOGRAPHY 239

Wandrey, Irina. 2003. "Fever and Malaria 'For Real' or as Magical-Literary Topos?" In *Jewish Studies Between the Disciplines: Papers in Honor of Peter Schäfer on the Occasion of His 60th Birthday*, edited by Peter Schäfer, Klaus Herrmann, Margarete Schlüter, and Giuseppe Veltri, 257–66. Leiden: Brill.

Wazana, Nili. 2007. "A Case of the Evil Eye: Qohelet 4:4–8." *JBL* 126, no. 4: 685–702.

Weber, Max. 1947. *The Theory of Social and Economic Organization*. Translated by Alexander Morell Henderson and Talcott Parsons. New York: Free Press.

Weingarten, Susan. 1999. "Was the Pilgrim from Bordeaux a Woman? A Reply to Laurie Douglass." *JECS* 7, no. 2: 291–7.

Weissenrieder, Annette and Gregor Etzelmüller. 2015. "Christus Medicus: die Krankenheilungen Jesu im Dialog zwischen Exegese und Dogmatik." *Zeitschrift für Dialektische Theologie* 31, no. 3: 64–89.

Weksler-Bdolah, Shlomit. 2014. "The Foundations of Aelia Capitolina in Light of New Excavations along the Eastern Cardo." *IEJ* 64, no. 1: 38–62.

Welles, C. B. 1938. "The Inscriptions." In *Gerasa, City of the Decapolis: An Account Embodying the Record of a Joint Excavation Conducted by Yale University and the British School of Archaeology in Jerusalem (1928–1930) and Yale University and the American Schools of Oriental Research (1930–31, 1933–1934)*, edited by Carl H. Kraeling, 355–494. New Haven, CT: American School of Oriental Research.

Wendt, Heidi. 2016. *At the Temple Gates: The Religion of Freelance Experts in the Roman Empire*. New York: Oxford University Press.

Westenholz, Joan Goodnick. 2000. *Images of Inspiration: The Old Testament in Early Christian Art*. Jerusalem: Bible Lands Museum Jerusalem.

Wickkiser, Bronwen L. 2006. "Chronicles of Chronic Cases and Tools of the Trade at Asklepieia." *ARG* 8: 25–40.

Wickkiser, Bronwen L. 2008. *Asklepios, Medicine, and the Politics of Healing in Fifth-Century Greece: Between Craft and Cult*. Baltimore: Johns Hopkins University Press.

Wilken, Robert Louis. 1983. *John Chrysostom and the Jews: Rhetoric and Reality in the Late Fourth Century*. Transformation of the Classical Heritage 4. Berkeley: University of California Press.

Wilkinson, John. 1978. *Jerusalem as Jesus Knew It: Archaeology as Evidence*. London: Thames & Hudson.

Wilkinson, John. 1999. *Egeria's Travels*. 3rd ed. Warminster: Aris & Phillips.

Wilkinson, John. 2002. *Jerusalem Pilgrims before the Crusades*. 2nd ed. Warminster: Aris & Phillips.

Williams, Frank, ed. 2009. *The Panarion of Epiphanius of Salamis, Book I*. 2nd ed. Nag Hammadi and Manichaean Studies. Leiden: Brill.

Wintermute, O. S. 1983. "Jubilees: A New Translation and Introduction." In *The Old Testament Pseudepigrapha*, edited by James H. Charlesworth, 2:35–142. Garden City, NY: Doubleday.

Wolff, Samuel R. 1993. "Archaeology in Israel." *AJA* 97, no. 1: 135–63.

Wortley, John, ed. 1992. *John Moschus: The Spiritual Meadow*. Kalamazoo, MI: Cistercian Publications.

Yarnold, Edward. 2000. *Cyril of Jerusalem*. London: Routledge.

Yeung, Maureen W. 2002. *Faith in Jesus and Paul: A Comparison with Special Reference to "Faith That Can Remove Mountains" and "Your Faith Has Healed / Saved You."* Wissenschaftliche Untersuchungen zum Neuen Testament 2, no. 147. Tübingen: Mohr Siebeck.

Zertal, Adam. 1977. "A Samaritan Ring and the Identification of 'Ain-Kushi." *Qad* 10, nos. 38–9: 84–6 (Heb.).

Zertal, Adam. 1979. "The Samaritans in the District of Caesarea." *Ariel: The Israel Review of Arts and Letters* 48: 98–116.

Ziv, Yehuda. 1987. "The Green Ones: A Legendary Hero Embraces Three Traditions." *Eretz* 2, no. 4: 37–44.

Index of Ancient Sources

Page numbers in *italics* refer to illustrations, and those with the suffix 'n' refer to notes. Abbreviations are expanded on pp. xii–xvi.

Hebrew Bible

Genesis
1:6 *53*, 56
18 72
28 82n

Exodus
7–12 183
7:9 184
7:11 184
13:9 194n
13:16 194n
15:3 32–3, 40–1, *43*, 53, 56n
15:26 40–2, *43*, 53, 54–5, 186
16:29 188
25:17–22 50n
28:36 51
28:36–8 51n
30:30 134
37:1–9 50n
38:8 42n, *43*, 53

Numbers
6:24 66
6:24–6 52
7:89 50n

10:35 40n, 43
10:35–6 42, *43*, 53
10:36 40, 56
14:14 42n, *43*, 53

Deuteronomy
6 33, 52n
6:1–9 41–2
6:2 66
6:4 31–2, 40, *43*, 53, 56
6:4–9 32, 65–7, 194
6:8–9 193
11:18 194
18 183
26:19 86n
33:26 40, 42n, 43, *43*, 53, 56, 61, 62, 63
33:29 42n

1 Samuel
4:4 50n
16:12–13 135
16:14 123
16:23 124

2 Samuel
6:2 50n

1 Kings
17–18 88
17:17–23 89
18 184n
18:36–40 89
18:41–6 167n
19:16 135

2 Kings
2 89
5:1–14 86n
13:20 165n
19:15 50n

1 Chronicles
13:6 50n

Job
38:12–13 55

Psalms
3 132n
3:1–3 190
19 121
41:4 205
46 50–1, 54
46:8 (45:8 LXX) *53*, 55

242 CONTESTED CURES

46:12 (45:12 LXX) *53, 55*
80:1 50n
91 131
91 (90 LXX) 190
91:1 (90:1 LXX) 33, 53,
    57, 62n
94:1 (93:1 LXX) *53, 55*
99:1 50n
116:6 (114:6 LXX) *53, 55*
145:6 59

Proverbs
6:20–2 194

Isaiah
1:6 138
6:3 58
37:16 50n
51:13 59
51:15 *53, 55, 56, 58*

Jeremiah
17:19–27 191n
31:35 *53*

Daniel
3:6 *53, 55, 56*
10:13 29n
10:21 29n
12:1 29n

Amos
4:13 *53, 55, 56, 58*

Deuterocanonical Books and Pseudepigrapha

3 Enoch
48D 49

Jubilees
10:7–14 126–7

Letter of Aristeas
158–60 194
159–60 65n

Testament of Solomon
125n
1.5–7 126n
7.5–6 136
13.6 136n
15.14 126
18.2 136
18.23–5 137n
18.27–8 137n
18.34 142–3
18.39 30
18.5 137n
Tobit 125n

2 Maccabees
12:40 185

Dead Sea Scrolls

1QH[a] Thanksgiving Scroll
1QH[a] XX.11 121n

1QS Rule of the Community
1QS III.13 121n
1QS IX.12 121n

1QSb Rule of the Blessings
1QS28b 121n

4Q4QpapLXXLev[b]
4Q120 32n

4QExorcism ar
4Q560 132

4QIncantation
4Q444 132n

4QS[b]
4QS IX.1 121n

4QSongs of the Maskil
4Q510–11 121, 131, 132,
    133n, 144

6QHymn
6Q18 132n

8QHymn
8Q5 132n

11Apocryphal Psalms[a]
11Q11 123, 190
11Q11 IV.3–14 131

11Psalms Scroll[a]
11Q5 XXVII.9–10 123

Damascus Document
CD 11:7–9 191n
CD 11:16–17 189n

New Testament

Matthew
8:3 154n
8:5–13 155n, 168n
8:15 154n
8:16 155n
8:28–34 119n, 129n, 155n,
    173n
9 112
9:2–8 154n
9:20–2 111, 154n, 159n,
    164n
9:25 154n
9:29 154n
10:8 151n
12:9–14 154n
14:35–6 154n
15:21–8 155n, 168n
16:13–20 156n
17:1–18 156n
17:14–21 155n, 159n
17:20 155
20:34 154n
23:5 204n
24:5 195n

Mark
1:21–6 129n
1:23–6 155n

INDEX OF ANCIENT SOURCES   243

1:31   154n
1:32–4   155n
1:41   154n
2:1–12   154n
3:1–6   154n
3:9–10   154n
5:1–20   119n, 129n, 155n,
    173n
5:5   154n
5:7   152n
5:25–34   159n, 164n
5:27–9   154n
5:41   154n
6:54–6   154n
7:24–30   155n, 168n
7:32–5   154n
8:23   154, 160n
8:27–30   156n
9:2–8   156n
9:14–29   129n
9:17–29   155n, 159n
9:19   155
9:23–4   155
9:27   154n
10:46–52   154n
13:22   195

Luke
4:24–7   156
4:31–6   129n
4:33–5   155n
4:38–9   154n
4:40   154n
4:40–1   155n
5:13   154n
5:17–26   154n
6:6–11   154n
6:18–19   154n
7   173
7:1–10   168n
7:1–17   155n
8:26–39   119n, 129n, 155n,
    173n
8:43   159n
8:43–4   154n
8:43–8   164n
8:54   154n
9:18–20   156n

9:28–36   156n
9:37–43   155n, 159n
10:1–12   151n
10:34   138
13:11–13   153
13:13   154n
17:11–19   154n
18:35–43   154n
21:8   195n
22:21   154n
24:13–34   81n

John
5   95, 98, 101n, 102, 109
5:2   97
5:2–9   94n
5:3b–4   94n, 95
5:8–9   154
9:1–3   108n
9:1–7   109
9:6   154, 160n
9:6–7   108n
11:38–44   155n

Acts
2:22   158n
5:12   158n
5:15–16   164n
6:8   158n
7:36   158n
7:54–60   109n
8:6   197
8:9   197
8:11   197
8:13   197n
15:12   158n
19:11–12   164n
19:13–15   130

1 Corinthians
8:4–6   34
9:11–14   151n
12:9   138n, 150n
12:30   138n

Philippians
4:15–18   151n

1 Timothy
5:17–18   151n

James
5   137–8
5:13–16   144–5
5:14   122
5:17   138

Jude
9   29n

Revelation
1:8   63n
12:7   29n
21:6   63n
22:13   63n

Rabbinic Literature and other Hebrew Texts

Mishnah
ʿAbodah Zarah 3:4   187
Berakot 5:5   168, 169
ʿErubin 4:3   188n
ʿErubin 5:7   188n
Šabbat 6:2   191n
Šabbat 6:10   191n
Šabbat 7:2   189n
Šabbat 8:1   138n
Šabbat 8:3   16n, 191n
Šabbat 14:3–4   189n
Šabbat 16:1   192
Šabbat 22:6   189n
Sanhedrin 10:1   55n, 186,
    190
Soṭah 7:1   32
Soṭah 9:15   167
Taʿanit 3:8   167n

Tosefta
ʿErubin 4:16   188n
ʿErubin 5:2   83n
Ḥullin 2:22–3   185n
Šabbat 4:5   191n

244 CONTESTED CURES

Šabbat 4:9 17n, 191–2
Šabbat 5:8 191n
Šabbat 7:23 190
Šabbat 12:8–13 189n
Šabbat 13:4 192, 193
Taʿanit 2:13 167n

Jerusalem Talmud
ʿAbodah Zarah 2:2
  (40c–41a) 185n
ʿAbodah Zarah 4:4
  (43d–44a) 187n
Berakot 5:5 (9d) 169
Demai 1:3 (21d–22b) 170n
ʿErubin 5:7 (22d–23a)
  188n
ʿErubin 10:11 (26c) 17n,
  21, 132, 190
Ketubbot 12:3 (34d–35b)
  88n
Qiddušin 3:12 (64c–d) 188
Šabbat 4:2 (6d–7a) 188
Šabbat 5:4 (7b–c) 191n
Šabbat 6:2 (8a–b) 17n, 121,
  190, 191n
Šabbat 6:9 (8c–8d) 186
Šabbat 8:3 (10d) 16n
Šabbat 14:3 (14c) 190
Šabbat 14:4 (14c–15a)
  182n, 185
Šabbat 16:1–2 (15b–c) 192n
Šabbat 18:2 (16c) 188
Soṭah 7:1 (20d) 32
Taʿanit 3:9–10 (66d–67a)
  167n

Babylonian Talmud
ʿAbodah Zarah 55a 186,
  187
Berakot 8a 83n
Berakot 10b 124n
Berakot 34b 169–70
ʿErubin 61a 188n
Ḥullin 106a 189n
Menaḥot 42b 193
Šabbat 39b–40a 188n
Šabbat 40b 188
Šabbat 53a–b 191n

Šabbat 61a–b 191n
Šabbat 67a 186n
Šabbat 109a–b 189n
Šabbat 109b 89n
Šabbat 115a–b 192n
Taʿanit 19a 167n
Taʿanit 23a–b 167n
Taʿanit 24b–25a 167n

Midrash
Leviticus Rabbah 10:4 171
Midrash ha-Gadol 81, 86n
Midrash Rabbah Numbers
  20:14 171n
Pesikta de Rab Kahana 22.2
  171

Other
Sepher ha-Razim 122–3,
  127, 136

Greek and Roman Literature

1 Clement
59.4 145

Acts of Pilate
1.1 199n

Ammianus Marcellinus
19.12.14 206

Antony of Choziba
Life of George of Choziba
  2.8 163
Miracles of the Most Holy
  Mother of God at
  Choziba 6 165n

Apostolic Constitutions
Const. ap. 122, 140n, 145
Const. ap. 8.29 135
Const. ap. 32 207

Apostolic Tradition
Trad. ap. 122, 140
Trad. ap. 5.2 134

Trad. ap. 16 207
Trad. ap. 20.3–8 134
Trad. ap. 21.9–10 134

Athanasius
De amuletis (frag) 206

Barsanuphius
Letters 71–153 161n
Letter 90 158–9
Letter 753 142, 145

Bede
Hist. Eccl. 1.30 93n

Bordeaux Pilgrim
Itinerary 585 104n
Itinerary 589 100n

Canons of Hippolytus 145

Cassius Dio 65.8 175n

Codex Theodosianus 206

Cyril of Jerusalem
Catch. 1.9 134n
Catch. 1.10 200–1
Catch. 1.13–14 134n
Catch. 13.36 205
Catch. 19.8 201
Catch. 20.3 139
Homily on the Paralytic 2 97

Cyril of Scythopolis
V. Abr. 9 165
V. Cyriac. 9 128
V. Euthym. 10 161–2
V. Euthym. 12 164n
V. Euthym. 47 165
V. Euthym. 49 165n
V. Euthym. 51–3 165n
V. Euthym. 56 165n
V. Jo. Hes. 21 128
V. Sab. 45 128
V. Sab. 46 128n
V. Sab. 62 164
V. Sab. 63 128

INDEX OF ANCIENT SOURCES · 245

V. Sab. 68 161n
V. Sab. 79 168n

Diogenes Laertius
Lives of Eminent Philosophers
 8.69 174n

Egeria
Itinerary 16.1, 3 86n
Itinerary 46.1 134n

Epiphanius
De Fide 24.3 205
On Measures and Weights
 14 86n
Pan. 1.5 205
Pan. 13.6 205
Pan. 30.4 120n
Pan. 30.6 120n
Pan. 30.7–8 75n
Pan. 30.10 119, 155n

Eucherius
Letter to Faustus 127.8
 100n

Eunapius of Sardis
V. Soph. 459 75n

Eusebius
C. Hier. 23 197
C. Hier. 26 197
C. Hier. 31 197
Dem. ev. 3.5.125 197
Dem. ev. 3.6.126 197
Dem. ev. 3.6.127 202
Dem. ev. 3.6.130–3 197
Hist. Eccl. 7.18 112
Onomasticon 240 100,
 101

Greek Magical Papyri
PGM 118, 125n, 141
PGM IV.1227–64 133
PGM IV.3007–86 132n,
 135, 143
PGM VII.211–14 132n
PGM VII.218–19 132n

Gregory of Nazianzus
Orationes 40.17 204n

Gregory the Great
Ep. 76 93n

Historia Augusta
V. Hadr. 25 174n
V. Hadr. 26 86n

Iamblichus
V. Pyth. 28:135 174n

Irenaeus
Adv. haer. 1.23.1 198
Adv. haer. 1.23.4 196n
Adv. haer. 2.31.2 197n
Adv. haer. 2.32.5 197n

Isaac of Antioch
De magis. 205

Jerome
Comm. Isa. 18.65 202
V. Hil. 14 159–60
V. Hil. 15 160
V. Hil. 24 149, 157, 158n
V. Hil. 30 141
V. Hil. 32 142
V. Hil. 33 206
V. Hil. 38 158
V. Hil. 42 158n
V. Hil. 44 142

John Chrysostom
Adv. Iud. 1.1 202
Adv. Iud. 1.6 202
Adv. Iud. 8.5 182
Adv. Iud. 8.5–8 204
Adv. Iud. 8.8 182
Catech. illum. 2.5 203
Hom. 3 in 1 Thess. 3 203
Hom. 8 in Col. 5 203, 204, 205
Hom. 12 in 1 Cor. 7 204
Hom. 12 in 1 Cor. 13–14 205

John Malalas
Chronographia 12.3 105

John Moschos
Prat. 157
Prat. 1 160n
Prat. 28 160n
Prat. 40 165n
Prat. 56 164n
Prat. 82 164n
Prat. 131 169n
Prat. 176 119–20

John Rufus
Plerophoria 18 101
V. Petr. Ib. 101
V. Petr. Ib. 25 158n
V. Petr. Ib. 60 163n
V. Petr. Ib. 98 158n
V. Petr. Ib. 105 158n
V. Petr. Ib. 127 163n
V. Petr. Ib. 132 163n

Josephus
Against Apion 2.10 111
Ant. 2.284–6 184n
Ant. 4.212 66n
Ant. 6.166 124
Ant. 6.168 124, 198n
Ant. 6.213–14 124
Ant. 6.214 198n
Ant. 6.45 198n
Ant. 8.45–7 125
Ant. 8.49 125
Ant. 14.19 167n

Justin Martyr
Dial. 69 184n
Dial. 69.1 199
Dial. 85.3 125n, 198
I Apol. 26 198
I Apol. 56 198

Lucian
Lover of Lies 16 129, 151n

Marinus of Neapolis
V. Procli. 19 114n

Origen
C. Cels. 1.32 182n
C. Cels. 1.6 129–31, 196

246   CONTESTED CURES

C. Cels. 1.68   150n
C. Cels. 2.49   195n
C. Cels. 2.50   196
C. Cels. 2.8   199
C. Cels. 3.24   199
C. Cels. 3.27   196n
C. Cels. 4.33   199
C. Cels. 7.8   151
C. Cels. 7.9   151
Commentary on John   97
Orig. Hom. Lev. (trans.
    Rufinus)   137–8

P. Berol. 17202   146–7

Philo
Spec. 4.137–9   194n
Spec. 4.141–2   194n

Philostorgius
Hist. Eccl. 7.3   112n

Philostratus
V. Apoll. 1.9   173n
V. Apoll. 4.20   173n
V. Apoll. 4.45   172–3
V. Apoll. 43   173n

Piacenza Pilgrim
Itinerary 7   78n, 85n
Itinerary 10   86n

Itinerary 24   86n, 109n
Itinerary 25   109n
Itinerary 27   101n, 102n
Itinerary 30   75n

Plutarch
Life of Pyrrhus 3.4   175n

Porphyry
V. Pyth. 29   174n

Pseudo-Athanasius
Homily on the Sower 15   101n

Pseudo-Clement
Hom. 9   199–200

Rufinus
Orig. Hom. Lev. 2.4   137–8

Sacramentary of Serapion
Prayer VII (22)   145
Prayer VIII (30)   138, 145
Prayer XVII (4)   145n
Prayer XVII (5)   141n
Prayer XXII (15)   139–40
Prayer XXIX (17)   140–1,
    146

Socrates Scholasticus
Hist. Eccl. 7.4   120n

Sophronius
Anacreonticon 20.81–94   101n
Miracles of Cyrus and John
    46   109n, 160n

Sozomen
Hist. Eccl. 2.4   71–2
Hist. Eccl. 5.21   92–3, 112n,
    114

Strabo
Geographica 16.2.45   81n

Suetonius
Vesp. 7   175n

Supplementum magicum
vol 1, no13   132n

Tacitus
Hist. 4.81   175n

Theodore of Mopsuestia
*Commentary on the Gospel
    of John*   97

Theodosius
*Topography of the Holy
    Land* 8   101n

Vita Melaniae
59   109n

Subject Index

Page numbers in *italics* refer to illustrations, and those with the suffix 'n' refer to notes.

Abraamius, 165
Aelia Capitolina, 3, 98, 100, 102, 110
Akiba, Rabbi, 186, 187–8
Akko, 63, 187
Aleppo, silver *lamella*, 55
amulet users
  named, 15–16, 24, 25–6, 38, 48–52, 58–9,
    61–3
  ownership, transfer of, 24, 46, 73
  self-understanding of, 16, 22–3, 33–6,
    44–6, 60–1, 192
  transgression of elite limits, 64, 67, 148,
    202, 208
  unnamed, 23–4, 34, 36, 38, 39, 73
amulets
  Christian elite rhetoric on, 198, 201,
    202–8, 209
  commissioned or premade, 24, 46, 48,
    64, 73
  Jewish elite rhetoric on, 185, 186, 190,
    191–4, 209
  types of, 16–18, *17*, 25n
  see also gemstone amulets; jewelry
    amulets; *lamellae*; papyri amulets
aniconism, 35, 36, 64
Antoninus Pius, 87–8, 90, 171
Apollonia (Arsuf), 26, 34
Apollonius of Tyana, 172–4, 197
Apostolic Constitution, 122, 135, 145, 207

Apostolic Tradition, 122, 134, 140, 207
apotropaic devices, 29–30, 66, 120–2,
    131–2, 136, 139–40, 190
Aramaic inscriptions *see* inscriptions,
    Aramaic and Hebrew
Aristaenete, 159–60, 165
Ark of the Covenant, 42, 50, 51, 56
Ashkelon, 31, 33, 35n, 113, 120
Asklepios
  Dora, 111
  healing cult of, 8, 9, 74, 76, 85, 89–90,
    199–200
  Paneas, 112–13
  Pool of Bethesda, 99, 100, 101, 102–3,
    110, 210
  Shuni/'Ein Tzur, 105, 106, 107

baptism, 119, 120, 128, 133–4, 139, 201, 205
Barsanuphius and John, correspondence,
    142, 158–9, 160–1
basilicas, 72, 101, 102, 110–11
Bethesda *see* Pool of Bethesda
biblical inscriptions *see* inscriptions,
    Aramaic and Hebrew; inscriptions,
    Greek; inscriptions, Samaritan;
    inscriptions, bilingual; *see also tefillin*
blindness, 108, 109, 154, 160, 174–5
boēth(e)i ("help") inscription *see*
    inscriptions, Greek

248 CONTESTED CURES

Bordeaux Pilgrim, 100, 104–6, 107
bracelets *see* jewelry amulets

Caesarea
    bracelets, 62–4, *62*
    diversity of population, 1, 2, 23, 107
    gemstones, 20, *21*, 22n, 23, 30, 31
    pendants, 31, 57, 190
    rings, 26, 31, 43
    Shuni/'Ein Tzur, 107
Celsus, 129–30, 150–2, 195, 199
charaktares, 18, *19*, 45–6, 49, 60, 61–2
charismatic wonderworkers, 149–77
    Apollonius, 172–4, 197
    Christian ascetics, 127–8, 141–2, 157–66,
        206
    compared to ritual practitioners, 119,
        138, 150–3, 158, 161, 211
    Elijah, 85–9, 138, 145, 156, 199
    Hadrian and Vespasian, 174–5
    Jacob of Kefar Sama, 11, 182, 186
    Jesus, 149, 150–1, 153–7
    in rabbinic texts, 166–72
Christ, inscriptions, 25, 26, 31, 56, 203
Christian elite rhetoric, 195–208
    amulets, 198, 201, 202–8, 209
    healers, 148, 158
    healing sites, 72, 79–80, 93–4, 201, 210
    Jesus' miracles, legitimacy of, 195–7,
        211–12
    Judaism, 182–3, 198–9, 200, 201–2, 204,
        205, 209
    magic, 195–201, 205–7
    Maioumas festival, 105, 107
    polytheist traditions, 198, 199–200, 201,
        205, 209
Christians, 3–7, 11
    amulet use, 22–3, 25–6, 31–6, 44, 46,
        59–60, 203
    charismatic wonderworkers/ascetics,
        127–8, 141–2, 157–66, 206
    conversions linked to healing, 119–21,
        159–62, 164–5
    exceptionalism, 129–30, 172
    Hammat Gader, 79–80, 81, 85, 90–1
    healing sites, other, 71–2, 106, 107,
        109–14

Pool of Bethesda, 94, 100–3, 154, 210
ritual practitioners with official
    authority, 117, 120, 122, 138, 143–4,
    147–8
Christogram, 60
churches, 72, 75, 90, 95, 98–9, 101, 102–3,
    109, 110–11
Codex Theodosianus, 206, 207
coins, 85, 106, 107, 110, 113, 114
communal identity
    elite rhetoric, 4n, 6, 9, 11, 181–3, 202,
        208
    between Jews and Christians, 5
    porosity of, 46, 57, 61, 64, 67, 148, 182,
        208
    at shared sites, 71–4
communal settings, 121–2, 132, 143–7
communitas, 73–4
Constantine, 3, 5, 72, 206
copper *lamellae*, 55, 57–60, *58*
Coptic language, 133
Cornelius Repentinus, 87–8
cross, 22n, 60, 82, 128, 141, 204, 205
cult of the saints, 110, 165
cults
    coexistence of, 71–4, 89–91, 93–4, 106–8,
        110, 114
    continuity of practice, 93, 98, 108, 110,
        111
    elite rhetoric on, 93, 182–3, 186–8, 201
    incubation rituals, 79–80, 81, 90–1, 103,
        111, 113
    see also Asklepios
Cyril of Jerusalem, 97, 139, 200–1, 205
Cyril of Scythopolis, 127–8, 157, 161–2,
    164–5

David (biblical king), 123–4, 134
Dead Sea Scrolls, 32n, 121, 123, 131–2,
    133n, 144, 189n, 190, 191n
demons *see* exorcism and demons
Dora, 110–11
dreams, 79–80, 89, 91, 175, 200, 201;
    see also incubation; visions

Edfu papyrus, 65–6
Egeria, 86, 134

SUBJECT INDEX 249

Egypt
  afterlife, 22
  amulets, 8, 16n, 18, 33n, 56, 146n
  exodus from, 41, 54–6, 183–5, 211
  healing sites, 74
  magic, 184–5, 186, 196, 199
  see also PGM (*Greek Magical Papyri*),
    Sacramentary of Serapion
'Ein Tzur *see* Shuni/'Ein Tzur
Eleazar ben Dama, 185
Elijah, 78, 85–9, 138, 145, 156, 199
Elisha, 86, 135, 156
elite rhetoric
  amulets, 16, 23, 36, 39, 43–4, 64
  charismatic wonderworkers, 149–50, 158
  creates communal identity, 4n, 6, 9, 11,
    181–3, 208
  freelance ritual practitioners, 118, 148
  magic, 9, 118, 150, 158, 184, 195–201, 205–7
  see also Christian elite rhetoric; Jewish
    elite rhetoric
Emmaus, 92–3, 114, 210
Epidauros, 173n
epilepsy, 128, 154n
Epiphanius of Salamis, 75, 119, 120–1, 155,
  205
Eucharist, 90, 138, 145, 147
Eudokia, Empress, 86–7, 210
Eusebius, 101, 111–13, 196–7, 202, 209
Euthymius, 161–2, 164–5
'Evron, 57–60, 58
exorcism and demons
  amulets, 30, 55
  Apollonius, 173–4, 197
  David, 123–4
  Eleazar, 125–6
  elite rhetoric on, 187, 190–1, 196–201,
    205, 211
  Euthymius, 161, 164
  Jesus, 129–30, 173
  Noah, 126–7
  oil/anointing, 128, 139–40, 141
  pre-baptismal exorcism, 133–4, 139, 201
  ritual words, 118, 119, 120–2, 128–37,
    190–1
  Solomon, 30, 100–1, 123, 124–6
eye, much-suffering, 29–30, 34, 36

faith, 121, 122, 130, 131, 155, 161–3, 166, 176
female supplicants, 75, 83, 99–100, 107, 171
fertility rituals, 10, 104, 105, 107
fevers, 1, 48, 51, 55, 58, 132, 136, 140–1,
  154, 159, 169, 174, 203–4, 212;
  see also malaria

Gadara, 75, 78, 79, 81, 83, 85, 188
gemstone amulets, 16, 17, 18, 18, 19, 20–5,
  27, 30–1, 36, 53–4, 54, 61–2, 73, 110, 114
genizah, 122, 192–3
gentiles, 7, 112, 188, 193–4, 198
George of Choziba, 162–3
Gihon spring, 108, 110
God
  as creator, 55, 58–9, 132, 135
  names of, 49–50, 51, 55–6, 58, 59, 135
  relationship with Israel, 40–2, 50, 54, 56,
    183–4
  source of charismatic power, 158–9,
    162–4, 166, 176
Greek inscriptions *see* inscriptions, Greek
Greek Magical Papyri see PGM
Gush Halav pendant, 28–32, 29, 34, 36

Hadrian, 3, 81, 174–5
hagios topos see inscriptions, Greek
Hammat Gader, 75–90, 76
  incubation rituals, 78–80, 81, 82n, 89–91
  inscriptions, 76–7, 80, 82, 83–4, 86–7
  Piacenza Pilgrim, 78–80, 81, 85–6, 90
  ring, 24–6, 25, 27–8, 36, 203
  Sabbath restrictions, 82, 188–9
  synagogue, 24, 27, 75, 82–4, 90
Hammat Tiberias, 73, 74, 82–4, 85
Ḥanina ben Dosa, 167–70
Hebrew inscriptions *see* inscriptions,
  Aramaic and Hebrew
heis theos see inscriptions, Greek
Helios image, 33
Hilarion, 141–2, 157, 158, 159–60, 165, 206
hip pain/sciatica, 20–1, 22n
historiolae, 31, 55, 56, 128–9, 130, 131, 135, 146
ho nikōn ta kaka see inscriptions, Greek
Holy Rider image, 30–1, 34, 36, 57, 62, 63,
  64, 190
Ḥoni the Circle-Maker, 152, 156n, 167

250 CONTESTED CURES

Horvat Kanaf *lamella*, 55
hot springs, 74–91, 92–3
   Christian elite rhetoric on, 72, 79–80,
     93–4, 201, 210
   inscriptions, 73, 76–7, 80, 82–4, 86–7
   Jewish elite rhetoric on, 82, 187–9, 211
   sacredness of, 75–80, 84, 92–3, 113
   see also Hammat Gader, Hammat
     Tiberias
Hygieia, 85, 87, 88, 110
hygi(ei)a (health) rings, 26–7, 36

Iaō Sabaōth, 28–9, 58, 59, 63
Iidentity, 1n; *see also* communal identity;
   otherness
idols/idolatry, 34, 185, 186–7, 201, 202–4, 207
images *see* much suffering eye; Holy
   Rider; reaper gemstones
imposition of hands, 137–8, 143, 147
incantations, 129, 130, 150, 196, 199, 205
incubation, 8, 78–80, 81, 82n, 89–91, 93,
   111, 113
infertility, 10, 104, 105, 107, 171
inscriptions, Aramaic and Hebrew
   absent from some amulet types, 67,
     191–2
   amulets, 15, 16, 19, *19, 20*, 32, 38, 48, 50–2
   biblical, 33, 53, *53*, 54–5
   with Greek, *19, 20*, 57–60, *58*
   at Hammat Gader, 83
   see also inscriptions, bilingual

inscriptions, bilingual, 57–64, *58*
   with biblical quotations, 53, *53*, 57
   Greek–Hebrew, *19, 20*, 57–60, *58*
   Greek–Samaritan, *19, 20*, 31, 33, 44,
     61–4, 73
inscriptions, Greek
   biblical, 53, *53*, 57, 190
   boēth(e)i ("help"), 25, 26–9, 31, 36, 48,
     61, 203
   hagios topos ("holy place"), 77, 80, 84
   at healing sites, 73, 76–7, 80, 82, 83–4,
     85–7, 99, 100, 113
   with Hebrew, *19, 20*, 57–60, *58*
   heis theos ("one god"), 16, 26, 31–6, 61,
     62–3

ho nikōn ta kaka ("who conquers evil"),
   32, 33, 62–3
hygi(ei)a (health), 26–7, 36
nomina sacra, 22n, 25, 203
pseudo-inscriptions, 28, 54n
reaper gemstones, 20–1, 23
with Samaritan script, *19, 20*, 31, 33, 44,
   61–4, 73
see also inscriptions, bilingual
inscriptions, Samaritan
   amulets as *tefillin*, 66–7, 194, 210
   biblical, 34–6, 38, 39–40, 42–3, *43*, 53–4,
     53, 56
   with Greek, *19, 20*, 31, 33, 44, 61–4, 73
   pendants, 42–4, *43*, 46, 61–2, 194
   polygonal rings, 38, 39–40, 42, 194
   pseudo-inscriptions, 28, 45, 61–2
   see also inscriptions, bilingual
Irenaeus, 196n, 197n, 198
Isaac of Antioch, 205
(i)schiou/(i)schiōn (hips), 20, 21
Ishmael, Rabbi, 182, 185
Israel, relationship with God, 40–2, 50, 54,
   56, 183–4

Jacob of Kefar Sama, 11, 182, 186
Jerome, 101–2, 141–2, 145, 157–61, 201, 206
Jerusalem, 35, 52, 63, 93–103, 108–10;
     see also Aelia Capitolina; Pool of
     Bethesda; Pool of Siloam; Temple,
     Jerusalem
Jesus
   ascetics linked to, 158–60
   demons addressed by, 129–30, 173
   Emmaus, 92–3, 114
   Jesus ben Pandera, 182, 185
   name invoked, 11, 119, 121, 130, 132–3,
     185, 196
   oil from Jesus' cross, 128, 141
Jesus' miracles
   Celsus' view of, 150–1, 195–6
   Christian elite rhetoric on, 195–7,
     211–12
   paralytic healed at Pool of Bethesda, 94,
     101, 102, 103, 114, 154
   other healings, 108, 111–12, 153–7, 159,
     164

jewelry amulets, *17*, 18–19, *18, 20*, 24, 54, *54*
   bracelets, 62–4, *62*, 67, 191–2
   pendants, 28–36, *29*, 34, 36, 42–4, *43*, 46,
      57, 61–3, 190
   rings, 24–6, *25*, 27–8, 36, 38, 39–45, *39,
      43*, 67, 125–6, 192, 194
Jewish elite rhetoric, 183–94
   amulets and tefillin, 185, 186, 190–4,
      209
   Christian cures, 182–3, 185–6
   healing sites, 82, 187–9, 211
   magic, 184
   Maioumas festival, 105
   miracles, legitimacy of, 183–7, 191
   Sabbath restrictions, 82, 138, 188–93,
      209
Jewish revolts, 3, 98, 105
Jews, 2–7, 10, 11
   amulet use, 15–16, 22–3, 31–3, 36, 38,
      51–2, 59–60
   charismatic wonderworkers, 166–72
   conversions to Christianity, 119–21
   sacred sites, 71–2, 80, 82–4, 90–1, 107,
      109, 110, 188–9
John Chrysostom, 122, 182, 201, 202–4,
   205, 209
John Moschos, 119, 120–1, 122, 139, 148,
   157, 158, 163–4
John Rufus, 101, 157, 163
Josephus (Christian convert), 119, 120–1,
   155
Josephus (historian), 66, 111, 123–6, 167,
   184
Judah ha-Nasi, Rabbi, 88–9, 188
Julian, 35, 206
Justin Martyr, 198–9

Ketef Hinnom scrolls, 52, 53, 65–6
Khirbet Kusieh octagonal ring, 38, 39–42,
   39
Kyrios, 26, 31, 56, 135

lamellae, 15–16, 17, 17n, 18, *18*, 19, *20*, 24n,
   27n, 23–4, 38, 46, 47, 48–52, 54, *54*, 55,
   57–60, *58*, 73, 141, 193
lamps, 77, 78, 81, 82
Latin language, 99, 100

leprosy, 78, 80, 85–6, 109
literacy, 23, 28, 45–6, 50
Lucian of Samosata, 129, 151–2, 155–6

"magic," 8–9, 17n, 118, 126, 127, 135–6, 143,
   148, 150–1, 184, 195–201, 205–7, 211
Maioumas festival, 104–5, 106, 107
malaria, 1, 48, 55, 58, 141, 159, 212; *see also*
   fevers
Mamre, 71–3, 74, 75, 91
Masada ring, 26, 27n
maskil, 121, 122, 143–4, 147, 151
Michael (archangel), 29, 30, 63
miqveh, 96–9, 101, 102–3, 108–9, 114, 210
miracle, 86, 89, 120–1, 138, 141–2, 145,
   156, 158, 159–60, 163–71, 173, 175,
   183–7, 191, 195–8, 200, 206, 211;
   see also Jesus' miracles
Moses, 41, 42, 156, 183–5, 196, 197, 199, 211
Mount Gerizim, 34, 113
Mount Syna, 104, 105–6, 114
much-suffering eye (*polypathēs ophthalmos*),
   30, 34, 36

Nablus gemstone, 61–2
Nahariya pendant, 44, 46
Nirim amulets, 15–16, 17n, 27n, 38, 51, 55,
   73, 193
Noah, 126–7
nomina sacra, 22n, 25, 203

oil, 127–8, 134–5, 137–44, 145, 147, 165
Origen, 97, 130–1, 137–8, 195–6, 199, 211
otherness, 4, 7, 31, 72, 198

pagan, 7, 107, 113, 182, 188, 196, 198, 200,
   202, 205–7, 209, 210
Paneas, 111–13, 114
papyri amulets, 16, 18, 48, 56, 65, 146n
paralysis, 94, 101, 102, 103, 114, 154
pendants *see* jewelry amulets
Peter the Iberian, 157, 163
PGM (*Greek Magical Papyri*), 118, 132–3,
   141
Piacenza Pilgrim, 5, 22n, 27, 72, 78–80,
   81, 85–6, 90, 93, 96, 100, 101, 102,
   103, 108, 109, 210

pilgrimage, 73–4, 86, 100, 104–6, 107, 110–11, 134, 165
Pinchas ben Yair, Rabbi, 170
polygonal rings, 38, 39–45, *39, 43*; *see also* jewelry amulets
Pool of Bethesda, 93–103, *96*
 Jesus, 94, 101, 102, 103, 114, 154, 158
 miqveh, 96–9, 101, 102–3, 108–9, 114, 210
 Serapis–Asklepios, 99, 100, 101, 102–3, 110, 210
Pool of Siloam, 108–10
prayers
 amulets, 28, 32, 42, 45, 55, 56
 charismatic wonderworkers, 161, 162–3, 166, 167–70, 171–2, 173
 communal, 143–7
 Jewish daily prayers (*Shema*), 32, 42, 65, 66
 Jewish elite rhetoric on, 186
 Sacramentary of Serapion, 138–41, 143, 145–6, 161
 tefillin, 65–6, 190
prophetic knowledge, 169–70, 172, 173–4, 176, 199
pseudo-inscriptions, 28, 45, 54n, 61–2

Qumran, 121, 126, 147

rain miracles, 145, 167
Ramat Hanadiv, 105, 106
reaper gemstones, 20–3, *21*, 25, 27, 36
religion and magic, 8–9, 212
rings *see jewelry amulets*
ritual actions, 117–9, 120, 127–8, 134–5, 137–44, 145, 147
ritual authority, 100–1, 119, 121, 123–8, 130, 132–3, 134, 141, 185, 196
ritual healing, 6, 8–9, 72, 73, 90, 93–4, 98, 103, 108, 110, 111, 114, 117
ritual practitioners, 117–48
 compared to charismatic wonderworkers, 119, 138, 150–3, 158, 161, 211
 as freelancers, 117–18, 122–3, 132, 143, 147–8, 211
 with institutional authority, 117–18, 121–2, 138, 143–4, 147–8, 211

ritual words, 118, 119, 120–2, 123–4, 127–37, 131–2, 147, 155, 190
Roman army, 81, 87–8, 99n, 100

Sabas, 128, 164
Sabbath, 82, 188–9, 190–4, 209
Sabaōth, 28–9, 58, 59, 63, 135
Sacramentary of Serapion, 138–41, 143, 145–6, 147, 148, 161
Samaritan inscriptions *see* inscriptions, Samaritan
Samaritans, 3–5, 6, 39–46, 60–7, 183, 197–8
Sepher ha-Razim, 122, 127, 135–6
Serapis, 74, 85, 99–100, 101, 102–3, 175, 210
Shema, 32, 42, 65, 66
Shuni/'Ein Tzur, 93, 103–7, *104*, 114, 210
Simeon ben Gamaliel, Rabban, 168–70, 187
Simeon ben Yohai, Rabbi, 171, 190
Simon the magician, 197–8
Solomon, 30, 100–1, 123, 124–6, 127, 132
Songs of the Maskil, 121, 131–2, 143–4
Sozomen, 71–3, 75, 92–3, 114
speech miracles, 154, 156, 171, 176
synagogues, 156, 201–2
 genizah, 122, 192–3
 Hammat Gader, 24, 27, 75, 82–4, 90
 Hammat Tiberias, 83, 84
 Nirim, 15, 16, 38, 51, 55, 193
Syria, 17n, 55, 57n, 134, 135, 159–60

tefillin, 10, 65–7, 190, 192–4
Temple, Jerusalem, 3, 50, 51, 71, 96–8, 108, 126
Testament of Solomon, 30, 126, 136, 142–3, 148
Tetragrammaton, 32, 40, 49, 50, 56, 58, 59, 60, 186, 193
thermal-mineral springs *see* hot springs
Tiberias, silver *lamella*, 38, 46, 47, 48–52, 141
Tiberias *lamella* for Ina, 38, 46, 47, 48–52, 141
tombs, 22, 24, 28, 31, 34, 38, 44, 46, 51–2, 110, 165

toothache, 88–9, 132
touch miracles, 154, 156, 163–4, 166, 175, 176, 200

Umm Qais *see* Gadara

Vespasian, 3, 125, 174, 175
visions, 78, 89, 119, 162, 164; *see also* dreams
voces magicae, 48–9, 51, 61–2, 73, 133

votive offerings, 27, 77–8, 80–2, 84, 98–100, 102, 106, 107, 112, 113, 114

water, 10, 75, 103, 105, 106, 113, 114, 210
witchcraft, 182, 184, 200, 204
wonderworkers *see* charismatic wonderworkers

Yahweh, 29, 31–2, 40–2, 49–52, 56, 57, 135
Yose, Rabbi, 190–1